TISSUE AND ORGAN TRANSPLANTATION

Implications for Professional Nursing Practice

TISSUE AND ORGAN TRANSPLANTATION

Implications for Professional Nursing Practice

SUSAN L. SMITH, R.N., M.N., CCRN

Clinical Nurse Specialist
Emory University Hospital
Associate Professor
Nell Hodgson Woodruff School of Nursing
Emory University
Atlanta, Georgia

AACN

American Association of Critical-Care Nurses

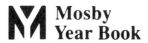
Mosby
Year Book

St. Louis Baltimore Boston Chicago London Philadelphia Sydney Toronto

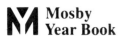

Mosby
Year Book

Dedicated to Publishing Excellence

Executive editor: Don Ladig
Developmental editor: Robin Carter
Project editor: Teri Merchant
Production editor: Mary Stueck
Designer: Liz Fett

Printed in the United States of America

Mosby–Year Book, Inc.
11830 Westline Industrial Drive
St. Louis, MO 63146

Library of Congress Cataloging-in-Publication Data

Organ and tissue transplantation: implications for professional
nursing practice / [edited by] Susan L. Smith; American Association
of Critical-Care Nurses.
         p.   cm.
      Includes index.
      ISBN 0-8016-5526-9
      1.   Transplantation of organs, tissues, etc.   2.   Transplantation of
organs, tissues, etc. – Social aspects.   3.   Transplantation of
organs, tissues, etc. – Nursing.   I.   Smith, Susan L. (Susan Lynn),
1950-   .   II.   American Association of Critical-Care Nurses.
      [DNLM: 1.   Critical Care – nursing.   2.   Tranasplantation – nursing.
WY   154   068]
RD120.7.0687   1990
617.9'5 – dc20
DNLM/DLC
                                                                                                  90-5986

GW/MV/MV   9   8   7   6   5   4   3   2   1

Contributors

THOMAS S. AHRENS, R.N., D.N.Sc., CCRN

Clinical Nurse Specialist, Barnes Hospital at Washington University Medical Center, St. Louis, Missouri

JUDY ELIZABETH BOYCHUK, R.N.

Program Coordinator, Clinical Specialist Program, Scimed Life Systems, Inc., Minneapolis, Minnesota

MARIA CIFERNI, R.N., B.S.N., CCRN

Head Nurse, Transplant Intensive Care Unit, Emory University Hospital, Atlanta, Georgia

JANE C. CLARK, R.N., M.N.

Clinical Nurse Specialist, Oncology, Emory University Hospital, Assistant Professor, Emory University School of Nursing, Atlanta, Georgia

JANICE Z. CUZZELL, R.N., M.A.

Skin and Wound Care Consultant, Woodland Hills, California

THOMAS F. DODSON, M.D., F.A.C.S.

Assistant Professor, Emory University School of Medicine, Atlanta, Georgia

DANNY HAWKE, R.N., B.S.N., C.P.T.C.

Executive Director, LifeLink of Georgia, Atlanta, Georgia

DELYNN HEBERLEIN, R.N., B.S.N.

Staff Nurse, Emory University Hospital, Atlanta, Georgia

MICHAEL A. HOOKS, Pharm. D.

Clinical Surgery Specialist, Emory University Hospital, Atlanta, Georgia

JAMES KRAFT, B.S., P.A., C.P.T.C.

Senior Transplant Coordinator, LifeLink of Georgia, Atlanta, Georgia

SUZANNE NICHOLSON MACDONALD, R.N., M.S.

Clinical Nurse Specialist, Cardiac Transplantation, The University of Arizona Health Sciences Center, Tucson, Arizona

JILL FELDMAN MALEN, R.N., M.S.

Clinical Nurse Specialist, Pulmonary, Barnes Hospital at Washington University Medical Center, St. Louis, Missouri

NANCY ALLEN NAUCKE, R.N., M.N.

Cardiac Transplant Coordinator, Emory University Hospital, Atlanta, Georgia

ANNA OMERY, R.N., D.N.Sc.

Assistant Professor, University of California, Los Angeles, School of Nursing, Los Angeles, California

JENNIE P. PERRYMAN, R.N., M.S.N.

Director, Center for Transplantation, Emory University Hospital, Atlanta, Georgia

LUANA C. POST, R.N., CCRN

Staff Nurse, Emory University Hospital, Atlanta, Georgia

CATHERINE POWERS, R.N., B.S.N., CCRN

Staff Nurse, Barnes Hospital at Washington University Medical Center, St. Louis, Missouri

ANNE MARIE RIETHER, M.D.

Assistant Professor, Emory University School of Medicine, Atlanta, Georgia

GEORGE RUTHERFORD, M.B.A., M.T. (A.S.C.P.)

Administrator of Emergency Services, Sparrow Hospital, Lansing, Michigan

SUSAN L. SMITH, R.N., M.N., CCRN

Clinical Nurse Specialist, Liver Transplantation, Emory University Hospital, Atlanta, Georgia

PAMELA U. STILLERMAN, R.N., M.S.

Clinical Nurse Specialist, Renal Transplantation, Emory University Hospital, Atlanta, Georgia

GAIL WALSH, B.S.

Program Coordinator, Georgia Lions Eye Bank, Atlanta, Georgia

JENNIFER S. WEBSTER, R.N., M.N.

Staff Nurse, Oncology/Hematology, Emory University Hospital, Atlanta, Georgia

BECKY G. WILLS, R.N., M.N., CCRN

Staff Nurse, Emory University Hospital, Atlanta, Georgia

Consultants

SHARON M. AUGUSTINE, R.N., M.S., C.R.N.P.

Transplant Coordinator, The Johns Hopkins Hospital, Baltimore, Maryland

DEBORAH CASWELL, R.N., M.N., CCRN

Clinical Nurse Specialist, University of California, Los Angeles, Medical Center, Assistant Clinical Professor, University of California, Los Angeles, School of Nursing, Los Angeles, California

SUZANNE CLARK, R.N., M.A., M.S.N., C.S.

Clinical Nurse Specialist, Psychiatry, Kaiser Permanente Medical Center, Los Angeles, California

JOLEEN KELLEHER, R.N., M.S.

Director of Nursing, Fred Hutchinson Cancer Research Center, Seattle, Washington

JOANN I. LAMB, M.S.N., R.N.-C.

Cardiac Transplant Nurse Practitioner, Columbia-Presbyterian Medical Center, New York, New York

JOAN MILLER, R.N.

Nurse Educator/Clinical Coordinator, Heart and Heart-Lung Transplantation Program, Stanford University, Stanford, California

MARY ANN PALUMBI, R.N., C.C.T.C.

Chief Coordinator/Director, Transplantation Services, Allegheny General Hospital, Pittsburgh, Pennsylvania

MARK S. SHAEFER, Pharm.D.

Assistant Professor, Pharmacy Practice, Clinical Pharmacist Liver Transplant and Surgery, University of Nebraska Medical Center, Omaha, Nebraska

ELIZABETH J. SCHEURER, R.N., CCRN

Cardiovascular Surgical Clinician, Abbott Northwestern Hospital, Minneapolis, Minnesota

MICHAEL SCHROYER, R.N., M.S.N.

Director, Organ and Tissue Bank, Rush-Presbyterian-St. Luke's Medical Center, Omaha, Nebraska

DEBORAH WRIGHT-SPHRITZ, R.N., M.S., CCRN

Instructor, Undergraduate Studies, University of Maryland School of Nursing, Baltimore, Maryland

LAUREL WILLIAMS, R.N., M.S.N.

Clinical Nurse Specialist, Certified Clinical Transplant Coordinator, University of Nebraska Medical Center, Omaha, Nebraska

Preface

The year is 2020. Ms. Jones is diagnosed, entirely by noninvasive means, with end-stage cirrhosis. She is scheduled for an elective liver "implant" in 6 weeks, which will allow time for her to undergo treatment to modify her immune system. The organ to be implanted is actually a "neo-organ," a shelf item, that has been constructed of liver cells fashioned around a synthetic scaffold. This neo-organ is grafted into the recipient and becomes vascularized over time. It is capable of performing the vital synthetic functions of a normal liver. The operative time is short, blood loss is minimal, and recovery is relatively uncomplicated. The neo-liver begins to function immediately. Preoperative education did not include information about rejection or the potential side effects of chronic immunosuppression because these, fortunately, are phenomena of the past. Ms. Jones is discharged on the fifth postoperative day, and the hospital bill is well within the amount reimbursed under the DRG for a liver implant.

This scenario is visionary, but no more so than the visions held by the pioneers of modern organ transplantation scarcely 30 years ago. The past 30 years have witnessed incredible progress in the field of organ and tissue transplantation. Dreams have turned into reality. "Transplant" has become a favorite media subject and a household word. It is probably safe to say that the potential of organ replacement is limited only by the number of body parts.

As vivid as is the past and as limitless as the imagination may seem about the future, reality is made more sobering by the factors presently limiting transplantation. These obstacles relate to surgical technique, rejection, a shortage of donor organs, and the expensive nature of transplantation.

Surgical technique

Historical events normally associated with other disciplines have had notable influence on the development of the field of organ and tissue transplantation as we know it today. In 1907 the death of a politician from a gunshot injury to the portal vein motivated Alexis Carrell to develop the technique of vascular anastomosis. During World War II the British government commissioned Peter Medawar to investigate skin grafting techniques as treatments for soldiers dying from burn injuries. Such were the beginnings of the myriad surgical techniques now performed for organ replacement.

It is now possible to remove, replace, or substitute for the heart, heart valves, lung, liver, kidney, pancreas, small intestine, adrenal cells, bone marrow, cornea, skin, bones, joints, ligaments, tendons, and blood vessels. Surgical techniques for solid organ replacement are essentially perfected, with the exception of the pancreas transplant. Major efforts at perfecting the surgical techniques of segmental and whole pancreas and islet cell transplant will continue. Not only are human organs and tissues transplanted in record numbers, but also natural elements and materials are being used increasingly to rebuild vital and nonvital body parts. Approximately 30,000 defective heart valves are replaced and 150,000 pacemakers are implanted each year. Thousands of prostheses are implanted each year to restore function or esthetics, including those for the eye, cochlea, chin, nose, mandible, shoulder, wrist, elbow, knee, femur, hip, breast, penis, testicle, and soft tissue. Dr. Barney Clark made medical history in 1982 when he was the first to receive a total artificial heart. William Schroeder was 52 years old when he was told he was too old to receive a human heart transplant. He was offered and accepted the total artificial heart instead. Today, with the technologic and clinical advances made, William Schroeder would probably be a candidate for a heart transplant.

Rejection

The phenomenon of graft rejection, an inherent property of human physiology, must be painstakingly overcome to broaden the applications of transplantation technology. Currently available immunosuppressant agents are toxic and far from perfect in preventing and controlling rejection. It is amazing, however, how much has been accomplished in this field in a relatively brief period.

Although Metchnikoff first conceived of specific immunosuppression with antilymphocyte globulins in the late nineteenth century, the major advances in immunosuppressant therapy have taken place in the last three decades. It was in the 1960s, almost 20 years after Sir Peter Medawar received a Nobel Price for his work with skin grafts, that prednisone, azathioprine, and antilymphocyte globulins were used clinically. The truly major advance during this time was made by Dr. Thomas E. Starzl when he combined the use of azathioprine and prednisone to treat rejection in kidney transplant recipients.

The 1970s held even greater promise. In 1972 Jean Borel serendipidously discovered the immunosuppressant Cyclosporin A from the soil fungi *Trichoderma polysporum* and *Cyclindrocarpon lucidurum* while searching for antifungal agents in southern Norway. This was the beginning of selective immunosuppression. Dr. Roy Calne was first to experiment in transplantation with this new agent, and in 1978 it was first used in human clinical trials. In 1981 Dr. Starzl ventured to use the combination of Cyclosporin A with prednisone. The impact on graft and patient survival was astounding. Cyclosporine, as it is called today, has been the essential factor

in the expansion of transplantation technology during the past decade.

Cyclosporine, however, was not the entire story of the 1970s. In 1975 Kohler and Milstein unleashed a virtual explosion in transplantation immunology with the development of the hybridoma technique for creating monoclonal antibodies. They too were awarded a Nobel Prize in 1984 for this discovery. The monoclonal antibody OKT-3 has further defined the concept of selective immunosuppression. In the next decade, transplant pharmacology will be based on the monoclonal antibody for prevention and treatment of rejection, use in diagnostic assays, cancer detection and elimination, and prevention and treatment of infection. A promising new immunosuppressant called FK 506, discovered in 1984, is currently in the initial stages of human clinical trials.

With the stage set by the availability of powerful immunosuppressant drugs, the 1980s were a decade not of discovery, but of perfection of surgical technique and patient management. Operations that until the 1980s were offered to only a handful of patients across the country on an experimental basis are now performed by the thousands. More than 250 hospitals in the United States now offer at least one transplant service. Future perspectives on overcoming the immunologic barriers will focus on modification of the immune system and achieving immunologic tolerance. With much-improved immunosuppression or the elimination of the need for it altogether, earlier transplantation in patients with terminal, but without end-stage disease, may be justified. These patients would probably have a shorter, less complicated, and less expensive postoperative course.

Shortage of donor organs

Arguments have been made to support the immune system as the greatest barrier to transplantation. In the transplanted patient this is evident. But the simple fact is that without donor organs, the role of the immune system is irrelevant. In the past decade there has been a tremendous surge in the number of organ transplants performed. Current success rates are impressive. In spite of these advances, however, many continue to die waiting for a donor organ to make a lifesaving operation possible. Of the approximately 2.2 million deaths in the United States each year, less than 50,000 result in organ or tissue donation. Society's support for transplantation clearly outweighs its support for donation.

Volunteerism has not been a successful mechanism for obtaining sufficient numbers of donor organs. In recent years various legislative initiatives, such as required request and presumed consent, have been implemented or proposed to address this problem. Early data indicate that these mechanisms are not successful either. Various other proposals, some of which are controversial, have been made for expanding the potential donor pool.

The redefinition of death has been proposed to include cerebral death, which would enable health professionals to declare anencephalics and those in chronic vegetative states dead, and therefore organ donors. In 1986 physicians at Loma Linda University astounded the transplantation community and beyond by transplanting the heart of a chimpanzee into a newborn with hypoplastic left heart syndrome. At present, xenografting, the transplanting of organs from another species, has not been successful and is not a viable alternative. The use of living-related donors is routine for kidney transplantation. In this case the risk to the donor is acceptable. Protocols now exist, however, for resection of partial liver and pancreas grafts from living donors. The mortality risks to the donors in these cases are unacceptably high. As older individuals are transplanted, organs from older donors will be used for transplant. Increasing the upper age limit for some donor organs to 65 would drastically increase the potential donor pool.

There is active research involving culture and purification of living cells for transplant as miniature organs to halt the progression of diseases or illnesses such as diabetes mellitus, Parkinson's disease, Alzheimer's disease, leukemia, hemophilia, spinal cord injuries, and burns. At present limiting factors to cell culture are quantity and quality of these cell cultures. Transplanting human fetal tissue to treat diseases such as Parkinson's disease has been of interest to investigators for approximately 50 years. Currently, largely as a result of the social and political issues related to elective abortion, there is a moratorium on federally funded research on the use of fetal tissue from elective abortions.

There have been few advances in the treatment of genetic diseases in the last 20 years. Gene transplantation for the treatment of genetic diseases is conceptually and technically feasible. This approach, however, is fraught with many technical problems.

All of these potential solutions to the donor shortage problem have generated complex economic, social, and ethical issues. Ethical issues have traditionally taken a back seat to technologic progress in transplantation. This can no longer be true. Society, directly confronted by these issues, will have to take a part in the resolutions. Society will demand a more active role in allocation of federal research dollars and the implementation of transplant technology.

Costs

The costs of the biomedical advances made in transplantation have been phenomenally high and are passed on to patients, with some procedures costing hundreds of thousands of dollars. This raises at least two issues: limited access to transplantation as a therapeutic option and the shifting of public health care dollars from less expensive programs to expensive transplant programs. Americans are underinsured, particularly for catastrophic illness. Some insurance companies continue to deny payment for transplant procedures, and federal assistance programs deny payment for the majority of extrarenal transplants. Will society continue to tolerate the use of large sums of public money for procedures that benefit a few, when these same funds could potentially improve the quality of life of many?

The all-important first steps have been taken. Intensive activity over the past 30 years has whetted humanity's appetite for and brought us closer to the ultimate cure. But is there an ultimate cure, as empiricism would imply? Or is organ transplantation merely a high-level palliative treatment, as long-term survival statistics might suggest? These questions are yet to be answered.

Features of the text

Tissue and Organ Transplantation: Implications for Professional Nursing Practice provides a comprehensive look at transplantation as it is practiced today, as it affects and as it is affected by society. The book is written in three parts. Part One provides a look back at the history of organ and tissue transplantation and examines a concept basic to understanding the major clinical problems of transplantation, the immunologic aspects. Part Two considers the issues created by the advances in transplantation technology, issues surrounding organ and tissue donation and recovery, and ethical and psychosocial issues. Part Three focuses on the practice of transplantation, with an emphasis on care of the transplant patient. We have attempted to present the full spectrum of the transplant experience, from the patient's perspective, beginning with the diagnosis of end-stage organ disease and moving toward the hope of regaining a quality life-style, and from the nurse's perspective, beginning with identification of potential organ and tissue donors and concluding with the delivery of quality care in the postoperative period. We welcome feedback from readers for future editions.

• • •

The accomplishments in organ and tissue transplantation have been called miracles. Indeed, thousands of lives have been touched by the gift of life. And there are many heroes. In *Many Sleepless Nights,* Lee Gutkind poignantly tells of the miracles and the pioneer heroes — the surgeons and scientists who laid the foundations, the organ procurement and transplant coordinators who make it happen, and the patients and families who allow it to happen.

This book is written for the silent heroes of transplantation — the nurses who not only witness the miracles daily, but also take an active part in fashioning them. In the words of Dr. Norman Shumway, "The problems come after surgery." For the measurement of success goes far beyond 1- and 5-year graft and patient survival rates. The surgical techniques, for the most part, have been perfected. The real challenges begin after the final sutures have been tied and continue sometimes for many days, at the bedside where the need for the blending of humanism with scientism is preeminent. Transplantation nursing is developing as a specialty in nursing practice. There is a specialized body of knowledge — organ function and dysfunction; chronic disease and its impact on individuals, families and society; transplantation immunology; transplantation pharmacology; organ and tissue donation and recovery; and the psychosocial impact of transplantation — that is unique and necessary to the care of the transplant patient. Much research in the basic and clinical sciences is still waiting to be done, and many answers to the questions about the field of transplantation are yet to be discovered. My colleagues in transplant nursing are hereby challenged to play an important role in the scientific inquiry into the field of transplantation, particularly to illuminate through alternative research methods lived aspects of the transplant experience.

Susan L. Smith

Acknowledgments

I wish to express my deep and sincere appreciation to the following individuals for their invaluable contributions:

Mary F. Woody, R.N., M.A., for her example of wisdom, and her encouragement and generosity in providing me with essential resources necessary to complete such an endeavor.

Cathy V. Wood, R.N., M.S.N., for her patience and constant support, and for providing me with the security that comes with knowing there is always someone there when you need them.

The nursing staff of the 5E ICU at Emory University Hospital for their many examples of perseverance and their inspiration, patience, and support.

Robin Carter for her constant encouragement and guidance.

Susan K. Collins for her expert assistance with manuscript preparation.

Craig Jones of LifeLink of Georgia, Inc., for his expert editorial assistance.

Richard Olson, M.D., for his expert editorial assistance.

J. Michael Henderson, M.D. and Thomas F. Dodson, M.D., for their expert editorial assistance and encouragement.

William J. Millikan, M.D., for his trust and collaborative support.

My contributors for sharing their expertise, and without whom this book would not have been possible.

Blakeman Eric Smith Sr. and Blakeman Eric Smith Jr. who have endured with me many late nights, early mornings, and lost weekends.

SLS

Contents

PART ONE

The Concepts

1

Introduction

Perhaps the most important single element in reshaping the day-to-day texture of hospital life was the professionalization of nursing. In 1800, as today, nurses were the most important single factor determining ward and room environment. Nursing, like professional hospital administration and changed modes of hospital financing, has played a key role in shaping the modern hospital.
CE Rosenberg

These are complex times: There are multiple forces at work that affect doctors, nurses, patients, the practice of medicine, and the delivery of health care. Never before have we had such an opportunity to help our fellow men and women, yet never before have we so struggled with the cost constraints and economic decisions that are inevitable in a nation with finite resources. Daily we face the effects of three competing issues: (1) the changing demographics of American society, with a steady rise in elderly people, an all-time high of people living below the poverty level, and a continued absence of health insurance for over 30 million people, (2) the changing nature of health care and health care delivery, with the ascension of the intensive care unit and high technology, expensive procedures and monitoring, and (3) the dramatic change in outlook for people with end-organ failure, with the present ability to replace those organs and provide a relatively normal life. As health care professionals involved in transplantation, we must confront each of these issues, not only so that we may become better informed, but also so that we can

play a role in the shaping of answers to the problems we face.

In some ways, we are doing better: A girl born in 1988 can expect to live about 78 years, and although boys still have a shorter life expectancy, they can expect to live about 71 years. Both of these figures reflect a 5-year increase in life expectancy over the past 30 years. In other ways, the statistics are disturbing and even alarming: According to the Federal Bureau of the Census, 32 million Americans are living below the official poverty level, a number unchanged from 1987.[2] According to the report by the Bureau of the Census, the gap between the richest and poorest individuals in this country is at an "all-time level." Adding to the alarm over the degree of poverty in our society is the fact that children make up a substantial proportion of the poor. A recent report by Bane and Ellwood has stated that 20% (one fifth) of our nation's children are in families with incomes below the poverty line.[3] The authors of this report, from the John F. Kennedy School of Government at Harvard University, stated, "There is increasing evidence that things may be getting worse for

3

those near the bottom." Our children carry our hopes and our dreams. Will they be able to improve themselves and their society when, at this early stage, they have so little opportunity? Will they be able to afford expensive health care?

From a health standpoint, two factors seem preeminent in trying to assess the future: the aging of our society and the lack of health insurance for many Americans. There are about 30 million Americans age 65 and older, according to 1987 census figures, and it is predicted that by the year 2010 more than 25% of the U.S. population will be at least 55 years old. Those 30 million Americans who are now age 65 and older presently make up about 12% of the U.S. population, but it is also predicted that by the year 2030 they will make up over 20% of the population.[4] Goldsmith further stated, ". . . American society will experience an unprecedented wave of health care cost pressure for both acute and chronic care."

What of those people with no health insurance? This figure is hard to pin down, but a frequent estimation is that approximately 37 million Americans have no health insurance. It has been estimated that another 27 million Americans have inadequate health insurance, so we are faced with approximately 64 million people, or a little over a quarter of the population, who are uninsured or underinsured.[5] Is it proper or fair to restrict access to transplantation to only those people who can afford to pay? And if we agree that in an ideal world ability to pay should *not* be a criterion for heart or liver or pancreas transplantation, then who *will* pay the bill for patients needing such expensive intervention?[6,7]

As we grapple with the problems of an aging society, and one in which poverty is endemic, we also must deal with the significant changes taking place in health care delivery. In a little less than 200 years, from the time of Thomas Jefferson and his inauguration as president in 1800, we have gone from a country with only two hospitals to one with thousands[1]; from a country where the majority of people lived in farms and villages to one where the great lights of our cities can be seen by orbiting spacecraft; and from a country in which people went to a hospital only

if they were critically ill or injured to one in which not only are limbs reattached, but also organs are replaced with increasing frequency and variety. In the midst of these changes, the role of nurses in the hospital and the increasing importance of the intensive care unit have been two major factors in the changes taking place in health care.

In the mid-1800s, nurses typically worked a 16-hour shift, or "from 5 in the morning to 9 in the evening."[1] This was before the advent of the acceptance of anesthesia, about 20 years before Lister's work on the use of carbolic acid and antisepsis, and about 80 years before the appearance of sulfanilamide and penicillin. Thus it is no wonder that the work was hard, the conditions terrible, the pay poor, and the outcome for the patient often even worse. However, with the establishment of the first three nursing schools in 1873, the seeds were planted for the educational and professional growth of the nursing profession.

The skills taught to nursing students at the Worcester Memorial Hospital at the turn of the century included ". . . the dressing of burns, blisters, and wounds, the application of leeches, minor dressings, and fomentations, the administrations of enemas and baths. Nurses were taught to pass catheters, manage helpless patients so as to prevent bedsores, manufacture bandages, apply splints and bandages—as well as to observe and report their patients' symptoms."[1] With the dramatic increase in knowledge and the potential for intervention in various disease processes, the nursing profession has likewise embraced both role and educational reform. As medicine has advanced, nursing education has advanced. As hospital systems have become more complex, nursing has responded by becoming an essential team member at all levels. While the impetus has been to become a "nurse executive," the underlying value system has been to maintain "humanism amid technology."[8]

The rise of the intensive care unit to its position of preeminence in health care is a relatively new phenomenon. The modern intensive care unit dates from the early 1960s and was formed initially to care for patients with cardiac disease.[9,10] The almost exponential expansion of knowledge in the intervening 30 years has mandated the specialization and proliferation of intensive care units. As of 1987, we had approximately 85,000 intensive care unit beds in the United States, and these were located in 7000 intensive care units in about 6000 hospitals.[11] Even with these extensive facilities, we face the dual crises of not enough nurses and too few beds. In 1981 it was reported that more than 90% of the hospitals in the United States had nursing vacancies in intensive care units.[12] It has been estimated that by the year 2000 at least 400,000 critical care nurses will be needed—twice the number working today.[8] And although it has been noted that we have more intensive care unit beds than any other country in the world, the *Wall Street Journal* and the *New York Times* have devoted articles to the "medical quandary," "wartime triage," and "crisis" resulting from overcrowded facilities in 1989.[13,14] Although we would not want to return to nursing as practiced at the turn of the century, a time of lye and leeches, it certainly was a simpler time.

In 1914 Alexis Carrell, 41 years old at the time, and speaking before the International Surgical Association, stated, "The surgical side of transplantation of organs is now completed as we are now able to perform transplantation of organs with perfect ease.... All our efforts must now be directed toward the biological methods which will prevent the reaction of the organism against foreign tissue."[15] Two years earlier Carrell had won the Nobel Prize for Physiology in Medicine, and his comments presaged the great struggles still being waged in the transplantation effort.[16] In 1954 the surgeons and physicians at the Peter Bent Brigham Hospital in Boston overcame the problem of transplanting "foreign tissue" by ingeniously transplanting a human kidney from Ronald Herrick into his *identical twin,* Richard Herrick.[17] Liver transplantation in humans was attempted by Tom Starzl in 1963, but after five consecutive failures, he halted his program until 1966. In 1967, still with relatively crude immunosuppression methods, Dr. Christiaan Barnard surprised the world medical community with his first heart transplant. The recipient, Louis Washkansky, lived only about 3 weeks. The fledgling efforts of these doctors and others awaited the discovery of new agents to combat rejection. That wait was relatively short: In 1969, Jean Borel began tests on soil brought back from southern Norway, and in 1972 he discovered that a polypeptide, cyclosporine, displayed immunosuppressive effects. Although the next decade would be devoted to evaluating the potential of this agent, the dream of combatting rejection was closer to becoming a reality.

As we approach the year 2000, the ability to transplant both tissues and organs has never seemed brighter. New agents to combat rejection, such as FK-506, promise even greater efficacy in fighting rejection with fewer harmful side effects.[18] Fresh attempts to solve heretofore insoluble problems are being made—witness the first reports of the transplantation of multiple abdominal viscera to overcome short bowel syndrome and secondary liver failure.[19,20] A cautionary note was sounded in a follow-up article by Dr. Francis Moore, who recommended that further such attempts should be delayed until laboratory and animal work had suggested a "palpable likelihood of success."[21] Ethics and economics are two fields that also have been strained by the development of transplantation, and as we approach the twenty-first century, we will be forced to confront issues, questions, and problems now not even thought of. With a limited supply of donor organs, we are already being asked to consider the propriety of using living donors for liver transplantation[22,23] or of using anencephalic newborns to supply multiple organs.[24]

In *Organ and Tissue Transplantation: Implications for Professional Nursing Practice,* Susan Smith and her colleagues have tried to look at transplantation not only from a medical perspective—"how we do it"—but also from the standpoint of how the transplantation of tissues and organs affects society as a whole. Nurses have a central role in health care and health care delivery. In these complex times, when many health care professionals find little time to pause at the bedside, to hold the patient's hand, in effect to say that "we care," the nurse has more responsibility for the patient's well-being than ever. To the extent that you are stimulated by this text, that you attempt to assimilate and understand the various demands on society and the nursing and medical professions that transplantation presents, then to that extent will Susan Smith and her colleagues have succeeded.

REFERENCES

1. Rosenberg CE (1987). *The care of strangers: the rise of America's hospital system.* New York: Basic Books, Inc.
2. Barringer F (Oct 19, 1989). 32 million lived in poverty in '88, a figure unchanged. *New York Times,* p. 16.
3. Bane MJ and Ellwood DT (1989). One fifth of the nation's children: why are they poor? *Science, 245,* 1047-1053.
4. Goldsmith JC (1986). The US Health Care System in the Year 2000. *Journal of the American Medical Association, 256*(24), 3371-3375.
5. Evans RW (1989). Money matters: should ability to pay ever be a consideration in gaining access to transplantation? *Transplantation Proceedings, 21*(3), 3419-3423.
6. Berwick DM and Hiatt HH (1989). Who pays? (Editorial). *New England Journal of Medicine, 321*(8), 541-542.
7. Garfunkel JM and Denny FW Jr (1989). Priorities for the use of finite resources: now may be the time to choose. *Journal of Pediatrics, 115*(3), 410-411.
8. Searle LD (1989). Milestones. The president's message. American Association of Critical-Care Nurses. *Heart and Lung, 18*(3), 23A-36A.
9. Brown KWG, MacMillan RL, Forbath N, Mel'Grano F, and Scott JW (1963). Coronary unit: an intensive-care centre for acute myocardial infarction. *Lancet,* August 17, *2,* 349-352.
10. Hughes WD (1963). An intensive coronary care area. *Diseases of the Chest, 44*(4), 423-427.
11. Baggs JG (1989). Intensive care unit use and collaboration between nurses and physicians. *Heart and Lung, 18*(4), 332-338.
12. Civetta JM (1981). Beyond technology: intensive care in the 1980's. Presidential address. *Critical Care Medicine, 9*(14), 763-767.
13. Otten AL (May 23, 1989). Intensive-care units are rejecting patients because of crowding. *Wall Street Journal,* vol CCXIII, no 100.
14. Rosenthal E (Aug 22, 1989). Crowding causes agonizing crisis in intensive care. *New York Times,* p. 5.
15. Cosimi AB (Jan 1989). Transplantation. *ACS Bulletin,* pp 41-47.
16. Friedman SG (1988). Alexis Carrell: Jules Verne of cardiovascular surgery. *American Journal of Surgery, 155,* 420-423.
17. Merrill JP, Murray JE, Harrison JH and Guild WR (1956). Successful homotransplantation of the human kidney between identical twins. *Journal of the American Medical Association,* 160, 277-282.
18. Starzl TE (1989). Transplantation. *Journal of the American Medical Association, 261*(19), 2894-2895.
19. Starzl TE, Rowe MI, Satoru T, Jaffe R, Tzakis A, Hoffman AL, Esquivel C, Porter KA, Venkataramanan R, Makowka L and Duquesnoy R (1989). Transplantation of multiple abdominal viscera. *Journal of the American Medical Association, 261*(10), 1449-1457.
20. Williams JW, Sankary HN, Foster PF, Lowe J and Goldman GM (1989). Splanchnic transplantation. *Journal of the American Medical Association, 261*(10), 1458-1462.
21. Moore FD (1989). The desperate case: care (costs, applicability, research, ethics). Editorial. *Journal of the American Medical Association, 261*(10), 1483-1484.
22. Raia S, Nery JR and Mies S (1989). Liver transplantation from live donors. Letter to the Editor. *Lancet,* August 26, *2,* 497.
23. Singer PA, Siegler M, Whitington PF, Lantos JD, Emond JC, Thistlethwaite JR and Broelsch CE (1989). Ethics of liver transplantation with living donors. *New England Journal of Medicine 321*(9), 620-621.
24. Peabody JL, Emery JR and Ashwal S (1989). Experience with anencephalic infants as prospective organ donors. *New England Journal of Medicine 321*(6), 344-350.

2

Historical Perspective of Transplantation

Susan L. Smith

THE PAST

Although advances in biomedical technology have focused much recent public and professional attention on lifesaving and life-extending organ transplant procedures, humanity's dream of longevity and yearning for rejuvenation are recorded in early Eastern and Western literature. In China, Hua To' (second century BC) and Pien Ch'iso (second century AD) are reported to have transplanted tissues and organs, including the heart.[1] In the West the patron saints of medicine Cosmos and Damian (285 to 305 AD) are reported to have transplanted the leg of a recently deceased man onto an amputee.[2] Given the scientific climate of the world during these times and the logical absurdity of the second example, these accounts are most likely mythical or legendary. A more credible account of autologous skin grafting by Sushruta for the purpose of plastic surgery of the face is recorded in the Indian Sanskrit text *Sushruta Shamhita* in the second or third century BC.[3]

The era of modern transplantation, however, began in the late eighteenth century when John Hunter successfully replaced a premolar in a man[3,4] (Fig. 2-1). Hunter, who is called the father of experimental surgery, believed that all living substances had the disposition to unite when brought into firm contact with one another. Following this line of thinking, Brown Sequard in the nineteenth century suggested that severed limbs might be sewn back on.[3,4]

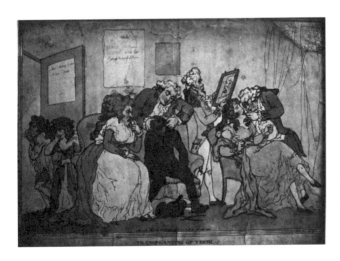

Fig. 2-1 Engraving by Thomas Rowlandson, "Transplanting of Teeth" (1787). (From the collection of William Hefland, New York. In Lyons AS and Petrucelli RJ (1989). Medicine: an illustrated history. St Louis: The CV Mosby Co.)

The immune system

The early focus of transplantation was technical: replacing lost limbs and teeth, transferring a body part from one animal to another. In the nineteenth century the focus changed, with one important exception, to the biologic aspects of transplantation. That exception is the work of Alexis Carrel on vascular anastomosis, which was a prerequisite to successful solid organ transplantation. Carrel began his work in 1902 and was awarded the Nobel Prize in 1912 for his technique for vascular suturing. Once this technique was mastered, solid organs could be transplanted from one animal to another.[5]

The biologic focus has been primarily concerned with the immune system. Although the earliest knowledge of immune mechanisms developed because of the need for an explanation of diseases that plagued humanity, organ and tissue transplantation provided the impetus for the scientific endeavors that revolutionized the field of immunology.

The earliest blood transfusions occurred in the seventeenth century.[3] The blood of animals was transfused into humans. The results were so devastating that the practice of blood transfusion was discontinued for approximately 150 years. In 1900 Landsteiner and Miller first recognized that humans could be grouped according to the presence of agglutinins in their sera. They eventually discovered ABO, Rh, and other red cell antigens and laid the foundation for histocompatibility testing.[6] In 1923 Williamson differentiated between autografting and homografting and made the observation that it was unfortunate that lower animals, such as dogs, did not possess a blood grouping similar to that of humans.[3] He predicted that tissue typing would someday be used in transplantation.

In the 1930s two scientists made significant contributions to transplantation immunology. George Snell, a molecular geneticist, while looking for a way to produce immunity to tumors, discovered the H_2 major histocompatibility system in mice.[3,7] In 1937 Peter Gorer identified the first histocompatibility antigen in humans.[3,4,8] He described the concept of "self versus nonself" when he realized that antigens on tissue cells are genetically determined and capable of eliciting foreign graft destruction.

It is primarily from the study of skin grafting that we have learned much about the immune system and the role of genetics in tolerance and rejection of foreign tissue. In 1943 Peter Medawar, an immunologist and zoologist investigating skin grafting in rabbits, differentiated between responses to homografting and autografting.[8] The observations were also made that skin grafts from a family member were better tolerated than those from an unrelated donor and that skin grafts from an identical twin were better tolerated than those from other family members. Medawar subsequently described the characteristics of the immune response: recognition, destruction, and memory.

The first evidence for leukocyte blood groups in humans was provided by Dausset in 1952.[3,9] He realized that individuals who had received numerous blood transfusions had leukoagglutinins in their sera, whereas those who had received few or no transfusions did not have isoagglutinins in their sera. This important observation led to the accurate conclusion that alloantibodies as well as autoantibodies exist.

Research in the 1960s was concentrated on transplantation antigens. Dausset discovered the HLA locus in humans when studying the sera of polytransfused patients and multiparous women.[3,4] In 1964 Terasaki et al[10] developed the methods for testing for the presence of preformed circulating cytotoxic antibodies, thus introducing microlymphocytotoxicity testing.

Rejection. In the last half of the sixteenth century the Italian physician Gasparro Tagliacozzi referred to what we now call rejection as the "force and power"[3]; and indeed the rejection response is forceful, and powerful drugs are required to overcome it. Tagliacozzi performed skin autografts, but refrained from tissue or organ allografting because of this force and power that he could not explain. Until the nineteenth century, transplantation was restricted to autografting techniques.

Beginning in the nineteenth century xenografting became the subject of experimentation, although it was recognized even then that autografting was a superior technique in terms of graft survival. The real problem of rejection began to be realized early in the twentieth century when allografting became the research model. In 1911 Eric Lexer in an address to the

German Medical Congress reported that allografts seldom lasted longer than 3 weeks.[3] Shortly thereafter in 1924 Holman recognized that a single donor's skin graft rejected more rapidly on the second application.[3] This observation was eventually referred to as the *second set* phenomenon and was to some researchers strong evidence that allografting was a useless and fruitless endeavor. But to others it represented the challenge of an as yet unexplained immunologic phenomenon. In the 1940s Peter Medawar collaborated with the plastic surgeon T. Gibson in skin grafting of rabbits in response to the need for human skin grafting of World War II burn victims in England. Reporting on the second set phenomenon, Medawar[11] stated, "If an initial skin graft was placed from Animal A to Animal B, it had a survival of about 7 days. If a second set of skin was applied in exactly the same fashion between the two animals, the second set of skin was rejected in about half that period of time." Medawar is credited with articulating this second set response as a reliable conceptual model for future research.

In the 1950s Morton Simonson[12] observed that acute rejection was not mediated by antibodies; Mitchison demonstrated that lymphocytes could indeed directly attack a foreign graft.[12] Merrill, Murray et al[13] defined the problem of solid organ transplantation in 1954, when a kidney transplanted from a healthy twin into the other twin suffering from chronic glomerulonephritis was not rejected. It was not until the 1960s and 1970s, though, that disparity at the major histocompatibility complex (MHC) was recognized as a genetic basis for rejection.

Immunosuppression. The birth of induced immunosuppression for transplantation is credited to John Loutit, who in the 1950s experimented with total body irradiation in rodents undergoing skin grafting.[14] In 1958 this form of immunosuppression was applied to humans by Murray in Boston and Hamburger in Paris.[3] This method, however, was not successful in preventing rejection and was complicated by the development of lethal infections.

Although other chemotherapeutic agents were being investigated for use in transplantation, it was the work by Schwartz and Dameshek[15] on the antimetabolite 6-mercaptopurine that dramatically changed the course of transplantation. From 6-mercaptopurine the Burroughs-Wellcome laboratory developed azathioprine (Imuran). In the early 1960s this new immunosuppressant drug was applied to kidney transplantation in the animal model by Calne[16] and to humans by Merrill et al[17] in 1962. Soon afterward Starzl[18] successfully combined azathioprine with a corticosteroid as an immunosuppressive regimen for transplantation. Since 1962 all transplantation of organs and tissues between unrelated individuals has been performed with pharmacologically induced immunosuppression.

The contributions of Starzl[19] to the field of transplantation immunology are notable. Starzl is credited with first combining prednisone and azathioprine for the prevention of allograft rejection. He was the first to recognize that ABO incompatibility is a contraindication to solid organ transplantation. He first described the histopathologic changes of solid organ rejection. He performed the first prospective randomized trial in clinical organ transplantation when investigating the role of thymectomy in long-term kidney graft survival. He also investigated the role of thoracic duct drainage in kidney graft survival.

Solid organ transplantation

Solid organ transplantation in humans has a relatively short history, spanning less than 40 years, but it is rich with the accomplishments of the early pioneers of each field. Although pioneered separately, the accomplishments in one field have consistently affected progress in the others.

Kidney transplantation. The kidney has been the prototype organ for the important developments in solid organ transplantation. There are several reasons for this.[14] First, the kidney has a relatively simple vascular supply. Second, the ability to visualize urine from the ureter provides immediate feedback on the functional status of the graft. Third, the kidney is a paired organ, which allows the use of either living donors or cadavers.

Ullman reported the first attempts at experimental kidney grafting in animals using prosthetic tubes for the anastamoses.[3] In 1906 Jaboulay transplanted kidneys from goats, sheep, and monkeys into humans. These attempts at kidney xenografting were unsuccessful.[4] It was not until 1936 that Voronoy performed the first human-to-human kidney transplant. He too, was unsuccessful. A true appreciation for and understanding of rejection and the role of immunosuppression were yet to be realized.

The first successful kidney transplant was performed in 1946 by Hume, Huffnagle, and Landsteiner when they anastomosed a cadaveric kidney graft to the upper extremity vessels of a patient in acute renal failure caused by septicemia.[3,4] The reason that this attempt was successful is that it was used as only a temporary measure to support the patient, whose renal function recovered within 2 days. Therefore, the graft was not in place long enough to succumb to acute rejection.

The development of dialysis made a major impact on kidney transplantation and on organ transplantation in general. Its beginnings, however, were auspicious. Kolff of Holland made the first dialyzer from sausage casing and tomato cans in 1944.[20] All the patients dialyzed by Kolf died. It was not until further work by George Thorn at the Peter Bent Brigham Hospital in Boston from 1947 to 1950 that dialysis became an acceptable therapeutic alternative. Not only were patients' lives being saved, but kidney disease could now be studied aggressively.[14]

With the advent of dialysis there existed a population of patients that could benefit from kidney transplantation. During the 1950s and 1960s the revolution in kidney transplantation was taking place. In 1951 Hume began cadaveric allotransplantation.[21] His initial attempts were not successful, which is not surprising, considering he did not use pharmacologic immunosuppression except for small doses of adrenocorticotropic hormone and cortisone. The first living-related donor kidney transplant was performed in 1953 by Michan in Paris.[3] Rejection destroyed the graft in 22 days.

Organ transplantation had a hallmark year in 1954, when Merrill and Murray performed the first successful human kidney transplant between monozygotic twins. The fact that the kidney did not reject led to the realization that there is a genetic basis for donor-recipient compatibility.

In the 1960s Scribner and Quinton developed the AV shunt as an access for hemodialysis.[4] Although the AV shunt is not in widespread use today, it was the gold standard for temporary dialysis access for approximately 20 years. During the first half of the 1960s the majority of kidney transplants were performed at Veterans Administration (VA) hospitals,[4] which began the first national hemodialysis program comprising a national network of regionalized health care. The VA financed the care of patients with end-stage renal disease. More than 40 dialysis centers and over a dozen transplant centers were established within the VA system.

End-stage renal disease legislation. What began as a relatively controlled form of treatment for patients with end-stage renal disease began to change in the late 1960s. In 1966 the Bureau of the Budget appointed a committee to analyze the implications to the federal government of the availability of dialysis and kidney transplantation.[22] The Bureau viewed transplantation as the ultimate treatment for end-stage renal disease and chronic dialysis as a "bridge" to transplantation. The Bureau recommended that a National Treatment Benefit Program be established under the Social Security Act.

It was not until 1970, however, that the treatment of kidney disease was targeted for federal support. In 1971, during hearings by the Ways and Means Committee of the House of Representatives, a patient was hemodialyzed before members of the committee. Legislation for financing of treatment for end-stage renal disease was introduced and in 1972 the End-Stage Renal Disease Program was enacted (Hartke Amendment, Section 299 I of the Welfare Reform Bill PL 92-603).[4] The purpose of the program was to provide access to lifesaving treatment for all in need and for whom treatment was prohibitively expensive. The program was federally funded within the Social Security Administration and entitled individuals who suffered from chronic renal failure and who required dialysis or transplantation to stay alive to financial support of those treatment options.

The expenses of dialysis and transplantation

for an unlimited number of patients were grossly underestimated. The initial yearly cost of $184 million grew to $2 billion for 70,000 beneficiaries in 1982. In 1991 the cost for an estimated 93,600 beneficiaries is $3.6 billion.[23]

Heart transplantation. The first attempts at heart transplantation were canine heterotopic procedures. In 1905 Carrell and Guthrie[24] transplanted a heart to the neck of the recipient. The real focus of the surgery was perfection of techniques of vascular anastomosis, rather than organ replacement. In 1933 Mann refined the technnique of heterotopic heart transplantation in dogs by placing the cadaver heart into the recipient's chest.[3] The attempt at successful canine transplantation was thwarted by allograft rejection. For the next two decades researchers met with a similar lack of success.

In the 1960s Lower and Shumway[25] at Stanford pioneered canine orthotopic heart transplantation and were the first to perform this procedure successfully. It was also in the 1960s that human heart transplantation was first attempted. In 1964 Hardy performed a cardiac xenograft. The heart from a chimpanzee was transplanted into a 68-year-old patient in cardiogenic shock.[3] The patient survived for 1 hour, because the donor heart was too small to support the larger recipient's volume. In 1967 Christiaan Barnard[26] made headlines worldwide after performing the first human-to-human heart transplant. The patient lived for 17 days. Other attempts were so disasterous that the practice was essentially abandoned until the mid-1970s.

The major barrier to successful cardiac transplantation was rejection. Shumway persisted with the study of cardiac rejection, and with the use of azathioprine and corticosteroids was able to perform over 30 successful heart transplants.[3] In 1974 Barnard performed the first human heterotopic heart transplant in a patient with pulmonary hypertension. Advances in immunologic monitoring and immunosuppressive therapy have allowed the clinical specialty of heart transplantation to be realized.

Liver transplantation. Not until the 1960s was there a glimmer of hope for a cure for end-stage liver disease. Until then the diagnosis of cirrhosis was a diagnosis of ultimate death from the consequences of portal hypertension. The first reported animal models of liver transplantation were in the mid-1950s. In 1955 Welch[27] performed the first heterotopic liver transplant in a dog. The first known efforts at experimental orthotopic liver transplantation were made by Cannon[28] in 1956 at the University of California at Los Angeles.

The years 1963 and 1967 are the landmark years for liver transplantation. In 1963 Starzl[18] performed the first liver transplant at the University of Colorado, but it was not until 4 years later that he performed the first successful human liver transplant, again at the University of Colorado. Thomas E. Starzl is the father of liver transplantation. From the late 1950s until the present he has pioneered every aspect of this procedure. Although liver transplantation has been most actively pioneered in the United States, the contributions of Sir Roy Calne, Professor and Chairman of the Department of Surgery at Cambridge University, are significant.

Liver transplantation represents a scientific revolution of the present decade. In 20 years liver transplantation has moved from a highly experimental procedure to one that is now accepted worldwide as a therapeutic option for patients with many types of liver disease. The number of centers performing liver transplantation in the United States now exceeds 50. In 1988 Iwatsuki et al[29] from the University of Pittsburgh reported on their experience in 1000 liver transplants using cyclosporine-steroid immunosuppression. Their overall survival rate in this group of patients is three times greater than in their previous experience using azathioprine-steroid immunosuppression before 1980.

THE PRESENT

The current status of organ transplantation reflects the early years of laboratory and clinical investigations. But just what is the current status? And what are the issues and problems?

The estimated need

In 1973 there were approximately 11,000 individuals in the United States with end-stage renal disease. Three thousand, or 27%, received transplants. By 1983 the number with end-stage renal disease had increased to approximately 72,000. Only 6000, or 8%, received transplants.[30] Currently there are approximately 80,000 patients receiving long-term dialysis and 8500 awaiting transplant.[31] The estimated number of individuals who could potentially benefit from a heart transplant is between 2000 to 75,000 per year.[31] At least 14,000 individuals die each year of conditions that could be treated with heart transplantation.[31] And the estimated need for liver transplantation is 5000 to 9500 per year.[31]

The lack of donor organs is the major rate-limiting factor in organ transplantation today. The discrepancy continues between the demand for donor organs for transplantation and the available supply. The estimated potential organ donor pool is 17,000 to 26,000 per year.[32] Yet with only about 4000 donors each year, only 15% to 20% of the potential is being realized.

Number of transplants performed

There has been a tremendous surge in the 1980s in the number of transplant procedures performed.[33] From 1982 to 1986 the number of kidney transplants increased by approximately 70%. The number of heart transplants doubled in the years 1985, 1986, and 1987. In the years 1982 through 1985, the number of liver transplants doubled and increased by 505 in 1986. In 1988 the number of solid organ transplant procedures was as follows[34]:

Kidney: 9123 (7278 cadaveric and 1845 living-related)
Liver: 1680
Heart: 1647
Pancreas: 243
Heart/lung en bloc: 74
Lung: 31 (21 bilateral and 10 single)

Success rates

Current success rates for graft and patient survival are impressive, particularly when compared with those in the era before the introduction of cyclosporine. Before cyclosporine was developed, 1-year kidney graft survival was 25% to 30%; currently it is 95% to 97%.[35] Before the advent of cyclosporine the 1-year patient survival rates for heart and liver transplantation were 63% and 35% respectively; currently they consistently exceed 70%.[36]

The cost of transplantation

In the last two decades the percentage of health care resources dedicated to high-technology medicine, such as dialysis and organ transplantation, has increased dramatically. To say that transplantation is costly is to make a grand understatement. The average cost for solid organ transplants, including the first year of treatment and followup, are as follows[31]:

Kidney transplant: $25,000 to $50,000
Heart transplant: $95,000 to $148,000
Liver transplant: $130,000 to $320,000

The real issue, however, is not the actual costs, but the fact that these expensive procedures are provided to a relatively small number of beneficiaries and at a high price to society, and that these life-saving procedures are cost prohibitive to some. The ethical question of who should be transplanted now has the added dimensions of "Who will pay and how much?" and "How many transplants should one person be offered?"

When the Social Security Act was amended in 1972 to cover the cost of dialysis and treatment for end-stage renal disease, the revolution in transplantation was not complete, nor is it today. It was not foreseen that the cost of this program alone would be in excess of $2 billion annually. Now there are thousands of patients and families with end-stage heart and liver disease who are asking, "What is so privileged about end-stage renal disease?" Although many federal and state task forces have convened to answer these and other pertinent questions related to the fiscal constraints of transplantation, there are, unfortunately, no answers at this time or on the horizon.

CONCLUSION

The history of organ and tissue transplanation is one of changing and emerging paradigms and scientific revolution. For advancement of the early field of transplantation, scientific and philosophical beliefs had to change. One of the most significant factors in the advancement of scientific medicine in the nineteenth century was the challenge to the theory of spontaneous generation in favor of the germ theory. Although this was to have no real significance to transplantation until well into the present century, it was a critical change in thinking, since infection remains today the major contributor to morbidity and mortality in transplant patients.

A conceptual revolution in the field of immunology took place that provided the foundation for combating rejection. The old world view was the Greek *humoralist* view that disease was caused by an imbalance in essential body humors. In the nineteenth century a new world view evolved, that of Virchow's cellular pathology view that disease is caused by abnormal cellular function. Until this time the possibility of cellular immunity had not been recognized. In the early part of this century the immunologic foundations were laid for the current practice of transplantation. The scientific revolution culminated in the 1960s and 1970s with the worldwide acceptance of kidney transplantation as a therapeutic option for patients with end-stage renal disease.

A great deal of pioneering by visionary scientists and clinicians alike has taken place to bring organ and tissue transplantation to its present status. Scientists and clinicians from multiple fields have joined together to construct the discipline of transplantation. Geneticists, pathologists, radiologists, immunologists, biologists, zoologists, engineers, and clinicians have not only contributed to the technology, but also have taken risks and suffered disappointments, as the early days of transplantation were fraught with many problems, tragedy among them.

Developments during World War II had widespread and lasting impact on clinical medicine, nursing, transplantation, and society in general, for it was in response to the casualties of that war that the biomedical advances in antibiotics, plasma fractionation, endotracheal positive pressure anesthesia, dialysis, and skin grafting were made.[14]

Factors that have changed the course of transplantation are numerous. The importance of the ability to vascularize foreign grafts has been discussed. With histocompatibility testing it is possible, to some extent, to predict a negative outcome and to increase the likelihood of a positive outcome. Artificial organ support— dialysis, mechanical ventilation, extracorporeal bypass—can keep patients alive long enough to receive transplants and can temporarily support vital organ function during and after transplant surgery. Technical advances in the 1970s and 1980s made it necessary to redefine death, and there has been a great deal of discussion and legislation directed at increasing the supply of donor organs for transplantation. Organ preservation techniques have been improved in some cases to the extent that kidney and liver transplantation can be elective surgical procedures. Widespread third-party reimbursement has made lifesaving procedures available to many. And last, but certainly not least, the development of powerful immunosuppressants has contributed most to the dramatic increases in graft and patient survival. In short, the field of organ transplantation has evolved, particularly in the last three decades, from one of highly experimental procedures to one of therapeutic options to patients with end-stage organ disease.

REFERENCES

1. Veith I (1949). Huang ti nei ching su wen: *The yellow emperor's classic of internal medicine.* (3). Baltimore: Williams & Wilkins Co.
2. MacKinney L (1965). *Medical illustrations in medieval manuscripts.* (p 87). Berkeley: University of California Press.
3. Flye MW (1989). *History of transplantation.* In Flye MW. Principles of organ transplantation. Philadelphia: WB Saunders Co.
4. Ferguson RM (1988). The evolution of solid organ transplantation. In Gallagher TJ and Shoemaker WC (eds). *Critical care. State of the art.* vol 9. Fullerton, Calif: The Society of Critical Care Medicine.
5. Guthrie CC (1912). Applications of blood vessel surgery. In Guthrie CC. *Blood vessel surgery.* (113). New York: Longmans, Green & Co.
6. Landsteiner K (1928). Cell antigens and individual specificity. *Journal of Immunology, 15,* 589-600.
7. Medawar P and Lehner T (1983). *Major histocompatibility system. The Gorer symposium.* London: Blackwell Scientific Publications.
8. Medawar P (1944). The behavior and fate of skin autografts and skin homografts in rabbits. *Journal of Anatomy, 78,* 176-199.
9. Miller WV and Rodey G (1981). *HLA without tears.* Chicago: American Society of Clinical Pathologists.

10. Terasaki PI, Marchioro TL and Starzl TE (1965). *Histocompatibility testing.* (83-95). Washington, DC: National Academy of Sciences.

11. Medawar PB (1945). A second study of the behavior and fate of skin homografts in rabbits. (A report to the War Wounds Committee of the Medical Research Council). *Journal of Anatomy, 69,* 157-176.

12. Simonson M, Buemann J and Gammeltaft A (1953). Biological incompatibility in kidney transplantation in dogs. I. Experimental and morphological investigations. *Acta Pathology Microbiology Scandinavia, 32,* 1-35.

13. Merrill JP, Murray JE, Harrison JH and Guild WR (1956). Successful homotransplantation of the human kidney between identical twins. *Journal of the American Medical Association, 160,* 277-282.

14. Moore FD, Birtch AG, Dagher F, Veith F, Krisher JA, Order SE, Shucart WA, Dammin GJ and Couch NP (1964). Immunosuppression and vascular insufficiency in liver transplantation. *Annals of the New York Academy of Science, 120,* 729-738.

15. Schwartz R, Stack J and Dameshek W (1959). Effect of 6-mercaptopurine on primary and secondary immune responses. *Journal of Clinical Investigation, 38,* 1394-1403.

16. Calne RY (1960). The rejection of renal homograft; inhibition in dogs by 6-mercaptopurine. *Lancet, 1,* 417-418.

17. Murray JE, Merrill JP, Harrison JH, Wilson RE and Dammin JG (1963). Prolonged survival of human kidney homografts by immunosuppressive drug therapy. *New England Journal of Medicine, 268,* 1315-1323.

18. Starzl TE, Marchioro TL and Waddell WR (1963). The reversal of rejection in human renal allografts with subsequent development of homograft tolerance. *Surgery, Gynecology and Obstetrics, 117,* 385-395.

19. Salvatierra O (1988). Renal transplantation — the Starzl influence. *Transplantation Proceedings, 20,* 343-349.

20. Kolff WJ and Berk HTR (1944). The artificial kidney: a dialyser with a great area. *Acta Medica Scandinavica, 117,* 121-134.

21. Hume DM, Merrill JP, Miller BF and Thorn GW (1955). Experiences with renal homotransplantation in the human: report of nine cases. *Journal of Clinical Investigation, 34,* 327-382.

22. Rettig RA (1980). *Implementing the end-stage renal disease program of Medicare.* (25-27). (Prepared for HCFA/HEW). Santa Monica, Calif: Rand Corp.

23. Blagg CR (1988). Lessons learned from the end-stage renal disease experience: Their implications for heart transplantation. In Mathieu D. *Organ substitution technology. Ethical, legal and public policy issues.* (175-197). Boulder: Westview Press.

24. Carrel A and Guthrie CC (1905). The transplantation of veins and organs. *American Medicine, 10,* 1101-1102.

25. Lower RR and Shumway NE (1960). Studies on orthotopic homotransplantation of the canine heart. *Surgical Forum, 11,* 18-19.

26. Barnard CN (1967). A human cardiac transplant. *South African Medical Journal, 41,* 1271-1274.

27. Welch CS (1955). A note on transplantation of the whole liver of dogs. *Transplant Bulletin, 2,* 54-55.

28. Cannon JA (1956). Organs (communication). *Transplant Bulletin, 3,* 7.

29. Iwatsuki S, Starzl TE, Todd S, Gordon RD, Esquivel CO, Tzakis AG, Makowka L, Marsh JW, Koneru B, Stieber A, Klintmalm G and Husberg B (1988). Experience in 1,000 liver transplants under cyclosporine-steroid therapy: A survival report. *Transplantation Proceedings, 20,* 498-504.

30. Mathieu D (1988). Organ procurement and recipient selection. Introduction. In Mathieu D. *Organ substitution technology. Ethical, legal, and public policy issues.* (33-51). Boulder: Westview Press.

31. Baily MA (1988). Economic issues in organ substitution technology. In Mathieu D. *Organ substitution technology. Ethical, legal and public policy issues.* (198-210). Boulder: Westview Press.

32. Task Force on Organ Transplantation (April 1986). *Organ transplantation: issues and recommendations.* Rockville, Md: Health Resources and Services Administration.

33. United States Department of Health and Human Services. Public Health Service (August 1987). *The status of organ donation and coordination service: report to the Congress for fiscal year 1987.*

34. United Network for Organ Sharing (1988). *UNOS Annual Report.* Richmond, Va: UNOS.

35. Held PJ (1987). Analysis of survival of patients undergoing dialysis. *Journal of the American Medical Association, 257,* 645-650.

36. Cosimi AB (1989). Transplantation. *American College of Surgeons Bulletin, 74,* 41-47.

3

Immunologic Aspects of Transplantation

Susan L. Smith

IMMUNE PHYSIOLOGY
Functions of the mature immune system

The word *immune* is derived from the latin term *immunis,* which translates as "free from taxes or free from burden."[1] And indeed our immune system functions to protect us from the burden of injury related to potentially harmful environmental substances and organisms. The mature immune system consists of millions of cells capable of performing three general types of functions: defense, homeostasis, and surveillance.

In providing *defense,* resistance to infection is facilitated by both nonspecific phagocytic mechanisms and more specific immune responses that not only destroy but also remember foreign antigens. Maintaining immunologic *homeostasis* encompasses keeping a balance between immune protective and destructive responses and the removal of senescent or dead immune cells from the body. Although the function of the immune system is inherently protective, there are conditions in which immune responses become destructive to the host, such as autoimmune diseases and anaphylactic reactions. *Surveillance* involves the recognition of microorganisms bearing foreign antigens. Some of the immune cells, lymphocytes in particular, are highly mobile and travel throughout the vascular and lymphatic systems in surveillance of potentially harmful antigens. Some types of cancer cells in particular are sought out and destroyed by immune cells.

Immunocompetence, then, is the possession of a mature immune system that can do at least three things: recognize, destroy, and remember foreign antigens.[2] A lack of this essential property of immunocompetence is termed *anergy,* which is manifested by an inability to mount an effective immune response to a foreign antigen.

The innate immune system. Immune responses, as we understand them today, can be classified into two major types of responses[1-5]: (1) *nonspecific* responses, which are also called natural or innate responses, and (2) *specific* responses, which are the acquired responses. Both types of responses play critical roles in host defense.

The innate immune system consists of natural or nonspecific mechanisms for the protection of an individual against foreign antigens.[1-5] These natural defenses are present from birth and do not necessarily require exposure to antigens to develop. Natural defenses, the body's first line of defense, consist of both anatomic and chemical barriers to microbial invasion.[1-5] Anatomic barriers include the skin, mucous membranes, and ciliated epithelia. Chemical barriers include gastric acid, lysozymes, natural immunoglobulins, and the interferons.

Anatomic and chemical defenses. The skin provides the initial physical barrier to external environmental antigens. The outermost skin layer, the stratum corneum, is the main barrier to microbial invasion.[6] Certain conditions influence the growth of potentially pathogenic organisms on the skin: pH, humidity, and temperature. Alterations in normal conditions related to these factors favor the development of infection. The normally acid pH of the skin inhibits growth of microorganisms. When the acid-base balance of the skin is altered in favor of a higher pH, this protective mechanism is lost. When water loss from epidermal cells exceeds intake, the stratum corneum can dry and crack, predisposing the host to microbial invasion. On the other hand, excessive moisture decreases barrier efficiency.[6]

Skin cells are constantly exfoliating, and in this process organisms are sloughed along with dead skin cells. In addition, the skin is colonized with "normal flora" that through various mechanisms prevent the colonization of potentially pathogenic organisms. Resident flora maintain the skin's pH in the acidic range and compete effectively for nutrients and binding sites on epidermal cells, making it difficult for nonresident flora to survive. Normal flora consist mainly of aerobic cocci and diphtheroids.[7] It is when normal flora are altered, such as occurs with long-term or broad spectrum antibiotic therapy and with the use of disinfectants or occlusive dressings, that potentially pathogenic organisms become "opportunistic." Opportunistic organisms take advantage of the lack of competition for nutrients and epidermal binding sites and multiply to cause potentially lethal infections.

Normal human epidermis contains dendritic antigen-presenting Langerhans cells and keratinocytes that secrete immunoregulatory cytokines.[8] Langerhans cells express macrophage-type surface markers and immune response-associated antigens.[9] These cells perform antigen presentation functions similar to macrophages that are necessary for T helper cell activation.

The sebaceous glands, mammary glands, respiratory epithelium, gastrointestinal (GI) mucosa, genitourinary (GU) mucosa, and conjunctivae all secrete a protective immunoglobulin called secretory IgA. Ciliated respiratory epithelial cells also facilitate the removal of bacteria and other foreign antigens from the respiratory tract, and the low pH of the gastric mucosa prevents bacterial growth in the stomach.

Leukocytes. Leukocytes develop along two major lineages: the *myeloid* lineage or the *lymphoid* lineage.[10,11] The myeloid lineage includes all leukocytes except the lymphocytes, and the lymphoid lineage is composed of T and B lymphocytes (see the box below). Myeloid cells make up the backbone of the natural or innate defense system. All cells of the myeloid lineage are either phagocytes or antigen-presenting cells (APCs).[10] Myeloid leukocytes can be further classified into two major groups: granulocytes and monocytes. The major function of both is phagocytosis.

Granulocytes, commonly referred to as polymorphonuclear granulocytes (PMNs) or "polymorphs," are produced in the bone marrow at the rate of approximately 80 million per day,[10] and their average life span is about 2 to 3 days. Sixty to seventy percent of all leukocytes are PMNs.[10-12] These cells are called "polymorphs" because their nuclei are multilobed; they are called granulocytes because they contain intracellular granules. Their intracellular granules contain hydrolytic enzymes, making the cells cytotoxic to foreign organisms. Furthermore, granulocytes are classified into three more distinct types: neutrophils, eosinophils, and basophils, according to the histologic staining reactions of the granules.

MYELOID AND LYMPHOID LINEAGE

Leukocytes begin as stem cells in the bone marrow and develop along two major lineages: the myeloid lineage and the lymphoid lineage.

Myeloid lineage
Polymorphonuclear granuloyctes
    Neutrophils (PMNs, segs, metamyelocytes)
    Eosinophils
    Basophils
Monocytes
    Phagocytic macrophages
    Antigen-presenting cells (APCs)

Lymphoid lineage
Lymphocytes
    T lymphocytes
       T cell subsets
    B lymphocytes

Neutrophils are the most abundant cells in the bone marrow and blood, comprising about 90% of all PMNs or granulocytes.[10] Three forms of neutrophils can be identified in the peripheral blood: segmented neutrophils or "segs," "bands," and metamyelocytes. Segmented neutrophils are fully mature, bands are slightly immature, and metamyelocytes are completely immature neutrophils. Neutrophils are strongly phagocytic; that is, they ingest microorganisms or other cells and foriegn particles and digest the ingested material within their phagocytic vacuoles.

In infection there is an increased demand for neutrophils. The bone marrow responds by releasing more neutrophils into the circulation, and in this process immature forms are released along with the mature cells. As a result the percentage of bands in the peripheral blood is increased. This condition, referred to as a "shift to the left," indicates acute inflammation. In more serious conditions metamyelocytes will also appear in increased numbers in the peripheral blood. The normal neutrophil count in the adult is between 1000 and 6000 mm^3 blood, or approximately 60% of the differential white blood cell (WBC) count.[10,12] Bands normally number about 600 mm^3 of blood, or approximately 0% to 5% of the differential WBC count.

Eosinophils are weakly phagocytic cells that are seen in increased numbers in the circulation specifically during parasitic infections and allergic hypersensitivity reactions. Eosinophils degranulate on antigenic stimulation and kill organisms extracellularly. The normal eosinophil count is about 200 mm^3 of blood, or between 2% and 5% of the differential WBC count.[10,12]

Basophils are responsible for anaphylactoid reactions to allergens. Like eosinophils, basophils are capable of releasing their cytotoxic granules when stimulated by certain antigens to effect extracellular killing. Basophils are morphologically identical to mast cells but can be differentiated from mast cells in that basophils are blood borne and mast cells reside in tissues outside the circulation. In other words, when a basophil migrates out of the circulation to reside in tissue, it becomes a mast cell. The normal basophil count is about 100 mm^3 of blood, or

about 0.2% of the differential WBC count.[10,12]

Polymorphonuclear granulocytes can be differentiated from monocytes by their multilobed nuclei and many intracellular granules. Monocytes are mononuclear cells that do not contain cytotoxic granules. They do however, release the prostaglandin PGE_2, which is a mediator of the inflammatory response. Blood-borne monocytes leave the bone marrow to become tissue macrophages for the purpose of phagocytizing foreign antigens. Macrophages are nonspecific accessory cells that play a role in primary host defense, control neoplasia, scavenge damaged or dying cells, and interact with lymphocytes to facilitate cellular and humoral immunity. The normal monocyte count is about 200 to 1000 mm^3 of blood, or about 5% of the differential WBC count.[10,12] A specific type of monocyte is the APC. APCs are formed in the epidermis, where they are called Langerhan's cells, and in the lymphoid system. APCs play an important role in linking the innate immune system with the acquired immune system. APCs carry foreign antigens that enter the host via the respiratory or gastrointestinal tract or via the skin through the lymphatic system and present them to lymphocytes in the lymph nodes and spleen, thereby triggering cellular and humoral immune responses.[10,13]

Auxillary myeloid cells also exist, including megakaryocytes (precursors to platelets) and mast cells, which have already been described. Platelets are also important in the initial phases of the inflammatory response.

Other mediators of innate immunity include null cells, killer cells, natural killer cells, the interferons, and acute phase proteins.[5,14] *Null cells* are also referred to as third generation cells because, although they are thought to be lymphoid cells, their exact lineage is unknown. They are neither T cells, B cells, nor macrophages. Null cells kill antibody-coated target cells. *Natural killer cells* are large granular lymphocytes that are activated by interferon to spontaneously kill tumor or virus-infected cells. Prior sensitization is not necessary for activation of natural killer cells.[14] *Interferons* are a group of proteins produced by virally infected cells and lymphocytes. Interferons are produced very early in infection and induce a state of immunity

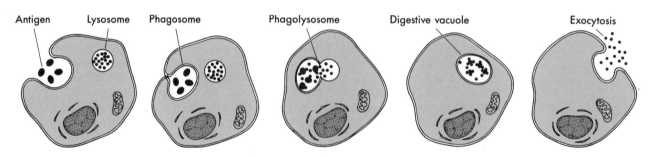

Fig. 3-1 Phagocytosis.

in surrounding noninfected cells by interfering with viral replication.[15] *Acute phase proteins* are a group of proteins that proliferate in the serum during acute infection. Acute phase proteins promote complement binding and opsonization.

Phagocytosis. Phagocytosis, which means "cell eating," is the first event of host defense when a foreign material enters the body. This process is carried out by a network of highly mobile phagocytes in the blood and other tissues that is collectively referred to as the reticuloendothelial system (RES). Phagocytes have surface receptors that allow them to seek out and attack nonspecific foreign organisms, engulf them, and ultimately destroy them. Phagocytosis is the process by which excess antigen and dead cells are removed from the body (Fig. 3-1). Phagocytosis is also essential in the initiation of cellular and humoral immune responses by T and B lymphocytes.[5] Phagocytes of the RES are strategically located in various body tissues (Table 3-1).

Inflammation. Inflammation is the body's attempt to restore homeostasis; it is the initial reaction to injury and the first step in the healing process. Wound healing cannot occur if the inflammatory response is fully inhibited. During the inflammatory response a series of cellular and systemic reactions are triggered that localize and destroy the offending antigen, maintain vascular integrity, and limit tissue damage.[2,16,17]

Tissue injury provides the initial stimulus for activation of inflammatory mechanisms and results in the cellular release of vasoactive substances such as histamine, bradykinin, and serotonin. The circulatory effects are vasodilation and increased blood flow to the affected site; increased vascular permeability, which

Table 3-1 Location of phagocytes of the reticuloendothelial system

Location	Type of cell
Bone marrow	Dendritic cells
Liver	Kupffer cells
Spleen	Sinus macrophages
Kidney	Intraglomerular mesangial cells
Lymph nodes	Sinus macrophages
Lung	Pleural and alveolar macrophages
Peritoneum	Peritoneal macrophages
Brain	Microglial cells
Synovia	Synovial A cells
Blood	PMNs, eosinophils, basophils, monocytes
Capillaries	Endothelial phagocytes

facilitates diapedesis of immune cells from the circulation to the tissues; and tenderness or pain. The clotting system is activated in an attempt to "plug up" the injury. Increased blood flow and capillary permeability lead to local interstitial edema and swelling. Leukocyte migration occurs as phagocytes are attracted (by a process called chemotaxis) to the affected site, and dying leukocytes release pyrogens that stimulate the hypothalamus to produce a state of fever. Pyrogens also stimulate the bone marrow to release more leukocytes, thus perpetuating the process.

And finally, the complement system is activated. The complement system consists of a complex set of approximately 20 interacting proteolytic enzymes and regulatory proteins found in the plasma and body fluids that attack antigens[18] (Fig. 3-2). Complement proteins are effector molecules that modulate inflammatory responses. Inflammatory cells, APCs, and lymphocytes have receptors for complement stimulation and activation. Conceptually, the complement system is similar to the coagulation system in that complement proteins react sequentially in a series of enzymatic reactions in a cascading manner. Several factors are responsible for activation of the complement system: the formation of insoluble antigen-antibody complexes, aggregated immunoglobulin, platelet aggregation, release of endotoxins by gram-negative bacteria, the presence of viruses or bacteria in the circulation, and the release of plasmin and proteases from injured tissues. Complement proteins can mediate the lytic destruction of cells, including red and white blood cells, platelets, bacteria, and viruses.

Complement activation, by itself, can initiate the inflammatory response. Complement is the mediator of the process called *opsonization,* which is the coating of antigen by complement fragments in preparation for destruction of the antigen by neutrophils or antibodies. Complement inactivators present in the liver and spleen "turn off" the complement cascade to prevent damage to normal tissue.

The inflammatory response can be altered or suppressed in many situations: the administration of corticosteroids and other immunosuppressive drugs, malnutrition, advanced age,

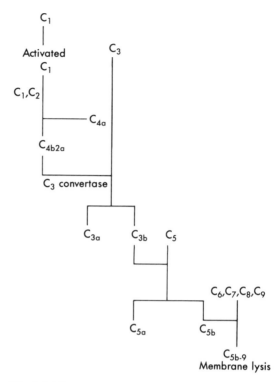

Fig. 3-2 The complement cascade. The human complement system consists of more than 20 plasma proteins, designated as components, that are activated by the formation of antigen-antibody complexes. Activation of the pathway occurs when C1 binds to an activator such as IgG, IgM, C-reactive protein, endotoxin, or virus. Complement activation results in an acute inflammatory-type response, opsonization, and lysis of antigen or antigen-bearing cells. (From Smith SL (1986). Physiology of the immune system. *Critical Care Quarterly, 9,* 7-13.)

chronic illness, and prolonged stress. Conversely, the inflammatory response can become exaggerated in conditions such as anaphylaxis and septic shock.

The body calls on the innate immune mechanisms as the first line of defense in ridding itself of threatening foreign antigens. However, if these mechanisms are not entirely successful, a second set of defenses, the acquired immune system, is activated to work in concert with the innate immune system. The acquired immune system is composed of lymphocytes and other lymphoid structures necessary for specific immune responses.

The acquired immune system. Maturation of the lymphoid system occurs during the fetal and neonatal periods,[13,16,19] when lymphoid stem cells differentiate into T or B lymphocytes. At this time the mechanisms for conferring genetic specificity to lymphocytes develop. This property of specificity is what differentiates the lymphoid cell from the myeloid cell, which can react with any antigen. The process of lymphopoiesis (lymphocyte origination and differentiation into functional effector cells) begins in the yolk sac and continues later in life in the thymus gland, liver, spleen, and finally the bone marrow, which is the primary site of lymphopoiesis in the full-term neonate.

Primary lymphoid tissue consists of "central" organs that serve as major sites of lymphopoiesis[13,20] (Fig. 3-3). Lymphoid stem cells, which originate in the bone marrow, give rise to the various components of the acquired immune system. Secondary lymphoid tissue is "peripheral" tissue that provides an environment for lymphocytes to encounter antigens and proliferate if necessary. Secondary lymphoid tissue

consists of the spleen, lymph nodes, bone marrow, liver, and mucosal associated lymphoid tissue (MALT) in the tonsils, respiratory tract, gut, and urogenital tract. Location of secondary lymphoid tissue is not coincidental, because all of these structures provide major portals for the entry of foreign microorganisms into the body. Once in secondary lymphoid tissues, lymphocytes may migrate from one lymphoid structure to another by vascular and lymphatic channel systems.

Lymphatic channels (Fig. 3-4) provide a major transit system for lymphocytes while they carry out specific functions related to immunologic surveillance. Both superficial and deep lymphatics empty into the large thoracic duct, which drains into the left subclavian vein. Lymph nodes are located at the junctions of lymphatic vessels and form a complete network for the draining and filtering of extravasated lymph from interstitial fluid spaces. Afferent lymphatics carry lymph to the lymph nodes, and efferent lymphatics serve as exit routes for lymphocytes from lymph nodes. The physiologic function of the spleen is not completely understood, but it is known that it has reticuloendothelial, immunologic, and storage functions. The spleen produces monocytes, lymphocytes, and IgM antibody–producing plasma cells.

Lymphocytes, the primary defenders of the acquired immune system, play a central role in regulating immune responses to all antigens; they are the only cells that have the intrinsic ability to recognize specific antigens. Lymphocytes have surface receptors that are specific for surface molecules, sometimes called epitopes, located on the surfaces of foreign proteins. T lymphocytes have receptors for class I and II antigens, and B lymphocytes have receptors for immunoglobulins.

Lymphocytes are the major components of lymph nodes. Only about 5% of lymphocytes are blood borne; the other 95% reside in the lymph nodes and spleen.[10] There are two major populations of lymphocytes: B lymphocytes (B cells) and T lymphocytes (T cells). B cells produce antibodies and mediate what is called the "humoral" immune response. T cells are involved in immunologic regulation and mediate what is called the "cellular" immune response.

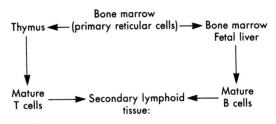

Fig. 3-3 Primary and secondary lymphoid tissue. Lymphocytes migrate by blood and lymphatic circulation from central organs of lymphopoiesis to secondary lymphoid tissue that provides the environment for maturation into functional effector cells and encountering antigens. Once lymphocytes migrate from primary lymphoid tissue, they circulate between the blood lymphocyte pool and the various secondary lymphoid organs.

For the sake of discussion, the two types of lymphocytes will be described separately, but in reality there is much interaction between them, and effective host defense is dependent on this interaction.

B lymphocytes (B cells). B cells are effector cells that mediate the humoral immune response through the production of antibodies,

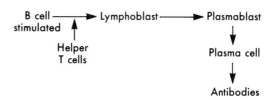

Fig. 3-5 Antigenic stimulation of B cells and subsequent antibody production.

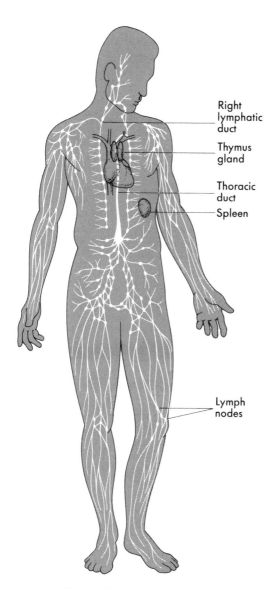

Fig. 3-4 Lymphatic channels.

which is their major function. B cells are important in defense against pyrogenic bacterial infections, and can destroy transplanted organs by mediating hyperacute graft rejection.[4,17,21] When a B cell is stimulated by a particular antigen, it differentiates into a lymphoblast. The lymphoblast differentiates into a plasmablast, which further differentiates into a plasma cell. Plasma cells, which are capable of producing antibody, release antibody until the antigen is destroyed (Fig. 3-5). Following exposure of a B cell to a specific antigen, the antibody it produces may combine with a toxic site on the antigen molecule or cause its removal by phagocytes. In addition, memory of the offending antigen is retained for at least several months.

Antibodies are also referred to as *immunoglobulins.* Immunoglobulins are specifically modified proteins present in serum and tissue fluids that are capable of selectively reacting with inciting antigens. The body produces several million antibodies that are capable of reacting with just as many antigens.[22] However, each is specific and can usually recognize only one antigen. When viruses or bacteria, for instance, enter the body, their structural surface features are recognized by the body as not belonging to it. Antibodies are then formed and attracted to these foreign structures for which they have identical matching receptors. In this way antibodies are able to bind with antigens, which is called antigen-antibody complex formation.

Antibodies can be divided into five major classifications: IgM, IgG, IgA, IgD and IgE.[3,23] *IgM* is the principle mediator of the primary immune response. IgM is a "natural" antibody; there is no known contact with the antigen that stimulated its production. About 10% of all antibodies are of the IgM type. *IgG* is the principle mediator of the secondary immune response, which requires repeated exposure to the same antigen. IgG is the major antibody against bacteria and viruses. About 75% of all antibodies are of the IgG type. *IgA* is the secretory immunoglobulin present in body secretions and offers natural protection against nonspecific foreign antigens. About 15% of all antibodies are of the IgA type. The function of *IgD* is not known, but about 1% of antibodies are of this type. Although only about 0.002% of antibodies are of the *IgE* type, IgE antibodies present on basophils and mast cells play a significant role in inflammatory and immune reactions.

Structurally, antibodies consist of four polypeptide chains, two heavy and two light chains (Fig. 3-6). The light chains have an adaptor component (Fab) that binds to antigen, and the heavy chains have an adaptor component (Fc) that activates complement. Using these adaptor components, the antibody forms a bridge between the antigen and a phagocyte, which facilitates destruction of the antigen. Mechanisms of antigen inactivation by antibody include agglutination, precipitation, neutralization, and lysis.

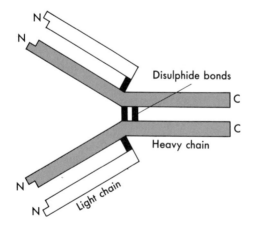

Fig. 3-6 Basic immunoglobulin structure. The unit consists of two identical light polypeptide chains and two identical heavy polypeptide chains linked together by disulphide bonds.

T lymphocytes. Under the influence of thymic hormones, immature T cells develop. During this immature phase of T cell development, reactivity of these cells to self-antigens is eliminated and tolerance to self-antigens occurs. Under continued thymic hormone influence, functionally active T cells develop. As mediators of the cellular immune response, T cells defend our bodies against viruses, fungi, and some neoplastic conditions and destroy transplanted organs by mediating accelerated and acute rejection responses.[4,17,22,24] T cell function is inhibited by viral and parasitic infections, malnutrition, prolonged general anesthesia, radiation therapy, uremia, Hodgkin's disease, and advanced age.

T cells are divided into four functionally distinct but interactive cell populations or subsets: cytotoxic, helper, supressor, and memory T cells. T cell subsets are differentiated by monoclonal antibodies that are specific to glycoproteins on the cell's surfaces. Many receptors are for self-proteins, but fortunately most of these are destroyed before reaching the circulation. In addition to being functionally distinct, these T cell subset populations have different surface antigens or "markers" that can be detected by monoclonal antibodies. *Cytotoxic* and *memory* T cells are referred to as "effector" cells, because they have a specific cytotoxic effect on antigen-bearing cells. Cytotoxic T cells bind to target cells and facilitate their destruction via substances known as *lymphokines* that stimulate inflammatory cells and via the production of cytolytic proteins.[25]

Lymphokines are one of the two soluble products of lymphocytes, the other being antibodies. Lymphokines and monokines released from monocytes are inflammatory and regulatory hormones of the immune system that serve a variety of functions, such as the recruitment of macrophages to antigen sites (chemotaxis), augmentation of T cell function in general, and inhibition of viral replication. Lymphokines carry molecular signals between immunocompetent cells for amplification of the immune response.[15] Their role in amplification of the T cell response is crucial to cellular immunity. A list of lymphokines can be found in the box on p. 23. Two of the most important lympho-

LYMPHOKINES: IMMUNE MEDIATORS RELEASED FROM ANTIGEN-ACTIVATED T AND B LYMPHOCYTES

Interleukin-1
Interleukin-2
Interleukin-3 (multi-colony stimulating factor)
Interleukin-4 (B cell stimulating factor)
Interleukin-5 (B cell growth factor)
Interleukin-6 (B cell differentiation factor)
Interferons (alpha, beta, gamma)
Tumor necrosis factor and lymphotoxin
Migration inhibitor factor
Macrophage activating factor
Chemotactic factor
Colony stimulating factors

kines are interleukin-1 (IL-1) and interleukin-2 (IL-2). IL-1 stimulates T cell proliferation, induces fever, stimulates the liver to produce acute phase proteins, and stimulates the release of prostaglandin. IL-2 (T cell growth factor) also stimulates T cell proliferation. The reaction of T cells with IL-1 is necessary for the production of IL-2.

Memory T cells are T cells that have been sensitized to a specific antigen and then cloned to remember the antigen.[25,26] Memory cells remain present in the body for many years and are therefore available for defense on repeated exposure to an antigen. Repeated exposure to an antigen that the host has been previously sensitized to will result in a more rapid and accelerated immune response than on the first exposure.

Helper and *suppressor* T cells are "regulatory" in nature. Helper T cells are active in lymphokine-mediated events. They produce multiple lymphokines that promote the proliferation and activation of other lymphocytes and macrophages. Although the B cell can produce antibody by direct interaction with surface antigen on a macrophage, the assistance of helper T cells is required for the majority of antibody production. They recruit cytotoxic T cells to antigen sites and interact with macrophages in the spleen and lymph nodes to facilitate antibody production by B cells.[25]

Specifically, helper T cells stimulate macrophage activating factor (MAF or gamma interferon), which causes macrophages to release interleukin-1. Interleukin-1 in turn promotes multiplication and activation of T and B lymphocytes. Helper T cells release migration inhibition factor (MIF), which keeps macrophages in the vicinity of the immune response. Interleukin-2 is also released by helper T cells, which causes activated T cells to proliferate. Helper T cells release B cell differentiation factor (BCDF), which causes B lymphocytes to stop producing IgM antibodies and begin producing IgG antibodies. Finally, helper T cells release B cell growth factor (BCGF), which causes the proliferation of B cells and IgG antibody production. Suppressor T cells produce a soluble factor that suppresses the cytotoxic response by effector cells and inhibits antibody production.[25] Helper and suppressor T cell activity is normally balanced to maintain immunologic homeostasis. Too much suppressor T cell function, for instance, will inhibit helper T cell function.

Lymphocyte responses

Antigen recognition by receptors. It is commonly understood that all cells express foreign antigens. Foreign cells, of course, express antigens that are genetically different from those of the host. It is through specific "receptors" on the surfaces of lymphocytes that B and T cells can be differentiated, and it is also through these receptors that B and T cells are able to recognize foreign antigens. During lymphocyte maturation, each B and T cell acquires specific cell membrane surface receptors that allow them to "match up" with certain foreign antigens. On B cell surfaces immunoglobulins function as receptors; the nature of T cell surface antigens is not entirely clear.[22] This matching between host lymphocytes and foreign antigens is the recognition phase of the acquired immune response. When this occurs lymphocytes are activated to differentiate, proliferate, and clone to mount an effective immune response against the offending antigen.

Specific genes are responsible for the receptors on lymphocytes and distinguish those which respond to particular antigens from those which do not. These genes, then, are responsible for the property of uniqueness that allows each individual to recognize antigens that are genetically different from themselves. No two persons are identical with respect to which antigens will incite an immune response; instead, the human population is extremely heterogenous in this respect.

The major histocompatibility complex. In humans the genetic factor that determines specific antigen recognition is called the *major histocompatibility complex* (MHC).[13,27-29] The MHC is the human leukocyte antigen (HLA) genetic complex located on the short arm of the sixth chromosome. The major function of the MHC is regulation of immune responsiveness. The HLA gene complex encodes cell surface molecules (antigens) that are highly immunogenic or antigenic against cells lacking the same genetic makeup. HLA molecules facilitate the distinction by the lymphoid system of self from nonself. HLA antigens are present on most cells in the body, including leukocytes and platelets, and are widely distributed in tissues and organs. They are not present on mature erythrocytes. These antigens are responsible for leukocyte reactions during blood transfusions and are important determinants of allograft rejection, hence the name "histocompatibility antigens."

The gene products of the MHC (HLA molecules or antigens) are divided into two classes on the basis of structure, tissue distribution, function, and the specific types of antigen

Table 3-2 Major histocompatibility complex (MHC) in humans

Chromosome six (HLA complex)						
Class II antigens				Class I antigens		
DR		DQ (DC)	DP (SB)	C	B		A
DR1	Dw1	DQw1	DPw1	Cw1	Bw4	Bw47	A1
DR2	Dw2	DQw2	DPw2	Cw2	B5	Bw48	A2
DR3	Dw3	DQw3	DPw3	Cw3	Bw6	B49	A3
DR4	Dw4		DPw4	Cw4	B7	Bw50	A9
DR5			DPw5	Cw5	B8	B51	A10
DRw6			DPw6	Cw6	B12	Bw52	A11
DR7	Dw7			Cw7	B13	Bw53	Aw19
DRw8	Dw8			Cw8	B14	Bw54	A23
DRw9					B15	Bw55	A24
DRw10					B16	Bw56	A25
DRw11	Dw5				B17	Bw57	A26
DRw12					B18	Bw58	A28
DRw13	Dw6				B21	Bw59	A29
DRw14	Dw9				Bw22	Bw60	A30
DRw52					B27	Bw61	A31
DRw53					B35	Bw62	A32
					B37	Bw63	Aw33
					B38	Bw64	Aw34
					B39	Bw65	Aw36
					B40	Bw67	Aw43
					Bw41	Bw70	Aw66
					Bw42	Bw71	Aw68
					B44	Bw72	Aw69
					B45	Bw73	
					Bw46		

expressed on their surfaces.[13,30] The two classes of HLA molecules are known as class I and class II antigens[13] (Table 3-2). Class I antigens (HLA A, B, and C antigens) are expressed on the plasma membranes of all nucleated cells, including T and B cells, platelets, and cells of the heart, kidney, and liver.[13,29,31] They function as surface recognition molecules for cytotoxic T cells. Cytotoxic T cells have receptors that recognize class I antigens and will be activated against an antigen only if they share at least one class I HLA determinant with the antigen. Antiviral and antitumor activity and acute graft rejection are facilitated by the recognition of "nonself" class I antigens on foreign cell surfaces by host T cells. HLA types A, B, and C express class I antigens.[13] Class I HLA molecules represent a problem for some patients awaiting transplantation, because they greatly decrease the number of compatible donors. Many individuals are exposed to class I HLA molecules through pregnancy, blood transfusions, or prior transplants. Those previously exposed develop antibodies to HLA class I molecules.

Class II antigens (HLA-DR, -DQ, and -DP antigens) have limited tissue distribution. They are normally expressed only on B cells, activated T cells, macrophages, monocytes, melanoma cells, Langerhans cells, and endothelial cells and dendritic cells in most nonlymphoid tissues.[13,29,31] Class II antigens serve as surface recognition molecules for the activation of interactions among macrophages, B cells, and T cells. Regulatory T cells have receptors that recognize class II antigens. Helper and suppressor T cells can recognize antigen only in the context of the class II molecules that they carry.

Inheritance of HLA antigens. There are five HLA loci: HLA-A, HLA-B, HLA-C, HLA-D, and HLA-DR. Each locus contains many individual alleles. The allelic specificities are designated by numbers following the locus symbol, e.g., HLA-A1 or HLA-B5. Those specificities not agreed on by the World Health Organization Committee on HLA Nomenclature are designated by the letter "w," e.g., HLA-Bw21.[32]

Because human chromosomes exist in pairs, it is possible to identify a total of ten HLA

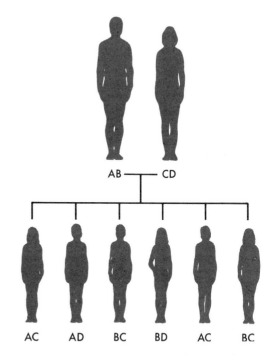

Fig. 3-7 Diagram of inheritance of HLA antigens in family group.

antigens in a given individual, five from each chromosome (HLA-A, -B, -C, -D, and -DR). The expression of HLA antigens on the individual's sixth chromosome is called a phenotype (Fig. 3-7). One haplotype, or half of the total HLA identity, is inherited from each parent. Therefore each individual has two haplotypes. The two inherited haplotypes represent the individual's genotype. Each offspring of the same biologic parents has a 25% possibility of having the same HLA type as a sibling, a 25% possibility of having a totally dissimilar HLA type as a sibling, and a 50% possibility of sharing one haplotype with a sibling.

The cellular immune response. Whereas B cells bind to soluble antigen on the surface of macrophages, T cells can recognize antigen only in association with an MHC antigen. The cellular immune response (Fig. 3-8) is, again, mediated by T cells. T cells recognize class I histocompatibility antigens only after they are

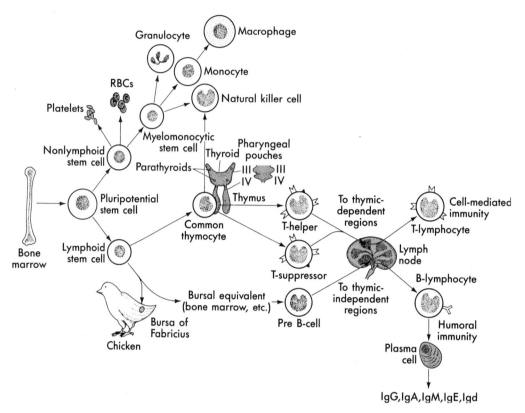

Fig. 3-8 Schematic representation of cellular and humoral mechanisms of the immune response. (Redrawn from Bellanti JA and Kadlec JV (1985). *Immunology III.* Philadelphia: WB Saunders Co.)

displayed on the surfaces of macrophages or APCs.[15] T cells are triggered by stimulation of antigen receptors on their cell surfaces. The cellular immune response can be summarized as follows:

1. Naturally, the presence of a foreign antigen is necessary to initiate the response.
2. Initially, macrophages encounter the antigen and begin to phagocytize it. Antigenic fragments complexed with MHC antigens are released, which are carried to T cells in the lymph nodes by APCs.
3. Resting virgin or memory T cells are activated when the antigen-APC complex binds with the T cell surface receptor.

4. APCs are stimulated to produce interleukin-1, which summons helper T cells.
5. Helper T cells are then responsible for a number of actions, including the release of interleukin-2, which causes the differentiation and proliferation of T cells. The helper T cells also stimulate antibody production by B cells.
6. Clonal expansion increases the sensitized T cell population approximately a thousand-fold.
7. Ultimately, the antigen-bearing cells are destroyed by the direct cytotoxic effect of effector T cells. Some sensitized T cells are returned to the lymphoid system with the

memory of the antigen for future challenge.

Examples of cellular immune responses include tumor cell surveillance, destruction defense against viral and fungal infection, acute organ rejection (a type IV hypersensitivity reaction), graft versus host disease (a type IV hypersensitivity reaction), and autoimmune diseases (type IV hypersensitivity reactions).

The humoral immune response. The humoral immune response (see Fig. 3-8) is mediated by B cells. Antigens trigger B cells by stimulating surface immunoglobulins. The humoral immune response can be summarized as follows:

1. Naturally, as with the cellular immune response, the presence of a foreign antigen is necessary to initiate the process. Unlike T cells, B cells can recognize antigen in its native configuration.
2. Initially, macrophages encounter the antigen and begin to phagocytize it. Antigenic fragments are released that are carried to B cells in the lymph nodes and spleen by APCs. Resting virgin or memory B cells are activated when antigen binds to surface immunoglobulin.
3. Interleukin-1 is released by APCs, and helper T cells stimulate the sensitization and clonal proliferation of effector B cells. B cells are activated to differentiate and produce antibody when antigen binds to their receptors.
4. Antigen-antibody complexes form and ultimately the antigen-bearing cells are destroyed.
5. As in the cellular immune response, some of the plasma cells with specific memory of the antigen are cloned and returned to the lymphoid system.

In addition, B cells can process and present antigen to T cells. Examples of humoral immune responses include resistance to encapsulated pyrogenic bacteria, such as pneumococci, streptococci, meningococci, and *H. influenzae,* and type II and III hypersensitivity reactions, including hyperacute organ rejection.

A first exposure of an antigen to an activated lymphocyte evokes a primary immune response. Repeated exposure of the identical antigen to activated lymphocytes evokes an accelerated secondary response. In the secondary immune response the latent period is shorter and the amount of antigen required to initiate the response is less.[22]

HISTOCOMPATIBILITY

The major limitation in transplantation technology is the potential for rejection of transplanted organs as a result of normal, protective host immune responses. Put another way, tissue transplanted from one individual to another will be rejected if the recipient's immune system recognizes the transplanted organ or tissue as foreign. Histocompatibility testing is used to minimize graft foreignness and reduce donor-specific immune responses to the transplanted organ. The type or types of histocompatibility testing performed will vary, depending on the exact organ or tissue transplanted. The reasons for this variability are that the immunogenicity of organs and tissues varies (see the box below), and the cold ischemic times for different organs and tissues vary considerably. In some cases this is a severely limiting factor; with heart transplantation (with a maximum cold ischemic time of 4 hours), for example, there simply is not enough time to perform HLA typing between donor and recipient.

IMMUNOGENICITY OF DIFFERENT TISSUES

The following tissues are listed according to their capacity to induce allogeneic reactions. Bone marrow is most immunogenic.
1. Bone marrow
2. Skin
3. Islets of Langerhans
4. Heart
5. Kidney
6. Liver

From Roitt IM et al (eds). (1989). Immunology, 2nd ed. St Louis: The CV Mosby Co.

The ABO and HLA systems have been identified as the major transplantation antigens in man. The ABO antigens are present in most body tissues as well as on red blood cells. Two categories of histocompatibility testing are routinely performed in preparation for organ and some types of tissue transplantation—*typing* and *matching* procedures.

Typing procedures

ABO typing. Basic ABO compatibility depends on the presence or absence of antigens on donor red blood cells and the presence or absence of specific antibodies to these antigens in the recipient's serum. Anti-ABO antibodies are of the IgM classification and cause agglutination, complement fixation, and hemolysis.

If an ABO-incompatible graft is transplanted, hyperacute rejection will occur (the possible exception being a liver graft). In kidney transplantation, preformed circulating cytotoxic antibodies in the recipient react with ABO isoagglutinins produced by the graft, and the graft quickly turns dark and soft as a result of diffuse thrombosis of the microvasculature.

Rho (D) antigens. Rho antigens are not expressed on endothelial tissue and therefore play no apparent role in graft rejection or survival. In other words, an organ from a donor with ABO type B positive can be safely transplanted into a recipient with ABO type B negative.

Minor red cell antigens. At least 15 different minor red cell antigen systems have been identified in humans. The most important of these appears to be the Lewis system.[29] Transplant recipients who are highly sensitized to minor red cell antigens as a result of numerous blood transfusions may experience antibody-mediated rejection responses (hyperacute or chronic rejection). For this reason, the potential recipient's blood is screened for the presence of antibodies to the known minor red cell antigens before transplantation.

Vascular endothelial antigens. Vascular endothelial antigens are known to occur but are not easily detected and therefore cannot necessarily be avoided. These antigens may stimulate antibody production in the recipient and trigger hyperacute rejection. Sensitization to these antigens occurs from exposure to monocytes through blood transfusions.

In the early 1970s there was some evidence that blood transfusions administered to kidney recipients before transplantation had beneficial effects related to increased graft survival. However, many centers have stopped this practice because of the relatively high incidence of patients who become sensitized to red blood cell antigens.

HLA typing (microlymphocytotoxicity testing). Microlymphocytotoxicity testing is used to detect class I antigens. HLA tissue typing is performed serologically by adding a standard panel of typing antisera, complement, and tryphan blue stain to purified lymphocytes and observing for lymphocytotoxicity. Cell death confirms that the test cells (recipient and donor cells) possess the antigens being tested for, namely HLA-A, -B, -C, and -DR antigens. Typing procedures identify the exact antigens that would be responsible for incompatibility between the donor and recipient tissue. Microlymphocytotoxicity testing is also used for cross-matching and antibody screening.

Matching procedures

Matching procedures provide an opportunity for donor and recipient antigens to interact and predict the degree of compatibility between donor and potential recipient. Pretransplantation cross-matching involves mixing the recipient's serum with potential donor lymphocytes to identify preformed antibodies in the recipient. Cross-matching can be done between the recipient and a specific potential donor or between the recipient and a panel of random potential donors.

White cell cross-match. The white cell cross-match is done to identify in the potential recipient the presence of preformed circulating cytotoxic antibodies to antigens on the lymphocytes of a specific donor. The recipient's serum is incubated with a specific donor's lymphocytes. A *positive* cross-match means that the recipient has cytotoxic antibodies in the serum against the donor's lymphocytes and is a good predictor of hyperacute rejection. A *negative* cross-match means that the recipient does not have these cytotoxic antibodies present.

Mixed lymphocyte cross-match. The mixed lymphocyte cross-match is also done to identify preformed circulating cytotoxic antibodies in the recipient. The potential recipient's serum is mixed with a randomly selected panel of donor lymphocyte samples to measure their extent of reactivity against the panel. This procedure is also referred to as percentage panel reactive antibody or PRA. A high level or percentage of reactivity suggests a low probability of finding a cross-match–negative donor. Because the development of antibodies may change over time, the potential renal transplant candidate is usually screened monthly.

Mixed leukocyte culture (reaction). The mixed leukocyte culture detects class II antigens and therefore measures donor-recipient compatibility between HLA-D loci. Because this test takes several days to complete, it is used only in preparation for living related donor kidney transplantation. HLA-D loci disparity can occur even when HLA-A and HLA-B loci are identical.

REJECTION

Transplantation of organs or tissue between genetically identical individuals is not hampered by the phenomenon of rejection. However, transplantation of organs or tissue between genetically nonidentical individuals of the same species (and different species) is plagued by rejection and its associated problems. Foreignness is equated with the presence on transplanted tissue of membrane antigens that the host does not have and therefore recognizes as foreign or nonself. If all other factors are optimal (e.g., donor management, the functional state of the donor organ, the surgical procedure, and intraoperative management of the recipient), the major reason for transplant failure is rejection.

The phenomenon of rejection is not fully understood. It is an immunologic response involving the recognition of HLA antigens on donor endothelial tissue cells by recipient lymphocytes or antibodies and subsequent destruction of the antigen-bearing graft. Transplantation of a vascular organ induces MHC sensitization by direct stimulation of circulating host immune cells (macrophages, RE cells) that encounter donor MHC antigens on allograft cell surfaces. The MHC epitopes are recognized, the antigen is processed by the RE cells and presented to the lymphoid system by APCs.

Both donor and host factors contribute to the immune response of rejection. The major donor factor is the expression of MHC antigens on the donor tissue and the presence of APCs within the transplanted graft. The major host factor is prior sensitization against ABO and HLA antigens expressed on the graft. In addition, microbial or other non-MHC antigens may stimulate antibodies that cross-react with MHC antigens.

Rejection is generally classified as one of four types: hyperacute, accelerated, acute, or chronic, according to temporal mechanisms and histopathologic characteristics.[33]

Hyperacute graft rejection

Hyperacute rejection occurs within minutes to hours of vascularization of the graft and is caused by the presence of preformed circulating cytotoxic antibodies, a humoral immune response. Hyperacute rejection is an antibody-mediated cytotoxic response to the fixation of antibodies to specific class I antigens on vascular endothelium, resulting in complement activation and massive intravascular coagulation. The initial event of hyperacute rejection is fixation of antibody to the graft. This is followed by entrapment of formed blood elements and clotting factors in the microvasculature of the graft and subsequent graft necrosis as a result of lack of tissue perfusion. Antibodies responsible for hyperacute rejection include antibodies to ABO blood group antigens, those produced against vascular endothelial antigens, and histocompatibility antigens. For example, if an ABO blood group O recipient receives a kidney from an ABO blood group A donor, once blood circulates through the transplanted kidney, antibody to the A antigen will combine with antigens on the endothelial cells of the kidney and will activate the complement system. The activated complement system causes chemotaxis for phagocytes and induces fibrin deposition. Recruited phagocytes degranulate and release hydrolytic enzymes that cause tissue destruction and rapid rejection of the kidney. Hyperacute rejection most commonly occurs while the patient is still in the operating room; the kidney frequently turns black before the surgical team's eyes. Antibody-to-transplant antigens can develop in recipients who have received multiple blood transfusions or prior transplants or who have had multiple pregnancies. Ensuring ABO blood group compatibility and avoiding positive lymphocyte cross-matches are universally accepted methods for prevention of hyperacute rejection.[34]

Until very recently hyperacute rejection was thought to occur only in transplanted kidneys and not in transplanted hearts or livers.[33] One reason that the kidney is prone to hyperacute rejection and the liver is not may be the difference in the microvascular structures (capillary versus sinusoidal system).[35] Currently there is no definitive evidence that it occurs in nonrenal transplanted organs. ABO compatibility and transplant antigen histocompatibility, however, is necessary for successful heart transplantation, but not for liver transplantation. Retrospective histocompatibility antigen typing and lymphocyte cross-matching have not shown these factors to be relevant to liver graft survival.[34]

Liver grafts are more tolerant of ABO and HLA incompatibility than are renal and heart grafts.[36] Therefore hyperacute rejection is less likely to occur after liver transplantation. Although the reason that hyperacute rejecton does not occur in liver grafts is not fully understood, it is speculated that the enormous cell mass of the liver is capable of absorbing circulating antibody.[37]

The major complication associated with ABO-incompatible liver transplantation is hemolysis.[38] A form of graft-versus-host reaction is caused by B lymphocytes in lymphoid tissue transplanted with the graft. Donor B lymphocytes produce antibodies to ABO antigens on recipient red blood cells, resulting in lysis or hemolysis.[34,38]

Acute graft rejection

Acute rejection occurs within a week to 3 months after transplantation; it is a cellular immune response involving mononuclear, cytotoxic, and helper T cells, monokines, and lymphokines (Fig. 3-9). Acute rejection occurs when antigen is trapped within recipient macrophages and cannot be cleared by the RE system. Quiescent, nonactivated helper T cells encounter specific

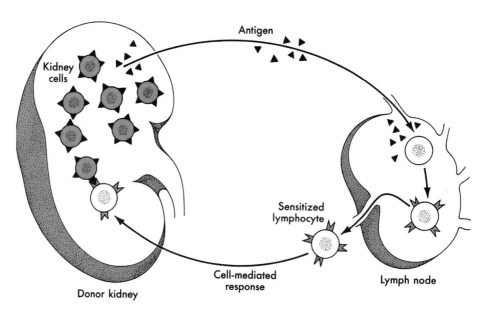

Fig. 3-9 Acute graft rejection. (Redrawn from Ortho Pharmaceutical Corp., Raritan, NJ.)

class II antigens displayed on the donor organ and change to activated cells that synthesize receptors for lymphokines that are simultaneously released from monocytes. Activated monocytes release the lymphokine interleukin-1, which causes clonal expansion of activated helper T cells. Monocytes also release the lymphokine interleukin-2, which activates and causes the clonal expansion of cytotoxic T cells. Acute graft rejection is also associated with viral infections in the transplanted organ. Antigens on the viruses may be similar enough to MHC antigens to stimulate an immune response.

Of the four types of rejection, acute rejection has the greatest clinical significance for critical care nurses, because it can be treated through pharmacologic interventions administered and monitored by nurses. A significant amount of time spent caring for an organ transplant recipient involves clinical assessment of the patient for rejection responses and administration of immunosuppressants to treat rejection. Diagnosis of acute rejection depends on the particular organ or organs transplanted but is generally based on clinical and laboratory evidence of graft dysfunction and biopsy findings. Patient responses to acute rejection vary, depending on the organ being rejected. These responses are addressed in the chapters on kidney (Chapter 11), heart (Chapter 12), liver (Chapter 15), and bone marrow (Chapter 17) transplantation.

Accelerated graft rejection

Accelerated rejection is primarily a cellular immune response, similar to acute rejection, but it occurs more rapidly. Assessment and diagnostic parameters are the same as for acute rejection.

Chronic graft rejection

Chronic rejection can occur at any time later than 3 months after transplantation. Chronic rejection is mediated by both T and B lymphocytes and is therefore a combination of cellular and humoral responses. Chronic rejection leads to insidious, progressive loss of graft function. There is no treatment for chronic rejection short of retransplantation for nonrenal transplant recipients. In extrarenal transplant recipients

this constitutes a potentially life-threatening situation in that retransplantation is ultimately the only therapeutic option; renal transplant recipients can, of course, resume dialysis.

Graft-versus-host reactions

Graft-versus-host disease (GVHD) is the principal limitation to histoincompatible bone marrow transplantation.[39] After bone marrow transplantation, GVHD can develop as either acute or chronic disease. Acute GVHD is characterized by cytolytic destruction of the recipient's skin, GI tract, and liver. Chronic GVHD is characterized by scleroderma-like changes in the skin, GI tract, and liver. GVHD is fully described in Chapter 17, Bone Marrow Transplantation.

INFECTION

Immunosuppression for the treatment of rejection of transplanted organs and tissues is associated with the development of infection in the host. The treatment of rejection and development of infection are in effect reciprocal processes, i.e., the greater the protection against rejection, the greater the risk of infection and vice versa. In the immediate post-transplant phase, finding the right balance involves daily assessment of patient responses and manipulation of pharmacologic regimens. Although specific etiologic and predisposing factors differ, depending on the organ transplanted, the major factor responsible for posttransplant infection is pharmacologic immunosuppression. Immunosuppression represents an alteration in normal protective responses and brings about a state of unresponsiveness of the immune system.

Opportunistic infections

The majority of infections that occur in organ transplant recipients are *opportunistic*. Opportunistic infections are a major cause of death in the immunocompromised patient.[40] Opportunistic infections are caused by organisms that are ubiquitous in the environment but that rarely cause disease in the absence of decreased host defenses. Normal protection from opportunistic organisms is from both innate and acquired immune mechanisms and normal flora. The immunosuppressed individual is vulnerable to both endogenous and external organisms. In general, opportunistic infections result from at least one of three basic mechanisms: (1) exogenous acquisition of a particularly virulent pathogen, e.g., meningococcal meningitis or pneumococcal pneumonia; (2) reactivation of an endogenous latent organism, e.g., herpes simplex, herpes zoster (shingles), or tuberculosis; and (3) endogenous invasion of a normally commensal or saprophytic organism, e.g., bacteria, viruses, fungi, or parasites.[41] The exact type of opportunistic infection (bacterial, viral, fungal, or parasitic) that occurs depends on the type and extent of immunologic alteration, whether it be cellular, humoral, phagocytic, or a combined defect, and organisms present in the internal and external environments. The administration of corticosteroids and other cytotoxic drugs to transplant recipients can result in massive depression of all phases of host defense including a breakdown of cutaneous and mucosal barriers.

Predisposing factors to infection in the transplant patient include the preoperative condition of the patient, i.e., presence of end-stage organ disease (uremia, cirrhosis, cardiomyopathy), nutritional status, and splenic function. Nosocomial factors that cause shifts in microbial flora include the surgical procedure itself, the hospital and critical care environment, the presence of multiresistant hospital organisms, the use of invasive procedures, the administration of antibiotics, and the administration of immunosuppressants to prevent graft rejection.

Nosocomial infections normally occur in one fourth to one half of patients admitted to an intensive care unit.[42] Most infections are caused by multiresistant strains of gram-negative bacteria.[42] In one study it was found that 50% of patients admitted to the ICU became colonized with gram-negative bacteria within 72 hours.[43] The most common nosocomial infections encountered in the ICU are urinary tract infections, pneumonia, and line-related sepsis.[44] Microflora that are abundant in the hospital environment quickly colonize patients' skin, oropharynx, and rectum, and it is these colonizing organisms that most often lead to actual infection.[44] Although fomites such as equipment

routinely used for assessing and treating patients are partially responsible as routes of transmission of organisms, the major route of transmission of iatrogenic infection is direct hand contact.

Although many infections are latent or reactivation infections, approximately 50% are acquired.[45] As shifts in the host's microbial flora occur, the characteristics of organisms colonizing the host change. More than 80% of acquired infections are caused by organisms that the immunosuppressed host was previously colonized with.[45] Organisms that normally colonize mucosae of the immunosuppressed host become pathogenic and penetrate the injured mucosae, establishing local infection that may disseminate to distant organs. The organism that most commonly colonizes the upper respiratory tract is *Staphylococcus aureus,* and organisms that commonly colonize the lower alimentary tract are *Escherichia coli, Klebsiella pneumoniae,* and *Pseudomonas aeruginosa.*

Normal protection from infection is provided by surface barriers such as the skin and mucous membranes, cellular immune mechanisms, and humoral factors. Very few organisms are capable of penetrating the keratin layer of the epidermis; most organisms that reach the host through the skin do so after iatrogenic breaks in the skin, usually for insertion of invasive devices. Few live organisms can be found between the esophagus and the large bowel. GI motility and pH and normal flora in the large bowel are responsible for maintaining this sterile environment. Administration of antibiotics, antacids, H_2 receptor blockers, and stasis of the GI tract interfere with this protective mechanism. Although the surface of the upper respiratory tract is covered by bacteria, the lower respiratory tract is sterile. Responsible protective factors include the cough reflex, cilia, and secretory IgA. The bladder, ureters, and kidneys are sterile, but bacteria colonizing the perineum extend a short distance into the urethra. The major offender in this sterile environment of the bladder is the urinary catheter.

Enteral nutrition is frequently necessary to provide adequate nutrients to critically ill or debilitated patients in the posttransplant period and may be favored over parenteral nutrition in hopes of avoiding fungal sepsis. Enteral formulas, however, are also superb microbiologic culture media and are easily contaminated. Contaminated enteral formulas have been responsible for gastroenteritis and sepsis.[46-51] Organisms that frequently contaminate enteral formulas include *Enterobacter cloacae, K. pneumoniae,* streptococci, *P. aeruginosa, Serratia* ssp., *Citrobacter* ssp., and *Bacillus* ssp.

Strict adherence to aseptic technique with procedures, equipment, and supplies and avoiding injury of tissue and mucous membranes are important in the prevention of infection in the compromised patient. The primary infection control measure, though, is thorough, consistent handwashing.

Bacterial infections. Gram-negative bacteria are ubiquitous in the environment. *P. aeruginosa, Serratia marcesans, Proteus rettgeri,* and *E. cloacae* are the four most common gram-negative organisms implicated in causing infection in the immunosuppressed host.[41] Most bacterial infections are caused by organisms that are already colonizing the patient and originate at sites of mucosal damage, ciliary dysfunction, or integumentary damage.[52] In other words, bacterial infections generally begin when bacteria are allowed to bypass local anatomic and mechanical defense mechanisms. In addition to the obvious example of a break in the skin as a result of tissue injury or the insertion of invasive catheters, loss of the gut mucosal barrier is another important mechanism of bacterial infection. The gut serves as a primary reservoir for life-threatening bacteria in immunosuppressed individuals.[52]

Legionella. The gram-negative bacillus *Legionella pneumophilia* is associated, in the majority of cases, with pathologic conditions limited to the lungs, causing bilateral bronchopneumonia and consolidation. *Legionella* is an aquatic organism commonly found in water sources. No cases of person-to-person transmission have been documented.[53]

Signs and symptoms include dyspnea, dry nonproductive cough, headache, chills, fever, diarrhea, myalgia, and arthralgia. *Legionella* infections are more severe in the transplant population, with the mortality rate being between 25% and 50%.[54-56] A definitive diagnosis of *Legionella* depends on positive cultures obtained by transbronchial or percutaneous needle biopsies or bronchial washings. Serologic diagnosis can be made by indirect and direct antibody assay techniques. A fourfold rise in titer by indirect technique or identification of antibodies in sputum, tissue, pleural fluid, or bronchoscopy specimens by direct technique is also considered diagnostic.

Legionella does not respond to beta-lactam antibiotic therapy. Treatment of *Legionella* infections is with erythromycin, doxycycline, trimethoprim or rifampin.

Nocardiosis. Nocardia species *(N. asteroides, N. caviae, N. braziliersis)* are often misclassified as either fungi or mycobacteria, but they are true bacteria.[57] *Nocardia* is found in soil and decaying vegetable matter worldwide. The organism enters the body by inhalation in most cases. Nocardial infections frequently involve the lung, but hematogenous spread is common, especially in the central nervous system. Sulfonamides are the recommended treatment for nocardiosis.

Viral infections. The viruses most responsible for infection in transplant recipients belong to the family of herpes viruses. Herpesviridae are divided according to their biologic properties into three families: *alpha* herpesviruses, which include herpes simplex virus 1 and 2 (HSV-1 and HSV-2) and varicella zoster virus; the *beta* herpesvirus, cytomegalovirus; and the *gamma* herpesvirus, Epstein-Barr virus.

Viruses are totally dependent on host cells for survival. After the virus enters the host cell it is uncoated, and the viral DNA enters the host nucleus, where it orders transcription of messenger RNA and synthesis of viral proteins in the cytoplasm. Viral proteins take part in DNA synthesis within the nucleus of the host cell. It is here that maturation of the virus occurs.

Viral infections can be of the primary ("de novo") or secondary (reactivation) type. Most viral infections seen in transplant recipients are of the secondary type, because most individuals have had a primary infection with a herpes virus (the species of virus most responsible for infection in transplant recipients), usually in early childhood. Gold[58] reports that by puberty 40% to 80% of individuals have been infected by a herpes virus and that by age 25 almost all adults have.

In primary HSV infection the virus enters the host organism through mucocutaneous surfaces and begins to multiply and migrate toward sensory ganglia. An individual who has experienced a primary infection will have antibodies to the virus in the serum and is said to be seropositive with respect to a particular virus. The individual who has never experienced a primary viral infection is seronegative with respect to a particular virus. A primary infection is an active infection in a previously seronegative recipient.

Secondary viral infections are called *latent* or *reactivation* infections. After the initial or primary infection, long-lasting humoral and cellular immunity is established and the virus establishes a latent and permanent residence in the host, either in the lymphocyte pool or the corresponding sensory ganglia. In latency, for example, the cytomegalovirus virus attaches to C3 receptors on B lymphocytes where viral proteins are produced, but complete viral replication is inhibited. The virus sets up residence in the cell, but outside of the chromosome, which prevents the virus from ever being fully "packaged" and allows for peaceful coexistence of the virus within the cell. Virus that is residing in a neuron or lymphocyte is in effect protected from antiviral antibodies, because antibodies do not penetrate human cells.

Although recurrence or reactivation of the latent virus occurs during or after therapeutic immunosuppression, the association between reactivation and decreased cellular immunity is unclear. During recurrence complete viral replication occurs. The differences between HSV infections in normal and in immunosuppressed individuals include both the severity and chronicity of disease. Even localized infections may be severe in the immunosuppressed individual.

Herpes simplex viruses. There is serologic evidence that approximately 90% of the population will be infected with an HSV at one time or another and that in the majority the virus will establish a latent and permanent residence.[59,60]

Reactivation occurs in 10% to 15% of the general population but is much more prevalent in transplant recipients. HSV-1 is responsible for most herpes infections above the waist, e.g., herpetic lesions of the lips (herpes labialis), face, and mouth. Recurrence sites are those innervated by the trigeminal nerve (eyes, nose, and mouth), and recurrence can lead to keratoconjunctivitis, blindness, and encephalitis.

HSV-2 is responsible for most herpes infections below the waist, e.g., herpes genitalis. Primary HSV-1 infections usually occur in childhood, and primary HSV-2 infections usually occur after puberty. Recurrence can lead to aseptic meningitis, transverse myelitis, and secondary fungal and bacterial infections. Crossover of both types of HSV does occur from autoinoculation and orogenital sexual contact.

Diagnosis of HSV infection can usually be made by direct observation of the characteristic lesions, but isolation of the virus in cell culture provides a definitive diagnosis. Scrapings from a vesicle can be stained (Tzanck smear) to reveal multinucleated giant cells containing intranuclear viral inclusion bodies. However, the Tzanck smear is also diagnostic for herpes varicella and herpes zoster.

HSV infections are prevalent in the transplant population. Pass et al[61] reported a 63% incidence of HSV recurrence in renal transplant patients within 1 month of transplantation. In bone marrow transplant patients, 15% of seronegative and between 70% and 80% of seropositive patients develop active HSV infections.[62-63] The most common manifestations of HSV infection in the immunosuppressed patient are mucocutaneous lesions of the oropharynx or genital regions.[64]

HSV-1. Most of the population develops antibodies to HSV-1 by the age of 50.[65] Following the primary infection, the virus establishes latency in the dorsal root of the trigeminal ganglion and recurs as herpes labialis. Although HSV-1 can occasionally extend below the oropharynx to involve the esophagus or trachea, resulting in focal necrotizing pneumonia and can disseminate through the bloodstream to involve the central nervous system, liver, colon, and adrenal glands, infection is usually localized and manifested by recurrent vesicles and shallow ulcerations. Herpetic lesions usually take approximately 10 to 14 days to heal.[66] Primary and secondary localized infections of the cornea can develop and are a major cause of blindness.[60] With immunosuppression small perioral lesions may enlarge and produce extensive and painful oropharyngeal ulcerations associated with gingivitis, stomatitis, and pharyngitis, and a rash indistinguishable from herpes zoster may develop.[66] Large, painful ulcerations can interfere with nutritional intake.

HSV-2. Primary HSV-2 genital infections are usually acquired during sexually active periods of life. A primary HSV-2 infection begins with local symptoms—soreness, itching, and discharge—and is accompanied by fever, general malaise, lymphadenopathy, neuralgia radiating to the thighs, buttocks, and groin, numerous clusters of painful vesicular lesions, and erythema on the penis, vulva, vaginal mucosa, or cervix. Herpetic vesicles break and form shallow ulcerations that take up to 3 weeks to heal. Genital herpes frequently flares up as a latent infection. Recurrent episodes are milder than the primary disease, with prodromal symptoms of tingling, itching, and burning.

Associated complications include aseptic meningitis, transverse myelitis, urethral stricture and dysuria, erythema multiforme, and secondary bacterial and fungal infections. Factors associated with recurrence of HSV-2 infection include fever, respiratory tract infection, sleep deprivation, menstruation, malnutrition, stress, hormonal imbalance, and mechanical friction from tight clothing.

HSV-2 infection can be diagnosed by observation of the characteristic lesions, but the only definitive diagnostic test is isolation of the virus in cell cultures. Often, however, a Tzanck smear of scrapings from the base of the vesicle is used for a simple, quick diagnosis.

TREATMENT OF HSV INFECTIONS. Prompt treatment of primary infections can reduce the amount of virus invading the ganglia and limit the reservoir of virus that can potentially be reactivated. Therapeutic goals include (1) containment of infection, (2) prevention of spread of lesions, particularly to other people, (3) rapid healing, (4) alleviation of symptoms, (5) prevention of bacterial superinfection, (6) prevention

of systemic disease, and (7) prevention of permanent blindness. Traditional attempts to treat reactivation infections have been unsuccessful, because the agents used acted on the virus only in the replicative phase. However, newer agents can treat (but not eliminate) reactivation infections. Two antiviral agents have been used with some success in the prevention and treatment of HSV infections: vidarabine and acyclovir.

Parenteral adenine arabinoside (vidarabine, ara-A) has been shown to be effective in the treatment of mucocutaneous HSV infection in immunosuppressed patients.[67] However, the period of viral shedding was not reduced as much as with acyclovir. Parenteral vidarabine has also been successful in the treatment of herpes simplex encephalitis and disseminated neonatal herpes. Intravenous administration of vidarabine requires a 12-hour continuous infusion, and this drug is more potentially nephrotoxic than acyclovir.[64]

Acyclovir is absorbed by herpes-infected cells and activated by HSV-coded thymidine kinase, which converts it to its active form, acyclovir triphosphate.[68] Acyclovir triphosphate inhibits HSV DNA synthesis. Acyclovir is currently the only treatment for mucocutaneous HSV infections. Oral or intravenous (IV) acyclovir is more effective than the topical preparation (5% ointment). Topical treatment is only useful for primary external cutaneous disease and must be started in the preeruptive phase to be most beneficial. It is not useful in treatment of secondary, intraoral, or intravaginal infection.

Topical acyclovir, when used, is applied to the affected area six times daily for 10 days. Symptomatic treatment of mucocutaneous lesions, however, also includes drying agents such as 4% zinc sulfate solution, antibiotic ointments to prevent bacterial superinfection, and topical anesthetics and analgesics for pain relief.

Oral acyclovir is very useful for the patient with normal GI absorption. Reduction in viral shedding and total healing time is comparable to that achieved with intravenous acyclovir in some patients.[64] Oral acyclovir, then, can be used to treat esophageal and gastric HSV infections. The drawback of oral acyclovir therapy is the dosing schedule. To maintain therapeutic levels at all times, the dosing schedule is approximately 200 mg taken five times daily for 10 days. Chronic acyclovir therapy, 200 mg three times daily for up to 6 months, is reserved for patients with more than six recurrences a year.[69] The most frequent side effects of short-term oral acyclovir therapy are nausea and vomiting. With long-term therapy, patients experience headaches, diarrhea, nausea, and vomiting.[70]

Intravenous acyclovir has been shown to significantly decrease viral shedding and total healing times in patients with HSV infections.[71-73] The intravenous dose of acyclovir is 5 mg/kg of body weight every 8 hours, when renal function is normal, for 5 to 7 days. The same dose can be administered every 12 hours if creatinine clearance is between 25 and 50 ml/minute.[74] It is recommended that IV acyclovir be infused over at least 1 hour to prevent precipitation of acyclovir crystals in the renal tubules. Aside from potential nephrotoxic effects, high-dose intravenous acyclovir is associated with neutropenia,[72] encephalopathy, lethargy, tremors, seizures, and phlebitis at the infusion site.[70] Close monitoring of renal function, liver function, neurologic status, and WBC count is necessary during administration of intravenous acyclovir.

Acyclovir has been studied extensively in the immunosuppressed patient population and found to be clinically effective for treatment of primary and secondary HSV-1, HSV-2, and varicella zoster infections. All reported studies that follow are double-blind, placebo controlled studies. Topical acyclovir therapy has not been shown to have an impact on length of disease but has decreased symptoms in immunocompromised patients with progressive cutaneous herpes.[67] Oral acyclovir preparation has been shown to be beneficial in decreasing viral shedding and facilitating healing of recurrent genital herpes lesions[75-77] and has been used successfully for prophylaxis against HSV infections in bone marrow transplant recipients.[78] Intravenous acyclovir has been used effectively for prevention and treatment of primary HSV infection in immunocompromised patients but is not as effective in treatment of latent infection.[62,72,73,79-82]

Cytomegalovirus. Cytomegalovirus (CMV) is the most common viral infection and a major cause of morbidity and mortality in transplant recipients. Steroids alone have limited ability to reactivate latent CMV infection, but with the advent of triple- and quadruple-drug therapy, CMV infections are common. Of all the immunosuppressants used, the antilymphocyte globulins (polyclonals and monoclonal) are associated with the highest risk of serious CMV infection.[83] CMV is found in oropharyngeal secretions, urine, cervical and vaginal secretions, semen, breast milk, and blood. CMV is transmitted in utero, during the first 6 months of life from exposure to mother's genital secretions and breast milk, and by oral and respiratory secretions in the preschool age-group. After congenital, perinatal, or early postnatal infection, the virus may linger for years in body fluids.[84]

In transplant recipients, sources of CMV infection include latent reactivation, virus present in the donor graft, and virus present in donor WBCs.[85] In the renal transplant population, the risk of a seronegative recipient contracting a primary CMV infection from a seropositive donor is 90% to 100%.[86] Between 35% and 80% of renal transplant patients have recurrent CMV infection.[86,87] This population becomes seropositive before transplantation through traditional routes of transmission and through exposure during hemodialysis and blood transfusions. Susceptibility is greatest during the first 3 to 4 months after transplant and is more common after treatment of a rejection episode.[88] Other precipitating factors include prolonged surgery and general anesthesia and the administration of antilymphocyte globulins (ALG, ATG, OKT-3), azathioprine (Imuran), and corticosteroids.[84] Attempts to prevent CMV infections include the administration of frozen red blood cells, blood from seronegative donors, attenuated CMV vaccine, and passive CMV immune globulin.[89]

The range of symptomatology for CMV infections is from the mild, subclinical case to life-threatening multiorgan disease. Subclinical infection is considered to be almost universal in the general population, as evidenced by findings of CMV antibodies in 86% of asymptomatic individuals.[90] Most cases of symptomatic CMV infection are self-limiting syndromes of episodic fever spikes (up to 39.4° C) for a period of three to four weeks, arthralgias, fatigue, anorexia, abdominal pain, and diarrhea.[87] CMV infections occur in both transplanted and nontransplanted tissues in the transplant recipient (e.g., CMV pneumonia and hepatitis). Reactivation infection is more frequent than primary infection in immunosuppressed patients, but primary infections are associated with more morbidity.[91]

Although one method of evaluating CMV is a serologic test, no single serologic test can distinguish an active from a latent infection.[92] All that will be revealed from a serologic test is antibody titers, which, as stated, most of the population will already have. However, a four-fold increase in CMV titer or conversion from IgM to IgG antibodies is an indicator of active infection. CMV infections are definitively diagnosed by tissue biopsy or bronchiole alveolar lavage (BAL).

CMV infections can disseminate and cause death. In disseminated CMV infection the lungs, liver, pancreas, kidneys, stomach, intestine, brain and parathyroid glands can be affected.[84] Mortality from CMV pneumonia in heart and heart-lung transplant patients in one series was 75%.[93] In bone marrow and kidney transplant patients CMV infection has been associated with peptic and colonic ulceration, hemorrhage, sepsis, and death.[94-96] Thrombocytopenia, leukopenia, and superinfections complicate this condition. CMV retinitis, manifested by decreased visual acuity and peripheral blindness, can occur and lead to retinal detachment and blindness.[84]

The patient with disseminated CMV infection poses certain problems relevant to critical care nursing practice. As a result of multisystem involvement, arterial hypoxemia, prolonged fever and superinfections, GI dysfunction, allograft dysfunction, coagulopathies, and neurologic dysfunction are commonly encountered. CMV infections also exacerbate the rejection process.[92]

CMV is resistant to acyclovir. However, a derivative of acyclovir, gancyclovir is effective in preventing replication of CMV. Gancyclovir has been used primarily in nonrandomized trials in bone marrow transplant patients and AIDS patients.[74] The recommended dose of intravenous gancyclovir for the patient with normal renal function is 2.5 mg/kg/day given in three divided doses every 8 hours, or 5 mg/kg/day given in two divided doses every 12 hours.[74] Although, like acyclovir, gancyclovir is potentially nephrotoxic, the most significant side effect by far is neutropenia, which usually manifests on about the tenth day of therapy. Therefore renal function and WBC and platelet counts are closely monitored during administration of gancyclovir. Therapy with gancyclovir may have to be discontinued if the WBC or platelet counts fall to life-threatening levels.

Epstein-Barr virus. The Epstein-Barr virus (EBV) is the same virus that is responsible for the syndrome of heterophile antibody-positive infectious mononucleosis in the general population.[66] Although EBV is associated with persistent infection, pneumonitis, and lymphoproliferative malignancies (lymphoma) in transplant patients, most infections are mild and associated with the characteristic symptoms of mononucleosis.[66] As with CMV, EBV infections can occur in both transplanted and nontransplanted tissues. Diagnosis of an EBV infection can be based on serial rises in antibodies to EBV, tissue biopsy, or BAL. Efficacious treatment of EBV infection has not been proven. Clinical trials with acyclovir are ongoing.

Approximately 10% to 15% of malignancies in transplant recipients are lymphomas (immunoblastic sarcomas) that invade the central nervous system, nasopharynx, liver, small intestine, and heart.[83] The EBV is implicated in the pathogenesis of these lymphomas. Cyclosporine, because it inhibits normal host defense mechanisms against EBV-induced oncogenesis, plays a role in the development of EBV infections and the development of lymphoma in the transplant population. If cyclosporine is discontinued in the patient with lymphoma, regression of the tumor usually occurs.[83]

Varicella zoster virus. The varicella zoster virus (VZV) is a highly communicable pathogen that causes chickenpox in childhood. Spread occurs by droplet infection or contact with involved mucocutaneous lesions.[34] The virus remains in a latent state in dorsal root ganglia and can be reactivated after years to produce the clinical syndromes of herpes zoster.[97] Varicella is the primary infection and herpes zoster is the secondary infection.

Approximately 5% to 10% of renal transplant recipients develop reactivation herpes zoster. Rarely is there dissemination, and the infection is self-limiting. Reactivation of herpes zoster is seen primarily as a vesicular infection in thoracic nerve dermatome distributions and is commonly referred to as *shingles*. A primary VZV infection in the transplant recipient can be devastating. The virus disseminates, causing hemorrhagic pneumonia and skin lesions, encephalitis, disseminated intravascular coagulation, and hepatitis.

Although herpes zoster is usually self-limiting, even in the immunosuppressed patient, dissemination to the skin can occur. In immunosuppressed patients visceral dissemination can also occur, most frequently to the lung.[66] Varicella or herpes zoster pneumonia is manifested by fever, dyspnea, and a nonproductive cough within 3 to 7 days of vesicular eruption. Varicella or herpes zoster encephalitis may also develop within the same time frame. Hepatitis and pancreatitis have also been associated with disseminated herpes zoster. Diagnosis of VZV is by rising antibody titer. Vidarabine has been used successfully in the treatment of varicella zoster and herpes zoster infections.[98-105]

Intravenous vidarabine is the first effective therapy for VZV infections.[106] In immunosuppressed patients with VZV infections, vidarabine has decreased dissemination and accelerated healing.[107] Acyclovir has been used in the treatment of herpes zoster infections. Although topical acyclovir is not practical for treatment of disseminated herpes zoster, oral and intravenous acyclovir have been shown to inhibit dissemination, lessen visceral complications, and decrease pain.[105]

Fungal infections. Fungi are unusual organisms in that although they can be responsible for fatal infections, they also provide a source of food for certain species and have been important in industry for baking, brewing, cheesemaking, and the production of penicillin.

Fungi of the *Candida* species are most common in immunosuppressed patients. *C. albicans* is the most commonly encountered organism, but *C. glabrata, C. tropicalis, C. pseudotropicalis, C. stellatoidea,* and *C. krusei* may also cause infection in this patient population. Other problematic fungi in the transplant population are *Aspergillis fumigatas, Cryptococcus neoformans,* and *Coccidioides immitus.*

Candidal infections

CANDIDA ALBICANS. In normal sterile fluids such as blood and cerebrospinal fluid, candidal growth is indicative of infection, but in specimens such as sputum, bronchial secretions, and urine that during collection pass through sites normally colonized with candida, growth alone is not diagnostic of candidal infection.[108] Fungi favor a warm, moist environment with an acid pH (4.0-5.0). Therefore primary sites of candidal growth are the mouth and vagina. The invasive potential of *C. albicans* depends, however, on the number of colonies and host resistance. Patients receiving immunosuppressants and/or broad spectrum antibiotics, diabetics, those with iron deficiency anemia, and hypothyroid individuals are more susceptible to invasion of adventitia by *C. albicans.*[109]

The hospital environment is particularly favorable to the growth of *C. albicans* in the immunosuppressed patient. Feeding tubes, nasogastric tubes, IV and central venous catheters, surgical drains, and urinary catheters have all been shown to support the growth of *C. albicans.*[110] Other important risk factors are malnutrition, surgical procedures, and length of hospitalization.[111]

ORAL CANDIDOSIS. There is an increased risk for the development of oral candidosis in the immunosuppressed transplant patient. Oral candidosis can contribute to nutritional deficiencies because of the associated pain and can lead to esophageal candidosis and fungemia. Oral candidosis, commonly referred to as *thrush,* presents as single or multiple wet, white lesions scattered over the tongue and oropharyngeal mucous membrane; the throat, tongue, and gums become red and sore.

Table 3-3 Drugs used to treat oral candidal infections

Drug	Dosage/route	Indication
Nystatin (Nilstat)	Oral suspension (100,000 units/ml) swish/swallow, qid	Oral thrush
Clotrimazole (Mycelex)	Oral troche (10 mg) 3 times/day	Oral thrush

Thrush can be avoided in many cases, except when severe neutropenia exists,[112] by topical application of the antifungal agent nystatin. Oral imidazole (clotrimazole) 10 mg three times daily has also been shown to be an effective prophylactic agent in severely immunosuppressed patients.[113] Patients receiving broad spectrum antibiotics, hyperalimentation, or immunosuppressants on a long-term basis should receive an oral-topical antifungal agent as a prophylactic measure. Frequent assessment of the oral cavity is an important component of the nursing care of the transplant recipient. Agents used for the treatment of oral candida infections are listed in Table 3-3.

CANDIDA ESOPHAGITIS. Candida esophagitis is most commonly seen in the neutropenic individual ($<500/mm^3$) but is not restricted to this situation.[114] Prolonged use of nasogastric or feeding tubes can lead to colonization of the esophagus with candida. Invasion of the esophageal mucosa is associated with retrosternal pain and sticking of food during swallowing that can interfere with the patient's desire to eat. Irregular mucosal ulcerations can be seen on endoscopy. Candida esophagitis is associated with broad spectrum antibiotic therapy and prolonged nasogastric intubation.[115] Untreated, candida esophagitis can lead to esophageal bleeding, perforation, and dissemination through the circulation to other organs and death. Candida esophagitis can be prevented with prophylactic oral antifungal agents (nystatin, clotrimazole), but may necessitate systemic treatment with amphotericin B.

URINARY TRACT CANDIDOSIS. Actual candidal infection of the bladder is rare; colonization of the bladder with candida is more common. However, candida can cause infection and obstructive uropathy in the severely immunosuppressed patient. In this condition, white flakes of yeast can be seen on gross inspection of the urine. Recommended treatment is removal of the urinary catheter and bladder irrigation with amphotericin B.

VULVOVAGINAL CANDIDOSIS. Vulvovaginal candidosis is caused by *C. albicans* in 60% to 70% of cases.[116] Itching is the most common symptom of vulvovaginal candidosis. Other signs and symptoms include a white, malodorous discharge and irritation. Pain is usually not a symptom unless vaginal adventitia is involved. Inspection in immunosuppressed patients of the vulvovaginal, perineal, perirectal, and anal areas for erythema, edema, and excoriations is an important component of the nursing assessment of transplant recipients.

Measurement of the vaginal pH may be helpful in the differential diagnosis of vaginal discharge, because *C. albicans* cannot thrive in an environment with a pH greater than 5.0. Trichomonas, however, does. A saline wet mount taken from the introitus and walls of the vagina is the easiest and most reliable diagnostic method. Tzanck smears, KOH wet mounts, and cultures can also be used to make the diagnosis. The differential diagnosis includes trichomonas, *Corynebacterium vaginale,* herpes genitalis, and allergic vulvovaginitis. The differential diagnosis of vaginal infections in female transplant recipients is crucial to their care. A false assumption that a vaginal infection is candida can lead not only to failure to eradicate the infection, but to dissemination and bacterial superinfection.

Before the development of clotrimazole, nys-

Table 3-4 Drugs used to treat vulvovaginal infections

Drug	Dosage/route	Side effects	Indication
Nystatin (Mycostatin, Nilstat)	Suppository (100,000 units) bid	Skin irritation, rare	Vaginitis
Clotrimazole (GyneLotrimin)	Suppository (100,000 units) bid	Skin irritation, occasional	Vaginitis
Miconazole (Micatin, Monistat-Derm, Monistat-7)	Topical cream	Skin irritation, occasional	Vaginitis

tatin was the treatment of choice for vulvovaginal candidosis. However, clotrimazole has been shown to be superior not only against candida but also against dermatophytes.[116] Clotrimazole is available as a 1% topical solution, a 1% vaginal cream, and a 100 and 500 mg vaginal tablet. The one-time dose of a 500 mg vaginal tablet has been shown to be as effective as dosing regimens using the 100 mg tablet, and the advantage in terms of patient adherence is obvious.[116,117] Agents used for treatment of local vulvovaginal infections are listed in Table 3-4.

DISSEMINATED CANDIDOSIS. *Candida* species are normally present in the bowel. Therefore, it is not surprising that the GI tract is usually the source of disseminated candidosis.[115] Under favorable conditions candida can penetrate through the gut mucosa and reach the muscles, kidneys, brain, lungs, liver, and pancreas through hematogenous spread. The result can be multiorgan dysfunction or failure. Lower GI candidosis can occur from the stomach to the anus, but is most common in the colon. Diarrhea is not usually associated with GI candidosis and the condition is difficult to diagnose. It can be suspected when the patient does not respond to antibiotic therapy and begins to deteriorate for no discernable reason. Dissemination to muscles is evidenced by an erythematous papular rash and tender, swollen muscle groups. Other signs and symptoms include persistant fever while the patient is receiving antibiotic therapy, negative blood culture results in the febrile patient, and pain in the eye or visual loss. Skin assessment is of utmost importance, because skin lesions may be the first sign of systemic infection, particularly candidal and cryptococcal

infections, and may appear weeks before central nervous system involvement. Treatment of disseminated candidosis is with systemic amphotericin B.

Aspergillis. *Aspergillis* species are ubiquitous in the earth, dust, and air. *Aspergillis* species cause clinical syndromes in immunosuppressed hosts that include pneumonia, brain abscesses, GI bleeding and skin lesions. *Aspergillis* pneumonia is difficult to diagnose, and the organisms tend to invade pulmonary blood vessels, causing clotting and infarction. Brain abscesses are diagnosed, after the development of neurologic signs, by biopsy. *Aspergillis* lesions of the lung and brain are best treated by surgical removal and systemic amphotericin B.

Cryptococcus. *Cryptococcus neoformans* is an encapsulated yeast found in the soil, pigeon feces, and the skin of fresh fruits and vegetables. Although the main portal of entry is the respiratory tract, cryptococcal pneumonia is rare. Cryptococcal fungemia with seeding to the central nervous system is, however, common. Treatment of cryptococcal infection is with systemic amphotericin.

Coccidioides. *Coccidioides immitis* is a soilborne fungus found in the deserts and cultivated areas of the North American southwest, Central America, and central South America. Infections occur after inhalation of the fungus. Dissemination occurs to the central nervous system, joints, liver, and skin. Treatment of coccidiodal infections is with systemic amphotericin B.

Histoplasmosis. *Histoplasma capsulatum* infections are most common in the United States along the Mississippi River valleys. It is also common in river valleys in South America. The mild form of histoplasmosis presents as an influenza-like syndrome, but in immunosuppressed patients dissemination can occur to the lungs, liver, spleen, central nervous system, and lymph nodes. Treatment of histoplasmosis is with systemic amphotericin B. *Aspergillis, Cryptococcus, Coccidioides,* and *Histoplasma* infections can originate in the hospital setting, but are more likely to be acquired from the external environment, such as when patients are directly exposed to large amounts of dry soil or dust, or bird excrement.

Parasitic infections. Although parasitic diseases such as malaria and schistosomiasis are epidemic worldwide, they are not considered opportunistic infections except in immunosuppressed individuals. On the contrary, protozoan parasites such as *Pneumocystis carinii* and *Toxoplasma gondii* almost never cause infection except in the presence of altered immunity.

Pneumocystis. P. carinii is an extracellular ameboid organism that is ubiquitous in the environment. Although it is most studied in the AIDS population, fatal *P. carinii* infections have occurred in organ transplant recipients. *P. carinii* affects the lung, occurring as *Pneumocystis carinii* pneumonia (PCP). The most common symptom in the transplant population is an abrupt onset of dyspnea associated with tachypnea at rest, hypoxia and cyanosis, fever and cough. However, as many as 50% of those with PCP will not have a cough as a presenting symptom.[115] On chest x-ray examination, diffuse bilateral alveolar infiltrates are seen, but this finding may lag as much as 48 hours behind the initial symptom of dyspnea.[115] A definitive diagnosis is made with BAL or transbronchial biopsy. Treatment of PCP is with trimethoprim sulfamethoxazole, pentamidine isethionate (Lomidine), or Bactrim.

Toxoplasmosis. T. gondii is an intracellular protozoan parasite that is also ubiquitous in the environment. It is usually acquired through ingestion of undercooked or raw meat, but exposure can also occur through cat feces, inhalation of dust containing oocysts, and food contaminated by cockroaches or flies. Toxoplasmosis can also be acquired after blood transfusions,[115] because it can remain dormant and undetected in its host.

T. gondii differs from *P. carinii* in that it affects multiple organs, especially the central nervous system and skeletal and cardiac muscles. The spectrum of clinical signs is vast, including mononucleosis-like symptoms and severe infection involving multiple organ systems. Treatment of toxoplasmosis is with pyrimethamine and sulfadiazine.

Treatment of opportunistic infections

While various treatment modalities have been described for opportunistic infections, attempts at prevention must precede treatment. Some common sense measures regarding the physical environment of the transplant recipient can logically make a positive impact on morbidity and mortality. The nursing profession has a long legacy regarding this important point. Florence Nightingale is credited with decreasing mortality from 42.7% to 2.2% at the Scutari Hospital near Constantinople in the Crimean War through sanitary reforms.[118] According to Nightingale, ". . . the greater part of nursing consists in preserving cleanliness."[119]

Hospitals, and ICUs in particular, harbor many potentially pathogenic organisms. In surgical ICUs, where transplant recipients are likely to be cared for in the immediate postoperative period, critical care nurses and physicians frequently come in direct contact with blood, pulmonary secretions, surgical drainage, feces, and urine. In addition to diagnostic equipment, these fluids serve as vectors (usually by the hands) for transmission of organisms from one patient to another.

As early as the mid-1850s Ignaz Semmelweis traced "blood poisoning" causing death in childbed fever victims to medical students who were carriers of infectious materials from the autopsy room to the labor rooms at Vienna General Hospital after only superficially washing their hands.[120] Before Semmelweis's investigations, 11.4% of delivering mothers died of childbed fever; after his findings and the implementation of thorough handwashing in chlorinated lime, mortality decreased to 1.27%. Although handwashing has long since been identified as the most effective measure for decreasing transmission of infection,[121] modern studies show that compliance among hospital

CDC RECOMMENDATIONS FOR HANDWASHING

Handwashing indications

1. In the absence of a true emergency, personnel should *always* wash their hands
   a. **Before** performing invasive procedures
   b. **Before** taking care of particularly susceptible patients, such as those who are severely immunocompromised and newborns
   c. **Before** and **after** touching wounds, whether surgical, traumatic, or associated with an invasive device
   d. **After** situations during which microbial contamination of hands is likely to occur, especially those involving contact with mucous membranes, blood or body fluids, secretions, or excretions
   e. **After** touching inanimate sources that are likely to be contaminated with virulent or epidemiologically important microorganisms; these sources include urine-measuring devices or secretion-collection apparatuses
   f. **After** taking care of an infected patient or one who is likely to be colonized with microorganisms of special clinical or epidemiologic significance, for example, multiply-resistant bacteria
   g. **Between** contacts with different patients in high-risk units
2. Most routine, brief patient-care activities involving *direct* patient contact other than that discussed above (e.g., taking a blood pressure), do not require handwashing
3. Most routine hospital activities involving indirect patient contact (e.g., handing a patient medications, food, or other objects, do not require handwashing)

Handwashing technique

For routine handwashing, a vigorous rubbing together of all surfaces of lathered hands for at least 10 seconds, followed by thorough rinsing under a stream of water, is recommended

Handwashing with plain soap

1. Plain soap should be used for handwashing unless otherwise indicated
2. If bar soap is used, it should be kept on racks that allow drainage of water
3. If liquid soap is used, the dispenser should be replaced or cleaned and filled with fresh product when empty; liquids should not be added to a partially full dispenser

Handwashing with antimicrobial-containing products (health-care personnel handwashes)

1. Antimicrobial handwashing products should be used for handwashing before personnel care for newborns and when otherwise indicated during their care, between patients in high-risk units, and before personnel take care of severely immunocompromised patients
2. Antimicrobial-containing products that do not require water for use, such as foams or rinses, can be used in areas where no sinks are available

Handwashing facilities

1. Handwashing facilities should be conveniently located throughout the hospital
2. A sink should be located in or just outside every patient room; more than one sink per room may be necessary if a large room is used for several patients
3. Handwashing facilities should be located in or adjacent to rooms where diagnostic or invasive procedures that require handwashing are performed (e.g., cardiac, catheterization, bronchoscopy, sigmoidoscopy, etc.)

From the Centers for Disease Control (1985). Guidelines: nosocomial infections in handwashing and hospital environmental control. Washington, DC: CDC.

personnel is poor with this simple, straightforward intervention.[42,122,123] Handwashing results in mechanical and chemical removal of transient (versus resident) microorganisms from the hands of hospital personnel. These pathogens, acquired through direct and indirect contact with colonized and infected patients, are responsible for the majority of nosocomial infections.[119] The absolute indications and the ideal duration and frequency of handwashing have not been established. However, recommendations from the Centers for Disease Control regarding handwashing practice in the acute care setting can be found in the box on p. 42.

The traditional approach to protecting the transplant patient from infection was the use of protective or reverse isolation. The patient was placed in a single room that may have been equipped with high efficiency particulate air (HEPA) filtration and positive pressure air flow.[124,125] HEPA filtration forces air in a unidirectional pattern through a filter that removes particles greater than 0.3 microns, thereby eliminating all bacteria, fungi, and large viruses from the air. The cost of such a device is in the range of $20,000 to $25,000. Contact with hospital personnel and family members was severely restricted, and anyone entering the patient's room was clothed in a sterile gown and gloves, disposable cap, mask, and shoe covers.[126] All equipment entering the room was wiped down with an antiseptic solution, as was the floor every 8 hours. It was the critical care nurse's responsibility to maintain this standard. All linen was sterilized and meals arrived on disposable, sterilized trays. Although the theoretic basis for this elaborate and time-consuming approach is loss of protective immune mechanisms, its efficacy, even in neutropenic patients (which most solid organ transplant recipients are not), has not been proven.

Today infection control protocols for transplant patients are much more relaxed in many ways. Protocols vary widely from transplant center to transplant center, and even from program to program within a given transplant center. For example, in one major transplant center in the southeastern United Stated, reverse or protective isolation is routinely used during the immediate postoperative period for all heart transplant patients, while handwashing is the technique routinely used for all liver transplant patients, even though this population is at higher risk for postoperative infection. Gamberg et al[126] did a retrospective review of the incidence of infection in heart transplant recipients before and after modifying a protective isolation protocol. They found no difference in the incidence of infection, morbidity, or mortality.

The recognition that many opportunistic infections are caused by latent or other internal organisms, has refocused the care of these patients. A clean, but not sterile, environment and frequent handwashing are cornerstones of the modern approach. There is an emphasis on keeping clean and maintaining the integrity of skin and mucous membranes, limiting the number and duration of invasive devices, and optimal nutritional and metabolic support. And last, but certainly not the least important, immunosuppression regimens have been modified to cause less morbidity in terms of opportunistic infection. With the use of traditional immunosuppressive regimens host defenses were universally altered and morbidity and mortality from infection was greater than it is today.

The advent of cyclosporine has allowed lower doses of corticosteroids and azathioprine to be used, and in some cases to be totally eliminated from the posttransplant immunosuppressive regimen. This has contributed to decreased morbidity and mortality from infectious complications.[53,127] However, because cyclosporine is a T cell–specific drug, and because T cells provide host defense against viral, fungal, and parasitic infections, these types of infections remain a complication after transplantation.[53,128,129]

REFERENCES

1. Smith SL (1986). Physiology of the immune system. *Critical Care Quarterly, 9,* 7-13.
2. Bellanti JA (1985). Introduction to immunology. In Bellanti JA (ed). *Immunology III.* (1-15). Philadelphia: WB Saunders Co.
3. Groenwald SL (1980). Physiology of the immune system. *Heart and Lung, 9,* 645-650.

4. Abernathy E (1984). How the immune system works. *American Journal of Nursing,* April, pp 456-469.
5. Bellanti JA and Kadlec JV (1985). General immunobiology. In Bellanti JA (ed). *Immunology III.* (16-53). Philadelphia: WB Saunders Co.
6. Baker H (1979). The skin as a barrier. In Rock A, Wilkinson OS and Ebling FJS (eds). *Textbook of dermatology,* 3rd ed. (289-298). Oxford: Blackwell Publishing.
7. Philpot CM (1988). The skin as a microbial barrier. In Marks RM, Barton SP and Edwards C (eds). *The physical nature of the skin.* (61-68). Lancaster, England: MTP Press Ltd.
8. Luger TA, Kock A, Danner M and Mickshe M (1985). Production of distinct cytokines by epidermal cells. *British Journal of Dermatology, 113* (Suppl 28), 145-156.
9. Breathnach SM (1988). The skin as an immunologic barrier. In Marks RM, Barton SP and Edwards C (eds). *The physical nature of the skin.* (53-60). Lancaster, England: MTP Press Ltd.
10. Boggs DR and Winkelstein A (1984). *White cell manual.* Philadelphia: EA Davis Co.
11. Roitt I, Brostoff J and Male D (1985). Cells involved in the immune response. In Roitt I, Brostoff J and Male D (eds). *Immunology.* (2.1-2.16). St Louis: The CV Mosby Co.
12. Fischbach F (1984). In Fischbach F (ed). *A manual of laboratory diagnostic tests,* 2nd ed. (1-104). Philadelphia: JB Lippincott.
13. McDevitt HO (1985). The HLA system and its relation to disease. *Hospital Practice,* July, 57-72.
14. Herscowitz HB (1985). Immunophysiology: cell function and cellular interactions in antibody formation. In Bellanti JA (ed). *Immunology III.* (117-159). Philadelphia: WB Saunders Co.
15. Dinarello CA and Mier JW (1987). Current concepts. Lymphokines. *The New England Journal of Medicine,* 317, 940-945.
16. Roitt I, Brostoff J and Male D (1985). Adaptive and innate immunity. In Roitt I, Brostoff J and Male D (eds). *Immunology.* (1.1-1.10). St Louis: The CV Mosby Co.
17. Jett MF and Lancaster LE (1983). The inflammatory immune response: the body's defense against invasion. *Critical Care Nurse,* September/October, 64-82.
18. Graziano FM and Bell CL (1986). The normal immune response and what can go wrong. *Medical Clinics of North America, 69,* 440-451.
19. Kemp DK (1986). Development of the immune system. *Critical Care Quarterly, 9,* 1-6.
20. Roitt I, Brostoff J and Male D (1985). The lymphoid system. In Roitt I, Brostoff J and Male D (eds). *Immunology.* (3.1-3.10). St Louis: The CV Mosby Co.
21. Murdock DK, Lawless CE and Scanlon PJ (1987). Rejection of the transplanted heart. *Heart and Lung, 16,* 237-246.
22. Herscowitz HB (1985). Immunophysiology: cell function and cellular interaction in antibody formation. In Bellanti JA (ed). *Immunology III.* (117-137). Philadelphia: WB Saunders Co.
23. Roitt I, Brostoff J and Male D (1985). Antibody structure and function. In Roitt I, Brostoff J and Male D (eds). *Immunology.* (5.1-5.10). St Louis, The CV Mosby Co.
24. Roitt I, Brostoff J and Male D (1985). Transplantation and rejection. In Roitt I, Brostoff J and Male D (eds). *Immunology.* (24.1-24.10). St Louis, The CV Mosby Co.
25. Bellanti JA and Rocklin RE (1985). Cell-mediated immune function. In Bellanti JA (ed). *Immunology III.* (176-188). Philadelphia: WB Saunders Co.
26. Roitt I, Brostoff J and Male D (1985). Cell-mediated immunity. In Roitt I, Brostoff J and Male D (eds). *Immunology.* (11.1-11.12). St Louis: The CV Mosby Co.
27. Roitt I, Brostoff J and Male D (1985). Major histocompatibility complex. In Roitt I, Brostoff J and Male D (eds). *Immunology.* (4.1-4.12). St Louis: The CV Mosby Co.
28. Carpenter CB (1986). Immunobiology of transplantation. In Garovy MR and Guttman RD (eds). *Renal transplantation.* (49-72). New York: Churchill Livingstone.
29. Braun WE (1986). Histocompatibility and renal transplantation. In Garovy MR and Guttman RD (eds). *Renal transplantation.* (15-27). New York: Churchill Livingstone.
30. Bach FH and Sachs DH (1987). Transplantation immunology. *New England Journal of Medicine, 317,* 489-492.
31. Traeger J, Monti LD and Piatti PM (1988). Immunologic aspects of pancreas transplantation. In Groth CG (ed). *Pancreatic transplantation.* (87-98). Philadelphia: WB Saunders Co.
32. Miller WV and Rodey G (1981). *HLA without tears.* Chicago: American Society of Clinical Pathologists.
33. Najarian JS and Foker JE (1969). Mechanisms of kidney allograft rejection. *Transplantation Proceedings, 1,* 184-193.
34. Gordon RD, Iwatsuki S, Esquivel CO, Tsakis A, Todo S and Starzl TE (1986). Liver transplantation across ABO blood groups. *Surgery, 100,* 342-348.
35. Iwatsuki S, Iwaki Y, Kano T, Klintmalm G, Koep LJ, Weil R and Starzl TE (1981). Successful liver transplantation from positive crossmatch donors. *Transplantation Proceedings, 13,* 286-288.
36. Ramsey G, Wolford J, Boczkowski DJ, Cornell FW, Laron P and Starzl TE (1987). The Lewis blood group system in liver transplantation. *Transplantation Proceedings, 19,* 4591-4594.
37. Rego J, Prevost F, Rumeau J-L, Modesto A, Fourtanier G, Durand D, Suc J-M, Ohayon E and Ducos J (1987). Hyperacute rejection after ABO-incompatible orthotopic liver transplantation. *Transplantation Proceedings, 19,* 4589-4590.
38. Angstadt J, Jarrell W, Maddrey S, Munoz S, Yang S-L, Mortiz M and Carabasi A (1987). Hemolysis in ABO-incompatible liver transplantation. *Transplantation Proceedings, 19,* 4595-4597.
39. Parkmann R (1988). Cyclosporine: graft versus host disease and beyond. *New England Journal of Medicine, 319,* 110-111.

40. Young LS (1981). Fever and septicemia. In Rubin RH and Young LS (eds). *Clinical approach to infection in the compromised host.* (75-122). New York: Plenum Medical Book Co.
41. Lauter CB (1976). Opportunistic infections. *Heart and Lung, 5,* 601-606.
42. Larson E (1985). Infection control issues in critical care. *Heart and Lung, 14,* 149-156.
43. Roderick MA (1983). *Infection control in critical care.* Rockville, Md: Aspen Publishers.
44. Yanelli B and Gurevich I (1988). Infection control in critical care. *Heart and Lung, 17,* 596-600.
45. Young LS and Rubin RH (1981). An overview of infection in the compromised host. In Rubin RH and Young LS (eds). *Clinical approach to infection in the compromised host.* (1-5). New York: Plenum Medical Book Co.
46. Anderson KR, Norris DJ, Godfrey MS, Avant CK and Butterworth CE (1984). Bacterial contamination of tube-feeding formulas. *Journal of Parenteral and Enteral Nutrition, 8,* 673-678.
47. Gill KJ and Gill P (1981). Contaminated enteral feeds. *British Medical Journal, 282,* 1971.
48. Fagerman KE (1986). Pharmacy admixture of enteral nutrient products. *American Journal of Hospital Pharmacy, 43,* 884-894.
49. Casewell MW (1981). Enteral feeds contaminated with Enterobacter cloacae as a cause of septicemia. *British Medical Journal, 282,* 973.
50. Baldwin BA, Zagoren AJ and Rose N (1983). Bacterial contamination of continuously infused enteral alimentation with needle catheter jejunostomy — clinical implication. *Journal of Parenteral and Enteral Nutrition, 8,* 30-33.
51. Schroeder P, Fischer D, Volz M and Paloucek J (1983). Microbial contamination of feeding solutions in a community hospital. *Journal of Parenteral and Enteral Nutrition, 7,* 364-368.
52. Dietch EA (1988). Infection in the compromised host. *Surgical Clinics of North America, 68,* 181-196.
53. Stampfer MJ and Tu RP (1988). Nosocomial legionnaire's disease. *Heart and Lung, 17,* 601-604.
54. Favor A, Frazier OH, Codey DA, Okereke OUJ, Radovancevic B, Powers P and Chandler L (1985). *Legionella* infections in cyclosporine-immunosuppressed cardic transplants. *Texas Heart Institute Journal, 12,* 153-156.
55. Gombert ME, Josephson A, Goldstein EJ, Smith PR and Butt KM (1984). Cavitary legionnaires' pneumonia: nosocomial infections in renal transplant patients. *American Journal of Surgery, 147,* 402-405.
56. Myerowitz RL (1983). Nosocomial legionnaires' disease and other nosocomial *Legionella* pneumonias. *Infection Control, 4,* 107-110.
57. Simon HB (1981). Mycobacterial and nocardial infections in the compromised host. In Rubin RH and Young LS (eds). *Clinical approach to infection in the compromised host.* (229-268). New York: Plenum Medical Book Co.
58. Gold E and Nankarvis GA (1982). Cytomegalovirus. In Evans AS (ed). *Viral infections of humans. Epidemiology and control,* 2nd ed. (167-186). New York: Plenum Publishing Co.
59. Klein RJ, Friedmain-Kien AE and Hatcher VA (1983). Herpes simplex virus infections: an update (Part I). *Hospital Medicine,* November/December, 1-11.
60. Klein RJ, Friedmain-Kien AE and Hatcher VA (1984). Herpes simplex virus infections: an update (Part II). *Hospital Medicine,* January/February, 1-8.
61. Pass RF, Whitley RJ, Whelchel JD, Alford CA, Reynolds DW and Diethelm AG (1979). Identification of patients with increased risk of infection with herpes simplex virus after renal transplantation. *Journal of Infectious Disease, 140,* 487-492.
62. Saral R, Ambinder RF, Laskin OL, Santos GW and Lietman PS (1981). Acyclovir prophylaxis of herpes-simplex-virus infections. A randomized, double-blind, controlled trial in bone marrow–transplant recipients. *New England Journal of Medicine, 305,* 63-67.
63. Meyers JD, Flournoy N and Thomas ED (1980). Infection with herpes simplex virus and cell-mediated immunity after marrow transplantation. *Journal of Infectious Disease, 142,* 338-346.
64. Meyers JD (1986). Advances in treatment of herpes simplex virus infections in the immunocompromised host. National Cancer Institute Grant #CA 30924, DHHS Grant #CA 18029. Burroughs-Wellcome Co. (Unpublished paper.)
65. Rawls WE and Campione PJ (1981). Epidemiology of herpes simplex virus type 1 and type 2 infection. In Nahmias AJ, Dowdle WR and Schinazi RE (eds). *The human herpesvirus: an interdisciplinary perspective.* New York: Elsevier.
66. Wong KK and Hirsh MS (1984). Herpes virus infections in patients with neoplastic disease, Diagnosis and therapy. *American Journal of Medicine, 76,* 464-468.
67. Whitley RJ, Spruance S, Hayden FG, Overall J, Alford CA, Gwalthey JM and Soong SJ (1984). NIAID Antiviral Study Group. Vidaribine treatment for mucocutaneous herpes simplex virus infection in the immunocompromised host. *Journal of Infectious Disease, 149,* 1-8.
68. Schnoeck CLE (1985). Acyclovir: a recently developed anti-herpes agent. *Critical Care Nurse, 5,* 8-10.
69. Krusinski PA (1988). Treatment of mucocutaneous herpes simplex virus infections with acyclovir. *Journal of the American Academy of Dermatology, 18,* 179-181.
70. Arndt KA (1988). Adverse reactions to acyclovir: topical, oral and intravenous. *Journal of the American Academy of Dermatology, 18,* 188-195.
71. Mitchell CD, Gentry SR, Boen JR, Bean B, Groth KE and Balfour HH (1981). Acyclovir treatment for mucocutaneous herpes simplex virus infections in the immunocompromised host. *Lancet, 1,* 1389-1392.
72. Wade JC, Newton B, McLaren C, Flournoy N, Keeney RE and Meyers JD (1982). Intravenous acyclovir to treat mucocutaneous herpes simplex virus infections after marrow transplantation: a double-blind trial. *Annals of Internal Medicine, 96,* 265-269.
73. Meyers JD, Wade JC, Mitchell CD, Levil MJ, Sergreti AC and Balfour HH (1982). Multicenter collaborative trial of intravenous acyclovir for the treatment of

herpes simplex virus infection in the immunocompromised host. *American Journal of Medicine, 73,* 229-235.

74. Reed EC and Meyers JD (1987). Treatment of cytomegalovirus infection. *Clinics in Laboratory Medicine, 7,* 831-851.

75. Nilsen AE, Aasen T and Halsos AM (1982). Efficacy of oral acyclovir in the treatment of initial and recurrent genital herpes. *Lancet, 11,* 571-573.

76. Reichman RC, Ginsberg M, Barrett-Connor E, Nyborny C, Connor JD, Redfield D, Savoia MC, Richman DD, Oxman MN, Dandliker PS, Badger GT, Ashihagn T and Polin R (1982). Controlled trial of oral acyclovir therapy of recurrent herpes simplex genitalis: a preliminary report. *American Journal of Medicine, 73* (Suppl 1A), 338-341.

77. Bryson YJ, Dillon M, Lovett M, Acuna G, Taylor S, Cherry JD, Johnson BL, Weismeier E, Growden W, Creigh-Kirk T and Keeney R (1983). Treatment of first episodes of genital herpes simplex virus infection with oral acyclovir: a randomized double-blind controlled trial in normal subjects. *New England Journal of Medicine, 308,* 916-921.

78. Gluckman E, Lotsberg J, Devergie A, Melo R, Nebout T, Lotsberg J, Zhao XM, Gomez-Morales M and Mazeron MC (1983). Prophylaxis of herpes infections after bone-marrow transplantation by oral acyclovir. *Lancet, 11,* 706-708.

79. Mindel A, Adler MW, Sutherland S and Fiddian AP (1982). Intravenous acyclovir treatment of primary genital herpes. *Lancet, 1,* 697-700.

80. Saral R, Armbinder RF, Burns WH, Angelopulos PA, Griffin DE, Barke PJ and Lietman PS (1983). Acyclovir prophylaxis against herpes simplex virus infection in patients wth leukemia. *Annals of Internal Medicine, 99,* 773-776.

81. Hann IM, Prentice HG, Blacklock HA, Ross MGR, Brigder D, Rosling AE, Burke C, Crawford DH, Brunfitt W and Hoffbrand AV (1983). Acyclovir prophylaxis against herpes virus infections in severely immunocompromised patients: randomized double blind trial. *British Medical Journal, 287,* 384-388.

82. Prentice HG (1983). Use of acyclvoir for prophylaxis of herpes infections in severely immunocompromised patients. *Journal of Antimicrobial Chemotherapy, 12* (Suppl B), 153-159.

83. Rubin RH (1988). Infectious disease problems. In Maddrey WC (ed). *Transplantation of the liver* (279-308). New York: Elsevier.

84. Schumann D (1987). Cytomegalic virus infection in renal allograft recipients. Indicators for intervention in the surgical intensive care unit. *Focus on Critical Care, 14,* (3) 40-47.

85. Betts R (1983). Cytomegalovirus infection epidemiology and biology in adults. *Seminars in Perinatology, 1,* 22-30.

86. Ho M, Suwansirikul S, Dowling JN, Youngblood LA and Armstrong JA (1975). The transplanted kidney as a source of cytomegalovirus infection. *New England Journal of Medicine, 293,* 109-1112.

87. Glenn J (1981). Cytomegalovirus infections following renal transplantation. *Review of Infectious Disease, 3,* 1151-1178.

88. Peterson RK, Balfour HH, Marker SC, Fryd DC, Howard RJ and Simmons RL (1980). Cytomegalic disease in renal allograft recipients: a prospective study of the clinical features, risk factors and impact on renal transplantation. *Medicine, 59,* 282-300.

89. Saliba F, Gugenheim J, Samuel D, Bismuth A, Mathieu D, Serres C and Bismuth H (1987). Incidence of cytomegalovirus infection and effects of CMV immune globulin prophylaxis after orthtopic liver transplantation. *Transplantation Proceedings, 19,* 4081-4082.

90. Hayes K (1985). Cytomegalovirus: the challenge of a common virus infection. *Medical Journal of Australia, 142,* 174-176.

91. Suwansirikul S, Rao W, Dowling JN and Ho M (1977). Primary and secondary cytomegalovirus infection. *Archives of Internal Medicine, 137,* 1026-1029.

92. Sinnott JT and Cancio MR (1987). Cytomegalovirus. *Infection Control, 8,* 79-82.

93. Dummer JS, Hardy A, Poosatter A and Ho M (1983). Early infection in kidney, heart and liver transplant recipients on cyclosporine. *Transplantation, 36,* 259-267.

94. West JC, Armitage JO and Mitros FA (1982). Cytomegalovirus cecal erosion causing massive hemorrhage in a bone marrow transplant recipient. *World Journal of Surgery, 6,* 251-255.

95. Cohen EB, Komorowski RA, Kauffman HM and Adams M (1985). Unexpectedly high incidence of cytomegalovirus infection in apparent peptic ulcer in renal transplant recipients. *Surgery, 97,* 606-612.

96. Foucar E, Mulkai K, Foucar K, David ER, Sutherland CT and Van Buren CT (1981). Colon ulceration in lethal cytomegalovirus infection. *American Journal of Clinical Pathology, 76,* 788-801.

97. Bastian FO, Rabson AS and Yee CL (1974). Herpesvirus varicellae: isolated from human dorsal root ganglia. *Archives of Pathology, 97,* 331-333.

98. Whitley R, Hilty M, Haynes R, Bryson Y, Connor JD, Soong S-J, Alford CA and National Institute of Allergy and Infectious Disease Collaborative Antiviral Study Group (1982). Vidarabine therapy of varicella in immunosuppressed patients. *Journal of Pediatrics, 101,* 125-131.

99. Whitley RJ, Ch'ien LT, Dolin R, Gallasso GJ and Alford CA (1976). Adenine arabinoside therapy of herpes zoster in the immunosuppressed. NIAID Collaborative Study. *New England Journal of Medicine, 294,* 1193-1199.

100. Whitley RJ, Soon SJ, Dolin R, Betts R, Linnemann C, Alford CA and National Institute of Allergy and Infectious Disease Collaborative Antiviral Study Group (1982). Early vidarabine therapy to control the complications of herpes zoster in immunosuppressed patients. *New England Journal of Medicine, 307,* 971-975.

101. Prober CG, Kirk LE and Keeney RE (1982). Acyclovir therapy of chickenpox in immunosuppressed children — a collaborative study. *Journal of Pediatrics, 101,* 622-625.

102. Peterslund NA, Seyer-Hansen K, Ipsen J, Esmann V, Schonheyder H and Juhl H (1981). Acyclovir in herpes zoster. *Lancet, 11,* 827-830.

103. Esmann V, Epsen J, Peterslund NA, Seyer-Hansen K, Schonheyder H and Juhl H (1982). Therapy of acute herpes zoster with acyclovir in the immunosuppressed patients. *American Journal of Medicine, 73* (Suppl 1A), 320-325.

104. Bean B, Braun C and Balfour HH (1982). Acyclovir therapy for acute herpes zoster. *Lancet, 11,* 118-121.

105. Balfour HH, Bean B, Laskin OL, Ambinder RF, Meyers JD, Wade JC, Zaia JA, Aeppli D, Kirk LE, Segreti AC, Keeney RE and the Burroughs Wellcome Collaborative Acyclovir Study Group (1982). Acyclovir halts progression of herpes zoster in immunocompromised patients. *New England Journal of Medicine, 308,* 1448-1453.

106. Huff JC (1988). Antiviral treatment in chickenpox and herpes zoster. *Journal of the American Academy of Dermatology, 18,* 204-205.

107. Levin MJ, Zaia JA, Hershey BJ, Davis LG, Robinson GV and Segreti AC (1985). *Journal of the American Academy of Dermatology, 13,* 590-596.

108. Kauffman CA and Jones PG (1986). Candidiasis. A diagnostic and therapeutic challenge. *Postgraduate Medicine, 80,* 129-134.

109. Carroll CJ, Hurley R and Stanley VC (1973). Criteria for diagnosis of candida vulvovaginitis in pregnant women. *Journal of Obstetrics and Gynecology of the British Commonwealth, 80,* 258-263.

110. Robertson WH (1984). *Volvovaginal candidiasis: current concepts of diagnosis and management.* West Haven, Ct: Miles Pharmaceuticals, 1-32.

111. Meunier-Carpenter FV, Kiehn TE and Armstrong D (1981). Fungemia in the compromised host. Changing patterns, antigenemia and high mortality. *American Journal of Medicine, 71,* 363-370.

112. DeGregorio MW, Lee WMF and Ries CA (1982). Candida infections in patients with acute leukemia: ineffectiveness of nystatin prophylaxis and relationship between oropharyngeal and systemic candidiasis. *Cancer, 50,* 2780-2784.

113. Cuttner J, Troy KM, Funaro L, Brender R and Bottone EJ (1986). Clotrimazole therapy for prevention of oral candidiasis in patients with acute leukemia undergoing chemotherapy. *American Journal of Medicine, 81,* 771-774.

114. Laudner JN, Lazarus HM and Harzig RH (1982). Bacteremias and fungemias in oncologic patients with central venous catheters. *Archives of Internal Medicine, 142,* 1456-1459.

115. Ruskin J (1981). Parasitic diseases in the compromised host. In Rubin RH and Young LS (eds). Clinical approach to infection in the compromised host. (269-334). New York: Plenum Medical Book Co.

116. Guess EA and Hodgson C (1984). Single-dose topical treatment of vulvovaginal candidiasis with a new 500 milligram clotrimazole vaginal tablet. *Advances in Therapy, 1,* 137-145.

117. Hughes D and Kriedman T (1984). Treatment of vulvovaginal candidiasis with a 500 milligram vaginal tablet of clotrimazole. *Clinical Therapeutics, 6,* 662-668.

118. Cohen IB (1984). Florence Nightingale. *Scientific American,* March, 128-137.

119. Nightingale F (1969). *Notes on nursing. What it is and what it is not.* The Dover Edition. New York: Power Publications, Inc.

120. Hempel CG (1966). *Philosophy of natural science.* Englewood Cliffs, NJ: Prentice-Hall, Inc.

121. Hospital Infections Program, Center for Infectious Disease, Centers for Disease Control (1985). *Guidelines for handwashing and hospital and environmental control.* Atlanta: Public Health Service, US DHHS.

122. Albert RK and Condie F (1981). Handwashing patterns in medical intensive-care units. *New England Journal of Medicine, 304,* 1465-1466.

123. Larson E (1983). Compliance with isolation techniques. *American Journal of Infection Control, 11,* 221-225.

124. King JG (1973). Air for living: comparison of HEPA and electrostatic air filtration. *Respiratory Care, 18,* 160-164.

125. Soots G, LeClerc H, Pol A, Savage C and Fieve R (1982). Airborne hazard in open heart surgery. Efficiency of HEPA air filtration and laminar flow. *Journal of Cardiovascular Surgery, 23,* 155-162.

126. Gomberg P, Miller J and Lough ME (1987). Impact of protection isolation on the incidence of infection after heart transplant. *The Journal of Heart Transplantation, 6,* 147-149.

127. Oyer PE, Stinson EB, Jamieson SW, Hunt SA, Pelroth M, Billingham M and Shumway NE (1983). Cyclosporine in cardiac transplantation: a 2½ year followup. *Transplantation Proceedings, 14* (Suppl), 330-335.

128. Brooks RG, Hofflin JM, Jamieson SW, Stinson EB and Remington JS (1985). Infectious complications in heart-lung transplant recipients. *American Journal of Medicine, 79,* 412-422.

129. Wajsczuk CP, Dummer JS, Ho M, Van Thiel D, Starzl TE, Iwatsuki S and Shaw B (1985). Fungal infections in liver transplant recipients. *Transplantation, 40,* 347-353.

4

Immunosuppressive Agents Used in Transplantation

Michael A. Hooks

The function of the human immune system is to protect the internal environment of the body from foreign proteins, cells, microorganisms, and other substances. To do this, the body must be able to discriminate between substances that are its own and those that are foreign. After the invader is identified, the immune system is then engaged and seeks to eliminate the foreign substance from the body. This is the event that leads to the rejection of many organ transplant grafts.

The rejection response is very complex and is not fully understood; however, rejection may be defined as the process by which the immune system of the host recognizes, becomes sensitized against, and seeks to eliminate the donor organ or tissue.[1] T lymphocytes and B lymphocytes are the two functional subpopulations of lymphocytes involved in rejection. T lymphocytes can further differentiate into two subunits: regulatory T lymphocytes (T helper cells and T suppressor cells) and effector T lymphocytes. Regulatory T lymphocytes function to amplify or suppress T and B lymphocyte responses. Effector T lymphocytes include the cytotoxic T lymphocytes, which play a key role in acute graft rejection.[2]

Fig. 4-1 illustrates the host response to a foreign transplanted graft. Helper T lymphocytes react with cell membrane proteins on the surface of the transplanted organ and become activated (activated T lymphocyte). Activated T lymphocytes subsequently secrete macrophage stimulating lymphokine.[3,4] Macrophages are then activated and secrete interleukin-1 (IL-1), which promotes the release of interleukin-2 (IL-2, T lymphocyte growth factor) from helper T lymphocytes. Helper T lymphocytes further differentiate into cytotoxic T lymphocytes, which attack the graft cell surface and destroy the graft.[4]

Billingham et al[1] illustrated in several studies that graft rejection is an immune response. These same investigators found that it was feasible to manipulate the immune system so that it would accept foreign grafts. The primary function of immunosuppression is to control the natural immune response of the host and thereby prevent or curtail rejection of the transplanted graft. It was not until 1950 that pharmacologic manipulation of the immune system was attempted.

The amount of time, effort, and money invested in trying to alter the immune system clinically is disproportional to the number of active agents available. This chapter will discuss those pharmacologic agents that have been shown to be of clinical value in organ transplantation.

HISTORY OF IMMUNOSUPPRESSION

The simple model of renal transplantation has long been used in the investigation of the efficacy of current immunosuppressive regi-

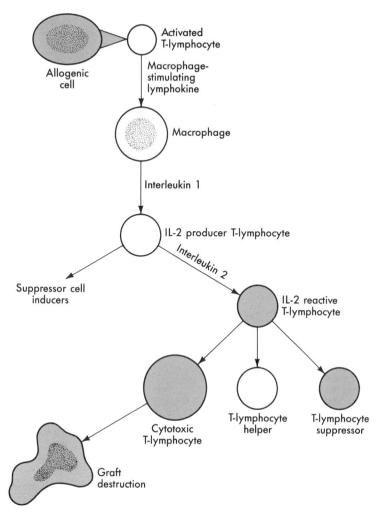

Fig. 4-1 Antigenic activation of the cellular immune response involving T lymphocytes with subsequent destruction of the graft.

mens. Table 4-1 shows the development and progression of immunosuppressive regimens. Investigations that began in 1962 saw the use of azathioprine as the sole immunosuppressive agent.[5] There were few long-term survivors in these studies, and since that time it has been recognized that cadaveric organ transplantation was not successful if azathioprine was the sole immunosuppressant.

In 1962 and 1963 it was demonstrated in renal transplants that the combination of azathio-prine and corticosteroids have additive and synergistic effects.[6] This double-drug therapy was soon adopted in several transplant centers and became the standard of therapy worldwide by 1964.[7-9] For more than a decade, however, the only satisfactory results were obtained in living-related donor transplants. The mortality and morbidity from cadaveric transplants were excessive, and the 1-year graft function was approximately 50%.[10]

The addition of antilymphocyte globulin

Table 4-1 Progression of immunosuppressive regimens used in transplantation

Immunosuppressive regimen	Year instituted	Deficiency of therapy
Azathioprine alone	1962	Ineffective, risky
Azathioprine with corticosteroids	1963	Suboptimal
Adjunctive thoracic duct drainage	1963	Required 20-30 days treatment before transplant
Adjunctive lymphocyte	1966	Suboptimal alone; however, immune globulin may be used as an adjunct in the treatment of acute rejection
Cyclophosphamide as substitute for azathioprine	1970	No advantage
Total body irradiation	1976	Risky
Cyclosporine alone	1978	Suboptimal
Cyclosporine with corticosteroids	1980	Presently used by most institutions
Adjunctive muromonab CD-3 (OKT-3)	1983	Presently used as rescue therapy
Triple therapy with azathioprine, cyclosporine, and corticosteroids	1984	Presently under evaluation

(ALG) as a third adjunctive immunosuppressive agent improved survival; however, the usefulness of ALG is limited. Because of the inability to standardize the drug product, and the numerous side effects, this drug is only used as a short-term adjunct.[11]

Other variations of immunosuppressive regimens have also been examined over the years. None of these techniques had a major impact on clinical transplantation. It was not until the late 1970s that the realm of immunosuppression began to change. With the advent of cyclosporine, newer immunosuppressive regimens were developed.

In 1976 Borel[12] reported studies of a new immunosuppressive agent called cyclosporin A. In 1979 the first major clinical experience with Cyclosporin A was reported.[13] Calne noted prolonged graft survival in his patient population when cyclosporin A was used as a single immunosuppressant regimen.[13] Currently, however, the combination of cyclosporine and corticosteroids is the therapy of choice for allograft transplantation. With the advent of newer research and investigation, many centers are now using triple-drug regimens (azathioprine, cyclosporine, and corticosteroids) as their immunosuppressive therapy. Triple-drug therapy will be discussed later in this chapter.

In the early 1980s Cosimi[14] began clinical trials using monoclonal antibodies raised against mature T lymphocytes. Since these initial investigations, other studies have shown that intractable rejection of renal grafts can be reversed with this monoclonal antibody.[15,16] In 1987 the monoclonal antibody CD-3 was approved by the Food and Drug Administration and marketed as Orthoclone OKT-3.

SPECIFIC IMMUNOSUPPRESSIVE AGENTS
Azathioprine

In 1951 6-mercaptopurine (6-MP) was found to have antipurine activity in *Lactobacillus casei*.[17] The antipurine activity causes an interference of nucleic acid synthesis during clonal expansion of cells resulting in a decrease in DNA synthesis and of precursor molecules. Schwartz et al[18] investigated the immunosuppressive activity of 6-MP on the immune response of rabbits when challenged with foreign antigens. This study showed an inability of the rabbit immune system to develop a response to the foreign protein in the presence of 6-MP. A number of purine antagonists have been studied; azathioprine, which is closely related to 6-MP, was found to have a superior therapeutic index for immunosuppression.[19] Azathioprine represents the basis of immunosuppressive treatment of human allograft recipients. In addition to anti-inflammatory actions, it has significant immunosuppressant action, even in very small doses. Azathioprine was first used in clinical organ transplantation by Murray[9] in 1963 and has since been shown to be a valuable immunosuppressant agent.

Mechanism of action. The exact mechanism of action of azathioprine is not fully understood. The action of azathioprine depends on several factors. First, azathioprine becomes active after conversion to 6-MP in vivo. The chemical reaction is primarily through nucleophilic attack by sulfhydryl-containing compounds (e.g., glutathione). Second, 6-MP is then metabolized to ribonucleotide thioinosinic acid, which becomes incorporated into nucleic acids causing chromosome breaks, suppression of guanine and adenine synthesis, and synthesis of fraudulent proteins.[20] The ultimate immunosuppressive effect is inhibition of RNA and DNA synthesis, leading to decreased immune cell proliferation.

Pharmacokinetic profile. Azathioprine is readily absorbed from the gastrointestinal (GI) tract after oral administration. The distribution of azathioprine is not fully understood, but it is known that the drug is rapidly removed from the blood. Both 6-MP and azathioprine are approximately 30% bound to plasma proteins; however, both compounds appear to be dialyzable.[21] Azathioprine is metabolized to 6-MP in vivo by sulfhydryl compounds such as glutathione in the liver. The metabolites and azathioprine are excreted renally, with only small amounts of intact parent compound seen in the urine. Because azathioprine is activated through hepatic pathways, one should be aware that a longer time may be needed for a therapeutic response to be seen in patients with liver dysfunction.

Therapeutic uses. Azathioprine is used as an adjunctive immunosuppressive agent for the prevention of rejection in solid organ transplants. The drug is used in conjunction with other immunosuppressive agents such as corticosteroids and cyclosporine. Maximum effectiveness of azathioprine occurs when the drug is administered during the initiation of the immune response. The effects of azathioprine and its active metabolite, 6-MP, may not be observed until several days after initiation of therapy and may have a residual effect several days after cessation of therapy.

Administration and dosage. Azathioprine is available in oral and intravenous (IV) dosage forms. Azathioprine dosages must be carefully adjusted and individualized according to patient response. The dosage of azathioprine must be adjusted in the presence of renal dysfunction and bone marrow suppression. The maximal oral dose used during severe renal impairment is 1.5 mg/kg of body weight per day.[22] Azathioprine is usually administered orally at a maintenance dose of 1 to 3 mg/kg of body weight per day; however, protocols that use triple-drug regimens may use lower doses of azathioprine. Oral azathioprine is available in 50 mg tablets and may be administered as a single dose or in divided doses.

Azathioprine in parenteral form is supplied in a 100 mg vial. The powder is reconstituted with 10 ml of sterile water for injection, yielding a solution containing 10 mg/ml. This solution may be given by direct IV injection or may be diluted in 0.9% sodium chloride of 5% dextrose for infusion. Intravenous infusions of azathioprine are usually administered over 30 to 60 minutes. Parenteral azathioprine may be used in patients unable to tolerate oral medications. The IV dose is the same as the oral dose (1 to 3 mg/kg of body weight per day).

Adverse reactions. Azathioprine is a toxic drug and must be used under close medical supervision. The principal toxic effect of azathioprine is bone marrow suppression. This is manifested by leukopenia, macrocytic anemia, and thrombocytopenia.[21,22] Hematologic effects are dose related and may be more severe in renal transplant patients who are experiencing graft rejection. A white blood cell (WBC) count of 3000/mm^3 to 5000/mm^3 is the parameter frequently used for decreasing the dose of azathioprine.[23] A rapidly diminishing WBC count, even if greater than 5000/mm^3, should be judged as a warning sign. The WBC count and hemoglobin level will drop first, followed by a decreasing platelet count in severe toxicity. The WBC count will usually return to normal when the dose of azathioprine is decreased.

Nausea, vomiting, anorexia, and diarrhea may occur in patients who are receiving large doses of azathioprine. These gastrointestinal effects may be avoided by giving azathioprine in divided doses or with meals. Other GI manifestations may include ulceration of the mucous membranes in the mouth, esophagitis, and steatorrhea.

A complication of azathioprine therapy possibly not related to cellular synthesis is hepatic damage.[23] This drug-related hepatitis is usually manifested by a low-grade jaundice, although a spectrum from slight abnormalities in bilirubin and liver enzymes to marked jaundice have been reported. The degree of liver damage is usually minimal but can be severe and lethal. It is not clear how much of the liver damage is the result of azathioprine itself or from commonly associated infections (e.g., hepatitis B, cytomegalovirus, and herpes simplex virus). Hepatitis from azathioprine toxicity is generally reversible if the drug is discontinued.

Other complications reported with the use of azathioprine include drug fever, rash, myopa-

Table 4-2 Azathioprine therapy: summary of side effects and nursing implications

Side effects	Assessment parameters	Nursing interventions
Cardiovascular: fluid and electrolytes		
Renal toxicity	Serum creatinine, BUN, Creatinine clearance Urine output Peripheral edema	Restrict fluids Administer diuretics Decrease dosage
Gastrointestinal		
Nausea, vomiting Anorexia Diarrhea Hepatotoxicity Pancreatitis	Appetite Elimination pattern Serum transaminases, phosphatases, bilirubin, coagulation factors serum amylase, lipase calcium	Administer oral dose with meals Consult with dietitian Institute enteral or parenteral nutrition
Hematologic		
Leukopenia Thrombocytopenia Macrocytic anemia	WBC count with differential and platelet count Red blood cell count Bleeding (oozing, hemorrhage) Signs/symptoms of infection Inspect mucous membranes for opportunistic infections	Increase attention to infection control measures Administer platelets Administer packed red blood cells Administer oral antifungal agent Administer antibiotics Decrease dosage
Neurologic		
None	None	
Psychologic		
None	None	
Dermatologic		
Stomatitis	Inspect mucous membranes	Maintain good oral hygiene

thy, and pancreatitis. Infection, which may be fatal, is a common hazard of therapy with azathioprine. Fungal, protozoal, viral, and uncommon bacterial infections may occur (see Chapter 3). When infection occurs, the dosage of azathioprine and other immunosuppressive therapy should be reduced as much as possible and appropriate therapy for infection instituted. Azathioprine is structurally similar to the xanthine oxidase inhibitor allopurinol. Xanthine oxidase is important in the conversion of azathioprine to its inactive metabolites. Since allopurinol inhibits this enzyme, dosage reduction of azathioprine (decrease in azathioprine dose by one fourth) is necessary when the patient is concurrently receiving allopurinol.[24] Table 4-2 summarizes the side effects and nursing implications of azathioprine therapy.

Corticosteroids

Corticosteroids, or glucocorticosteroids, exhibit a wide range of effects on almost every phase of the immune and inflammatory response in animals and humans. These agents, in pharma-cologic doses, have taken a major role in the treatment of many diseases, particularly those related to inflammatory or immune-mediated responses.[25,26] For more than three decades, the extraordinary ability of corticosteroids to prevent or suppress inflammation, whether the insulting agent is infectious, immunologic, or mechanical, has been examined.

The corticosteroids exert antiinflammatory activity. Corticosteroids include the primary endogenous glucocorticoid, cortisol, and exogenous therapeutic agents such as prednisone and methylprednisolone. The antiinflammatory effects of exogenous corticosteroids are similar to endogenous compounds.

Mechanism of action. Corticosteroids have a profound effect on the concentration of peripheral blood leukocytes. Lymphocyte, monocyte, and basophil counts will decrease in response to corticosteroids, while neutrophil counts will increase. The peak effects are seen within 4 to 6 hours after a dose of corticosteroid.

Fig. 4-2 illustrates the subcellular mechanism of action for the corticosteroids. It is felt that

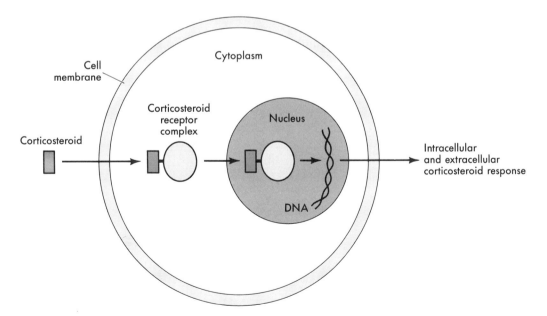

Fig. 4-2 The subcellular mechanism of action for corticosteroids involving a cytoplasmic receptor and incorporation into DNA, leading to transcription of specific messenger RNA for specific corticosteroid activity.

corticosteroids induce their effects on the cell through a glucocorticoid receptor.[27] Corticosteroids move freely through the cell membrane and react with a corticosteroid-specific receptor in the cytoplasm. On contact with the receptor, the steroid-receptor complex then translocates into the nucleus of the cell, where is attaches to DNA. The attachment to DNA causes transcription of specific messenger RNA, which produces cytoplasmic synthesis of proteins that mediate glucocorticoid activity.

Lymphocyte effect. A single dose of corticosteroids usually produces a rapid, transient lymphocytopenia within 4 hours. The peripheral lymphocyte count returns to normal within 24 to 48 hours.[28] This corticosteroid-induced lymphocytopenia is not a result of cell lysis, but rather a redistribution of circulating lymphocytes into other lymphoid compartments (e.g., spleen, lymph nodes, thoracic duct, and bone marrow).[29,30] The recirculating lymphocyte pool, which accounts for approximately two thirds of the body lymphocyte pool, consists mainly of T lymphocytes that migrate to and from the intravascular compartment and the lymphoid tissue. The nonrecirculating lymphocytes, which include some T lymphocytes and many B lymphocytes, live out their life span in the vascular compartment. Studies have shown corticosteroids to cause an emigration of recirculating T lymphocytes from the intravascular compartment to the lymphoid tissue with little effect on the distribution of B lymphocytes.[29] Fig. 4-3 illustrates this redistribution phenomena. The exact mechanism whereby corticosteroids cause a redistribution of lymphocytes is not known; however, it has been shown that alterations in the lymphocyte surface membrane result in changes in the lymphocyte circulation pattern.[31]

Monocyte effect. Because the monocyte-macrophage series of cells plays a major role in the induction and regulation of immune reactivity, the pharmacologic manipulation of these cells may have effects on the immune response as a whole. The corticosteroids have a wide range of effects on the cells of the mononuclear phagocyte series, which include the promonocytes in the bone marrow, the circulating monocytes, and their relatives, the tissue macrophages. Macrophages are intricately involved in the presentation of antigens to lymphocytes and in the subsequent removal of immune complexes. Corticosteroids can potentially modulate a wide range of monocyte functions, resulting in direct and indirect influences on inflammatory and immune responses. Quantitatively, corticosteroids produce a more profound depletion of monocytes, with cell counts dropping from 300 to 400 cells/mm³ to less than

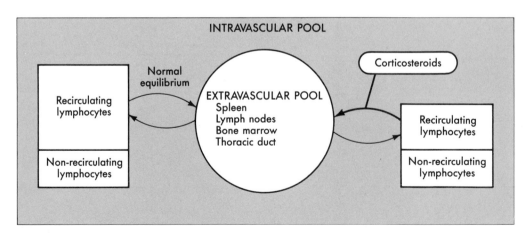

Fig. 4-3 Schematic representation of the lymphocyte redistribution phenomenon induced by corticosteroids. The recirculating lymphocytes are depleted from the intravascular compartment and redistributed into the extravascular lymphoid pool.

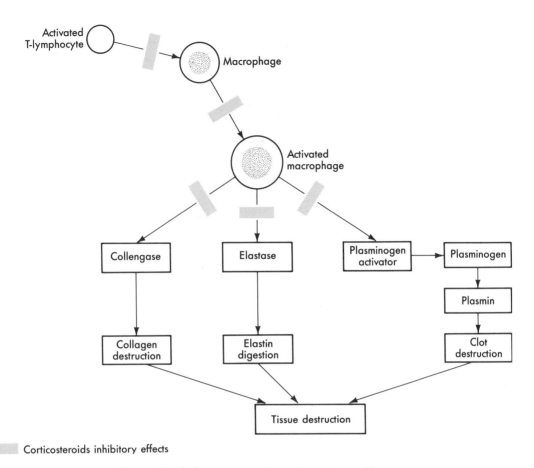

Fig. 4-4 Antiinflammatory actions of corticosteroids.

50 cells/mm³. This monocytopenia appears to be related to the redistribution phenomenon that is described for lymphocytes. However, monocytes appear to be more sensitive to redistribution than lymphocytes.[32] Corticosteroid-induced monocytopenia will inhibit the development of inflammatory reactions by inhibition of the response to chemotactic factors and macrophage activation factor, phagocytosis, pyrogen production, and secretion of collagenase, elastase, and plasminogen activator.[33] Fig. 4-4 illustrates the corticosteroid inhibition of tissue destruction associated with inflammation.

Neutrophil effects. A neutrophilia manifested by an increase of 2000 to 5000 cells/mm³ of blood also accompanies corticosteroid therapy. This corticosteroid effect causes an accelerated release of these cells from the bone marrow into the circulation and a reduction in migration out of the circulation. Corticosteroids inhibit the ability of neutrophils to adhere to the vessel walls, which is an essential step in the migration of cells from the circulation into the tissue. The net effect is a reduced number of neutrophils which may accumulate at the inflammatory site. This reduced accumulation of neutrophils, in addition to the reduced accumulation of monocytes, is one reason that host defenses are impaired in patients who receive daily corticosteroid therapy.

Eosinophil effects. One of the major effects of corticosteroids on eosinophils is a profound eosinophilia, which is manifested by a decrease in the eosinophil count to less than 25 cells/mm³.

As with monocytes and lymphocytes, it was initially thought that eosinophilia was caused by cell lysis; however, further study indicates that it is caused by a redistribution of the cells out of the intravascular compartment, similar to the effect of corticosteroids on lymphocytes. Chemotaxis is also affected and may result from the inhibition of cell response to chemotactic factors.

Other effects of corticosteroids. Corticosteroids have a negative effect on prostaglandin, probably as a result of reduction in the fatty acid precursors necessary for prostaglandin production. These agents may also act by blocking production of IL-1, which normally stimulates prostaglandin production.[34] Another effect of corticosteroids is complete inhibition of T lymphocyte growth factor or IL-2. IL-2 is produced by activated T lymphocytes and promotes proliferation of other T lymphocytes. Therefore T lymphocytes under the influence of corticosteroids lose their ability to proliferate and react to specific antigens.[35,36] Antibody production is not commonly suppressed at conventional doses in humans; however, high doses of corticosteroids given for long periods of time may lead to a decrease in antibody formation, particularly IgG.

Pharmacokinetic profile. Corticosteroids may be given by a number of routes: oral, topical, IV, intramuscular (IM), intraarticular, and by aerosol spray. Most corticosteroids appear to be readily absorbed when administered orally. Following IM administration, the absorption of the water-soluble salts, sodium phosphate and sodium succinate, is rapid, while the rate of absorption of the lipid-soluble salts, acetate and acetonide salts, is much slower. When abrupt onset of action is required, a water-soluble salt should be administered intravenously.

Studies have shown that corticosteroids are rapidly removed from the blood and distributed to muscles, liver, skin, intestines, and kidneys. Several authors have shown that tissue concentrations may be higher than plasma concentrations; thus circulating hormone may not accurately reflect concentrations in target organs. Corticosteroids vary in the extent of binding to plasma proteins. Hydrocortisone is extensively bound to plasma proteins, in particular transcortin (corticosteroid-binding globulin) and albumin. Prednisone, unlike other synthetic corticosteroids, has a high affinity for transcortin and competes with hydrocortisone for binding sites. Because only unbound drug is pharmacologically active, patients with hypoalbuminemia (serum albumin less than 2.5 gm%) may be more susceptible to corticosteroid effects than those with a normal serum albumin.[33] Corticosteroids cross the placenta and may be distributed into breast milk.

The main site of corticosteroid metabolism is the liver. Cortisone, prednisone, and methylprednisolone must first be reduced to their corresponding analogs, hydrocortisone, prednisolone, and methylprednisolone, to become pharmacologically active. Corticosteroids undergo glucuronic conjugation in the liver, and the inactive metabolites are then excreted renally. The precise effects of liver dysfunction on the metabolism of corticosteroids are not clear. Table 4-3 lists the plasma half-lives for some commonly administered corticosteroids.

Therapeutic uses. In physiologic doses, corticosteroids are used to replace deficient endogenous hormones. In pharmacologic doses, corticosteroids have both therapeutic and diagnostic applications. Corticosteroids are used in pharmacologic doses for their antiinflammatory and immunosuppressive properties. When corticosteroids are used for their antiinflammatory and immunosuppressive effects, the systemic agents with the least mineralocorticoid (sodium and water retention) activity should be used. Table 4-3 gives the antiinflammatory potency, equivalent dosage, and relative mineralocorticoid activity of commonly used corticosteroids.

Fig. 4-5 illustrates the antiinflammatory and immunosuppressive effects of corticosteroids. Circulating lymphocytes play a major role in the initiation and persistence of immunologic disease. They perform functions such as antigen recognition and memory, cell recruitment, direct cytotoxicity, production of lymphotoxins and other cytotoxic factors, and release of various immune mediators.[37] Sensitized lymphocytes are kept out of the peripheral circulation by corticosteroids by mechanisms already discussed, thus inhibiting the access of lymphocytes to target organs. Also, the effects of

Table 4-3 Clinical characteristics of commonly used corticosteroids

Drug	Antiinflammatory potency	Equivalent dosage* (mg)	Mineralocorticoid activity
Hydrocortisone	1.0	20.00	2+
Cortisone	0.8	25.00	2+
Prednisone	4.0	5.00	1+
Prednisolone	4.0	5.00	1+
Methylprednisolone	5.0	4.00	0
Triamcinolone	5.0	4.00	0
Betamethasone	20-30	0.60	0
Dexamethasone	20-30	0.75	0

*For example, prednisone is four times as potent as hydrocortisone (e.g., 5 mg of prednisone is equivalent to 20 mg of hydrocortisone).

corticosteroids on circulating monocytes and monocyte-macrophage functions are important in the mechanism of immunosuppression.

Administration and dosage. Corticosteroids may be administered orally, by oral inhalation, and by parenteral routes (IV, IM, subcutaneously, and intraarticularly). Corticosteroids used in immunosuppression are usually administered orally or parenterally. Because injections of slightly soluble corticosteroids may produce atrophy at the site of injection, IM injections should be administered deeply into gluteal muscle, and repeated injections at the same site should be avoided.

Dosage ranges for corticosteroids vary with the disease or condition for which they are being prescribed. Types of dosages used in various disease states include physiologic or replacement therapy (doses equivalent to the amount of corticosteroid normally secreted by the adrenal cortex per day) or pharmacologic therapy (any dose greater than physiologic dose). Pharmacologic therapy may be divided into several ranges: (1) maintenance or low-dose therapy: dosages slightly greater than physiologic (e.g., 5 to 15 mg of prednisone per day), (2) moderate-dose therapy: approximately 0.5 mg/kg of prednisone per day, (3) high-dose therapy: approx-

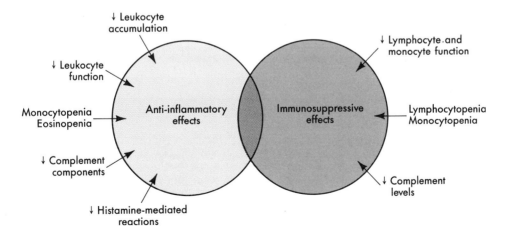

Fig. 4-5 The antiinflammatory and immunosuppressive effects of corticosteroids.

imately 1 to 3 mg/kg of prednisone per day, and (4) massive-dose therapy: approximately 15 to 30 mg/kg of prednisone per day. Typically, pharmacologic doses of corticosteroids are used in immunosuppressive regimens. The approximate dosage equivalents of the commonly used corticosteroids are shown in Table 4-3.

Long-term steroid therapy should not be initiated without first considering the risks of therapy. Some basic principles for steroid therapy include the following: (1) the objective is to maintain the patient on an alternate day dosing schedule, (2) a short-acting oral steroid should be used (prednisone is prescribed most often because it is inexpensive and has a short serum half-life), and (3) the minimum dosage to produce the desired response should be used.

Alternate-day therapy is the dosage regimen of choice for long-term corticosteroid therapy. The optimum alternate-day dose is usually 2½ to 3 times the minimum daily dose. The dose should be given in the morning to maintain the normal circadian cycle of morning peaks and evening troughs. Patients receiving corticosteroids in immunosuppressive regimens receive a slow decrease in dosage after transplanation; however, many transplant patients may not be able to be maintained on every-other-day therapy. For this reason, most patients will be maintained on a very low daily dose of corticosteroids. The box below illustrates a typical dosage regimen for a corticosteroid taper used in transplantation for the prevention of rejection.

Adverse effects. Complications of corticosteroid therapy are numerous and virtually any organ system in the body may be affected. It should be emphasized that when corticosteroids are used appropriately and judiciously, complications can be minimized.

Short-term or acute adverse effects, which usually occur with initiation of therapy, include

---

EXAMPLE OF A CORTICOSTEROID TAPER IN IMMUNOSUPPRESSION

Preoperatively: Adult
Methylprednisolone 1 g IV at induction of anesthesia

Postoperatively: Adult
Methylprednisolone 50 mg IV every 6 hours for 4 doses, then
methylprednisolone 40 mg IV every 6 hours for 4 doses, then
methylprednisolone 30 mg IV every 6 hours for 4 doses, then
methylprednisolone 20 mg IV every 6 hours for 4 doses, then
methylprednisolone 20 mg IV every 12 hours for 2 doses, then
methylprednisolone 10 mg IV every 12 hours
Once able to tolerate oral medications, the patient may be changed to:
Prednisone 20 mg orally daily

Preoperatively: Pediatric
Methylprednisolone 500 mg IV at induction of anesthesia.

Postoperatively: Pediatric
Methylprednisolone 25 mg IV every 6 hours for 4 doses, then
methylprednisolone 20 mg IV every 6 hours for 4 doses, then
methylprednisolone 15 mg IV every 6 hours for 4 doses, then
methylprednisolone 10 mg IV every 6 hours for 4 doses, then
methylprednisolone 10 mg IV every 12 hours for 2 doses, then
methylprednisolone 7.5 mg IV every 12 hours
Once able to tolerate oral medications, the patient may be changed to:
Prednisone 15 mg orally daily

central nervous system (CNS) effects, psychosis, pseudotumor cerebri, impaired glucose tolerance, and retention of salt and fluid. CNS effects may range from euphoria to depression, probably as a result of increased brain excitability. Insomnia, jitteriness, and increased appetite are common. Some patients may develop a "steroid psychosis," but this is rarely accompanied by suicidal tendencies. These CNS effects will usually subside when the dose is decreased. Fluid and salt retention may exacerbate congestive heart disease; however, dietary restrictions may improve the problem of fluid retention. Glucose intolerance may lead to "steroid-induced diabetes" or may aggravate preexisting diabetes mellitus. A personal or family history of diabetes mellitus demands an extra watchful eye when initiating corticosteroid therapy.

Long-term adverse effects of corticosteroid therapy are usually more insidious in onset and tend to subside more slowly when therapy is discontinued. These adverse effects are most likely to occur in patients who take corticosteroids daily for months or longer. The development of iatrogenic Cushing's syndrome with truncal obesity and "buffalo hump" associated with long-term corticosteroid use has been well documented. Other effects of long-term steroid use include acne, striae, and hirsutism. Growth retardation has also been shown to occur in prepubertal children. This phenomenon was a major side effect in pediatric transplantation before the introduction of cyclosporine therapy. Adjustment to alternate-day therapy at the lowest possible dose or withdrawal of corticosteroids altogether may help to reduce or reverse some of the complications.

There is general agreement that high doses of corticosteroids for more than 2 weeks at a time may predispose the patient to opportunistic infections such as those associated with *Aspergillus* species, *Pneumocystis carinii,* and herpes species. The appropriate antiinfective is the therapy of choice, as is reducing the dose of corticosteroid if possible.

One of the most common side effects of corticosteroid therapy is cataract formation. Glaucoma may be induced or aggravated by corticosteroid ophthalmic preparations.

Osteoporosis is a particularly troublesome

complication of prolonged corticosteroid therapy. In this type of osteopenia, there is a loss of bone matrix and bone mineral. This loss is caused by direct inhibition of bone formation and indirect stimulation of bone resorption resulting from inhibition of calcium absorption from the intestine. The resultant bone thinning can lead to spontaneous vertebral compression and bone fractures. Treatment of this condition includes reduction of corticosteroid dosage, physical therapy and activity to stimulate bone formation, and supplementation with vitamin D and calcium.

Several drug interactions with corticosteroids have been cited that may be of clinical importance. Drugs that induce liver enzyme systems, such as barbiturates, phenytoin, and rifampin, increase the metabolism of corticosteroids. Estrogens increase the effects of corticosteroids as a result of an increase in available transcortin, thereby decreasing the amount of steroid available for metabolism. Potassium-wasting diuretics, such as furosemide, bumetanide, and the thiazides, and other drugs that waste potassium, such as amphotericin B, may enhance the potassium-wasting effect of corticosteroids. Corticosteroids in combination with anticholinesterase agents may produce a pronounced muscle weakness.

Abrupt withdrawal of corticosteroids is dangerous. When corticosteroids are rapidly tapered, patients may exhibit withdrawal symptoms such as headaches, myalgias, and fatigue. These symptoms reflect mild adrenocortical insufficiency and are usually transient. They may be prevented or lessened by a more gradual tapering of corticosteroids. The abrupt withdrawal of high-dose corticosteroids may also cause cardiovascular collapse, resulting in hypotension and shock. Table 4-4 summarizes the side effects and nursing implications of corticosteroid therapy.

Lymphocyte immune globulin

Antilymphocyte sera (ALS) or globulin is a product of animal sera containing heterologous antibodies (immunoglobulin G, or IgG) to lymphocytes, while antithymocyte globulin (ATG) contains heterologous antibodies to thymocytes or T lymphocytes. For the purpose of

Table 4-4 Corticosteroid therapy: summary of side effects and nursing implications

Side effects	Assessment parameters	Nursing interventions
Cardiovascular; fluid and electrolytes		
Sodium retention	Serum electrolytes	Administer low-sodium, high
Potassium wasting	Serum calcium, phosphorus	potassium diet
Calcium and phosphorus	Serum albumin	Administer oral or parenteral
wasting	Intake and output	electrolyte replacement
Metabolic alkalosis	Acid-base status	Administer oral or parenteral
Fluid retention	Peripheral edema	calcium, phosphorus re-
Systemic arterial hyper-	Blood pressure	placement
tension		Administer antihypertensives
		Instruct patient about side
		effects
		Decrease dosage
Pulmonary		
None	None	None
Gastrointestinal		
Peptic ulceration (esopha-	Guaiac stools and vomitus	Administer oral corticoste-
gus, stomach, duodenum)	Serum amylase, lipase	roids with food
Pancreatitis	Serum calcium	Administer antacids, H_2 re-
Hepatitis	Serum transaminases, phos-	ceptor blockers
Increased appetite	phatases, bilirubin	Consult dietition
Diarrhea	Coagulation factors	Decrease dosage
	Peritoneal signs	
Endocrine		
Impaired glucose tolerance	Serum glucose	Insulin
Diabetes mellitus	Polydipsia, polyuria	Thyroid hormone replace-
Cushing's syndrome	Cushingoid character — moon	ment
Hypothyroidism	face, truncal obesity	Instruct patient about conse-
Impaired carbohydrate	buffalo hump, striae	quences of sudden corti-
tolerance	T_3, T_4	costeroid withdrawal
Adrenopituitary sup-	During period steroid with-	Avoid sudden withdrawal
pression	drawal or increased stress:	from corticosteroids
	headache, lethargy, weak-	
	ness, hypotension	
Osteoporosis	Assess patient complaints of	Administer calcium and vita-
	back or limb pain	min D supplements
Hematologic		
Neutrophilia, eosinophilia,	White blood cell (WBC)	Increase attention to infection
basophilia	count with differential	control measures
Lymphocytopenia	count	Administer oral antifungal
Opportunistic infection, im-	Inspect mucous membranes	agents
paired wound healing	for opportunistic infection	Administer antibiotics
Aseptic necrosis of femoral	Signs/symptoms of infection	
and humoral heads	Wound healing	

Continued.

Table 4-4 Corticosteroid therapy: summary of side effects and nursing implications—cont'd

Side effects	Assessment parameters	Nursing interventions
Neurologic		
Headache	Neurologic status	Analgesics for headaches
Insomnia	Sleep periods	Provide environment condu-
Vertigo		cive to sleep
Seizures		Initiate seizure precautions in
Increased intracranial		susceptible patient
pressure		Consult physical therapy
Muscle weakness		Decrease dosage
		Give dose in the morning if pos-
		sible
Psychologic		
Psychosis	Mental status	Consult psychiatrist if
Euphoria		necessary
Depression		Instruct patient about side
		effects
		Decrease dosage
Dermatologic		
Thin, fragile skin	Inspect skin	Administer topical antiacne med-
Petechiae, ecchymoses	Inspect mucous membranes	ication
Erythema		Avoid adhesive tape
Acne		Avoid skin trauma
Hirsutism		Counsel regarding options for
Stomatitis		dealing with hirsutism
Other		
Blurred vision		Consult ophthalmology depart-
Cataracts		ment

this discussion, these agents will be referred to as *lymphocyte immune globulin*. The immunosuppressive activity of lymphocyte immune globulin has been known since 1956; however, the immunosuppressive potency of lymphocyte immune globulin was not known until 1963, when it was demonstrated to prolong skin graft survival in rats.[38] Although in the animal graft model antilymphocyte globulin (ALG) and antithymocyte globulin (ATG) have proved successful in prolonging graft survival, their effectiveness in clinical immunosuppression has been difficult to evaluate. Lymphocyte immune globulin was first used in clinical transplantation by Starzl in 1965.[39] Early experience with lympho-

cyte immune globulin was unfavorable, with little evidence of improved outcome in transplantation.[40,41] However, as the use of lymphocyte immune globulin continued, noncontrolled and controlled trials began to show improved graft survival in renal transplant patients.[42-46] The use of lymphocyte immune globulin in combination with other agents has become universally accepted and has been shown to improve survival after cardiac transplantation.[47]

Typically, lymphocyte immune globulin preparations are produced by injecting an animal with human lymphocyte and allowing the animal to produce antibodies to the foreign antigen.

The animal serum is then separated and purified to yield the immune globulin.

Mechanism of action. Various lymphoid cells have been used in the preparation of lymphocyte immune globulin for human use. Initially, splenic and blood lymphocytes were used; however, these have been excluded from use because of excessive production of anti–red cell and antiplatelet antibodies. Thoracic duct cells have been used with good results; however, these are difficult to obtain. Thymocytes have been used most widely and successfully in the preparation of lymphocyte immune globulin. It should be noted that the immunosuppressive properties of ATG, because it consists of heterologous antibodies raised against thymocytes, are theoretically more specific than antilymphocyte globulin. For this reason, it is more desirable to use ATG in the clinical setting. Lymphocyte immune globulin for clinical use has been produced in horses, goats, rabbits, and cows.

Although several mechanisms of action have been proposed for lymphocyte immune globulin, there is now abundant evidence that the immunosuppressive effect of lymphocyte immune globulin is achieved by selective depletion of long-lived, circulating lymphocytes from the lymph nodes and spleen. There is also a similar reduction of small lymphocytes in thoracic duct lymph and the lymphoid organs.[48,49]

There is evidence in animal models that lymphocyte immune globulin depletes circulating lymphocytes in animals by coating and opsonizing the lymphocytes so that they are phagocytized by macrophages within the liver and lymphoid organs.[50] Chanard et al[51] suggested that this same process may occur in humans. In vitro studies indicate that lymphocyte immune globulin binding is generally nonspecific. The drug has been shown to bind to visceral tissues (thymus and testicular cell membranes), nuclear and cytoplasmic components of tissue (tonsils, kidney, liver), and extensively to bone marrow cells and peripheral blood cells other than lymphocytes.

Pharmacokinetic profile. Following IV administration, peak plasma levels of equine IgG vary, depending on the ability of the individual to catabolize foreign IgG. The distribution of lymphocyte immune globulin into body fluids and tissues has not been fully described. In vitro studies have shown that lymphocyte immune globulin binds to essentially all types of circulating lymphocytes, granulocytes, platelets, bone marrow cells and visceral tissues. Information dealing with the ability of lymphocyte immune globulin to cross the placenta is not available; however, since other immunoglobulins cross the placenta, it is suspected that lymphocyte immune globulin has this same property. The plasma half-life of lymphocyte immune globulin averages about 6 days. Approximately 1% of lymphocyte immune globulin is excreted unchanged in the urine.

Therapeutic uses. Lymphocyte immune globulin has been used in the prevention and treatment of rejection in allograft transplantation as an adjunct to other immunosuppressive agents such as azathioprine and corticosteroids to delay the onset of rejection.[52] There is significant evidence that lymphocyte immune globulin can prolong the graft survival of renal, hepatic, and cardiac allografts in experimental animals.[50] Studies have attempted to demonstrate the benefit of using lymphocyte immune globulin as an adjunctive therapy.[52,53] Despite the clear-cut potency of lymphocyte immune globulin, the initial results of adding lymphocyte immune globulin to clinical regimens failed to conclusively demonstrate improvement. These trials did demonstrate a reduced incidence and severity of early rejection and a greater ease of reversibility in reactions; however, statistically improved long-term graft survival has not been proved.[54,55] Past and recent studies using lymphocyte immune globulin as an adjunctive agent have shown a 10% to 15% improvement in functional graft survival, but no increase in patient survival.[54-57]

Recent studies have demonstrated lymphocyte immune globulin to be highly effective in the treatment of acute allograft rejection in both living-related and cadaveric kidney transplants.[58,59] Reversal of the first rejection episode appears to respond more frequently, more rapidly, and more completely to lymphocyte immune globulin than do subsequent rejection episodes. Immunosuppressive therapy that includes lymphocyte immune globulin generally appears to reverse the course of rejection 2 to 3 days earlier than regimens that do not include lymphocyte immune globulin.

Dosage and administration. Because of the risk of a severe systemic allergic reaction or anaphylaxis, an intradermal skin test is recommended by the manufacturer before the administration of therapeutic doses of lymphocyte immune globulin. The skin test procedure is performed by injecting 0.1 ml of a 1 : 1000 dilution of lymphocyte immune globulin in normal saline for injection. Only freshly diluted lymphocyte immune globulin should be used in the skin testing procedure. A control test of normal saline should be used to facilitate interpretation of the results of the skin test. The test site should be observed for 1 hour for the appearance of a wheal or erythema greater than 10 mm in diameter.

Lymphocyte immune globulin is administered by slow IV infusion. The available concentrate of lymphocyte immune globulin should be diluted with either 0.45% or 0.9% saline before administration. It is recommended that the final concentration of the infusion mixture not exceed 1 mg/ml. Patients should be observed throughout the administration period for signs and symptoms of allergic reactions. To prevent such reactions, patients are usually premedicated with an antipyretic and an antihistamine. Inline filters (0.22 microns) should be used with IV administration of lymphocyte immune globulin to avoid inadvertent administration of insoluble material. Lymphocyte immune globulin should be infused over at least a 4-hour period.

In the prevention and treatment of allograft rejection, lymphocyte immune globulin is administered concomitantly with other immunosuppressive therapy. For the prevention of graft rejection, it is recommended that a fixed dose, beginning within 24 hours of transplant, of 15 mg/kg of body weight be administered daily for 14 days, followed by alternate-day therapy of the same dose for 14 additional days.

For the treatment of allograft rejection, the recommended dosage of lymphocyte immune globulin is 10 to 15 mg/kg body weight administered daily for 14 days. If necessary, this regimen may be followed with alternate-day therapy of the same dose for 14 additional days. Therapy with lymphocyte immune globulin should begin promptly when the initial diagnosis of acute rejection is made.

Adverse reactions. Fever, which may be accompanied by chills, is the most prominent adverse effect of therapy with lymphocyte immune globulin. The exact mechanism is not known; however, it has been speculated that lymphocyte immune globulin may enhance the release of endogenous leukocyte pyrogens.[50] This febrile reaction tends to subside with the progression of therapy.

Anaphylaxis occurs in approximately 1% of patients treated with lymphocyte immune globulin and may occur at any time during therapy. Anaphylaxis is usually manifested by hypotension, respiratory distress, and pain in the chest, back, and flank. If any symptoms of anaphylaxis occur, the infusion should be stopped and appropriate actions taken. Lymphocyte immune globulin anaphylaxis can be managed with epinephrine, corticosteroids, assisted ventilation, and other supportive measures. It is recommended that epinephrine and corticosteroids be available on hand while the patient is receiving these products. Patients who exhibit a sensitivity to horse sera should not receive lymphocyte immune globulin.

Serum sickness reactions have occurred in patients receiving lymphocyte immune globulin. The symptoms of serum sickness usually develop within 6 to 18 days after initiation of therapy but may occur at any time during therapy and/or following discontinuation of therapy. The diagnosis of serum sickness is usually made on the basis of clinical presentation. The patient will exhibit such signs and symptoms as fever, malaise, arthralgia, nausea and vomiting, lymphadenopathy, and cutaneous eruptions.

Leukopenia and thrombocytopenia occur in approximately 10% to 20% of patients treated with lymphocyte immune globulin.[56] Acute thrombocytopenia induced by lymphocyte immune globulin is usually accompanied by a sequestering of platelets in the spleen and liver. Splenic entrapment of antibody-coated platelets may be the prominent mechanism for thrombocytopenia.[50]

An increased incidence of infection, particularly fungal and viral infections, has been reported with the use of lymphocyte immune globulin. It is, however, difficult to determine whether these infections result from the use of lymphocyte immune globulin per se or are the result of a general increase in immunosuppression. An increase in cytomegalovirus infections, over and above the number reported with conventional therapy, has been reported.[60]

Muromonab CD-3

Advances in immunosuppression and refinements in surgical procedures have led to improvement in patient and graft survival in allograft transplantation. An increased understanding of the mechanism of rejection has made it possible to plan a more rational approach to immunosuppression. One of the newest agents in the armamentarium for immunosuppression is muromonab CD-3 (Orthoclone OKT-3).

Muromonab CD-3 is a monoclonal antibody that has been shown to be effective in the treatment of allograft rejection. Muromonab CD-3 differs from early polyclonal antibody preparations such as the lymphocyte immune globulins in many ways. In contrast to the polyclonal product, which is produced from a mixture of numerous clones of antibody-producing lymphocytes, each molecule of the monoclonal product is identical to every other molecule, because each molecule is derived from a single antibody-producing clone. There is no lot-to-lot variation in the monoclonal preparation, as there is with the polyclonal preparation. In addition, the monoclonal nature of the preparation allows adequate immunosuppression to be achieved with a much smaller daily dose of immunoglobulin.

Monoclonal antibodies are highly specific antibodies derived from a single clone and are considered homogenous. Each molecule of the same monoclonal antibody is equally active against a specific antigen. As in the preparation of lymphocyte immune globulin, animals are used in the process of generating monoclonal antibodies. Monoclonal antibodies are manufactured using a hybridization technique. In this technique, a single antibody-producing B cell (each B cell produces only one type of an antibody) is coupled with a myeloma cell to produce a hybridoma that is capable of secreting a limitless supply of highly specific antibodies.

Typically, a mouse is first injected with a particular antigen. The B lymphocyte of the mouse's immune system then produces antibodies to the injected foreign antigen. Immunologically active B lymphocytes are then harvested from the mouse, either from the spleen or from ascitic fluid formed in the mouse. Single cell lines are isolated, harvested and then coupled with myeloma cells. These cells are allowed to proliferate in a medium and the antibodies are produced. Since each antibody molecule is produced by descendants of a single B lymphocyte, they will react with only one antigen and are termed *monoclonal.*

Mechanism of action. Muromonab CD-3 binds to all mature T lymphocytes in the peripheral blood. It is now recognized that the T lymphocyte has two molecules located on its surface which function primarily in antigen recognition. These antigen recognition structures are associated with three polypeptide chains called the *CD-3 complex.* The CD-3 complex transduces the signal for the T lymphocyte to react to the foreign antigen, proliferate, and attack the foreign matter. Muromonab CD-3 is a monoclonal antibody that specifically reacts with the T-3 complex by blocking the function of T lymphocytes (Fig. 4-6).

In the body, muromonab CD-3 acts in two phases.[61] During the first phase, which begins immediately after injection of muromonab CD-3, there is a depletion of circulating T lymphocytes. This depletion results primarily from opsonization in the liver and cytolysis. The second phase of muromonab CD-3 action involves antigenic modulation. As mentioned above, the CD-3 complex on the cell surface is removed, producing immunoincompetent T lymphocytes, but there is no further depletion of the T lymphocyte population.[62]

Therapeutic uses. Initially, muromonab CD-3 was indicated for the treatment of acute allograft rejection in renal transplant patients. The evaluation of muromonab CD-3 as specific therapy for rejection in human renal transplant

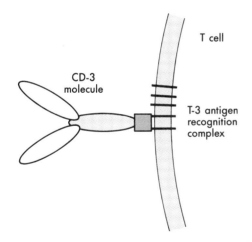

T cell

CD-3
molecule

T-3 antigen
recognition
complex

Fig. 4-6 Muromonab CD-3 reacts specifically with the T-3 antigen recognition complex, thereby blocking T lymphocyte effector cell function.

recipients began in 1980.[63] This study provided strong evidence that muromonab CD-3 produced significant results in the treatment of renal graft rejection. Subsequent prospective randomized trials produced similar results.[64] Muromonab CD-3 has also been of benefit in the treatment of steroid-resistant rejection in renal transplant patients who have received prophylactic cyclosporine.[65]

Muromonab CD-3 has also been used to treat acute rejection in hepatic and cardiac transplant patients. One study reported a reversal of rejection within 72 hours of initiation of therapy in 73% of hepatic transplant patients treated.[66] The most favorable results in hepatic transplant patients have been achieved in patients who experience rejection in the first 90 days after transplantation.[67] In the treatment of cardiac transplant rejection, muromonab CD-3 has been shown to be effective in the treatment of primary graft rejection and rejection unresponsive to steroids and lymphocyte immune globulin.[68]

Muromonab CD-3 initially was reserved for the rescue of transplant patients experiencing acute rejection of their allograft. Recently, however, muromonab CD-3 has been used prophylactically in patients with compromised renal function to prevent acute rejection in the early postoperative period. Studies by Bristow[68] and Norman[69] have shown muromonab CD-3 to be successful in preventing acute cardiac and renal rejection when used prophylactically. Millis[70] demonstrated a reduction in the number of early rejection episodes following liver transplantation by using muromonab CD-3 prophylactically.

Dosage and administration. The recommended dosage for muromonab CD-3 (Orthoclone OKT-3, Ortho Pharmaceutical Company) for the treatment of acute allograft rejection is 5 mg IV daily for 10-14 days. Treatment should begin immediately on diagnosis of acute rejection. The IV product should be inspected visually for particulate matter before administration. In the preparation of muromonab CD-3, the injection solution should first be filtered through a 0.20 to 0.22 micron low–protein binding filter to remove particular material. Muromonab CD-3 should be given as an IV bolus without the filter over 1 minute. This drug should not be administered by IV infusion or concomitantly with other drug solutions.

Following administration of muromonab CD-3, patients should be monitored closely for 48 hours. Intravenous methylprednisolone (1 mg/kg of body weight) may be given as a premedication to avoid some of the adverse effects of administration. Acetaminophen and an antihistamine may also be given as premedications to avoid early adverse reactions. Table 4-5 gives a sample protocol for the administration of muromonab CD-3. The doses of concomitant immunosuppressive agents should be decreased during therapy with muromonab CD-3.

Therapeutic monitoring of muromonab CD-3 is relatively new. Presently some institutions are monitoring peripheral T lymphocyte counts to measure the therapeutic benefit of muromonab CD-3. In some patients who do not have an adequate reduction in peripheral T lymphocyte counts, the dose of muromonab may be increased to 10 mg IV daily. Another means of assessing response to muromonab CD-3 is to monitor drug levels or monitor the appearance of antimurine antibodies.

Because muromonab CD-3 is a foreign protein, some patients may develop antibodies to

Table 4-5 Sample protocol for the administration of muromonab CD-3

Dose	≥ 30 kg IBW	5.0 mg IV
	< 30 kg IBW	2.5 mg IV
Premedication	1. 1 g methylprednisolone IV 6 to 12 hours before first dose or 1 g hydrocortisone IV 1 hour before first dose	
	2. Acetaminophen 10 grains and diphenhydramine 50 mg before each dose	
Precautions	1. Have crash cart outside patient's room for the first two doses.	
	2. Vital signs following the first 2 doses should be monitored every 15 minutes for the first 2 hours; then every 20 minutes for the next 2 hours; then follow routine monitoring procedures.	
	3. For subsequent doses, vital signs should be monitored per routine.	

the product. For this reason, patients should be tested for antibodies to muromonab CD-3 before a second course of therapy is planned. Currently, Ortho Pharmaceutical Company offers an immunoassay service to measure antibody titers for muromonab CD-3. Patients who are seronegative for muromonab CD-3 antibodies may theoretically receive a second course of therapy; however, those who are seropositive should not receive a second course.

Adverse reactions. Patients typically experience chills and fever for 45 to 60 minutes after the initial dose of muromonab CD-3. This reaction may be related to the abrupt lysis of circulating lymphocytes. Respiratory symptoms may be more severe in patients who are fluid overloaded. Cardiopulmonary arrest has been observed in patients with pulmonary edema before receiving muromonab CD-3. For this reason, a chest x-ray examination and body weight measurement within 24 hours of initiating muromonab CD-3 therapy is mandatory.[72] Muromonab CD-3 administration is not advised for patients who have had a greater than or equal to 3% increase in body weight during the week before beginning therapy.

Recently a syndrome of aseptic meningitis has been reported to be associated with the administration of muromonab CD-3.[73] This reaction is manifested by fever, headache, and neck stiffness. The cerebrospinal fluid had an elevated protein content and WBC count, but no infectious organism could be found. This syndrome was self-limiting without sequelae.

Cytomegalic (CMV) and herpes simplex viral infections are common during the 2 to 3 weeks after muromonab CD-3 administration. Herpes simplex infections usually manifest as herpes stomatitis, which responds to acyclovir therapy. Cytomegalovirus disease may manifest as hepatitis, pneumonia or enteritis. Typically these infections are diagnosed by biopsy or bronchoalveolar lavage (BAL) and are manifested by the presence of inclusion bodies within the infected cells. Therapies for CMV infections are currently under investigation but include the use of gancyclovir and intravenous immune serum globulin.

Most side effects occur after the first two doses of muromonab CD-3. Other side effects the patient may experience include headache and a flulike syndrome. These patients may also complain of acute joint pain for the first couple of doses. Diarrhea, sometimes quite severe, may also be experienced.

Cyclosporine

Cyclosporine is a molecule with unique biological properties. The name cyclosporine has been adopted by the United States Adopted Names (USAN) as the name of the early compound cyclosporin A. Cyclosporine is a neutral cyclic polypeptide consisting of 11 amino acids and is the major metabolic product of the fungus *Tolypocladium inflatum.*

The potent immunosuppressive properties of cyclosporine were demonstrated initially by Borel et al.[74] After 6 years of animal model evaluations, cyclosporine was used in clinical transplantation.[75] Cyclosporine has revolutionized immunosuppression for organ and tissue transplantation.

Mechanism of action. The most promising aspect of cyclosporine as an immunosuppressive agent is its apparent selectivity to lymphocytes. All other drugs with this claimed immunosuppressive action, except muromonab CD-3, show varying degrees of myelotoxicity, which limits their use. Further analysis of the action of cyclosporine has shown the selectivity to be within the lymphocyte compartment affecting mainly T lymphocytes and sparing B lymphocytes.[76]

Activation of T lymphocytes by foreign antigens requires the presence of at least two distinct sets of factors for clonal expansion and maturation.[36,77,78] The sequence of events in T lymphocyte proliferation is discussed in Chapter 3.

Early experiments showed that cyclosporine inhibits the responsiveness of T lymphocytes to Interleukin-2 (IL-2).[36] Later studies showed that in the presence of cyclosporine, T lymphocytes do not express receptors for IL-2.[79] Cyclosporine also causes IL-2–produced T lymphocytes to become unresponsive to IL-1, which renders them incapable of producing IL-2 receptors.[79-81] It is important to note that once T lymphocytes have been activated by antigens to express IL-2 receptors, cyclosporine no longer suppresses proliferation of T lymphocytes. This suggests that at some point after primary antigen exposure T lymphocyte effector action becomes cyclosporine resistant. This process is consistent with the observation that recurrent or ongoing (chronic) rejection is resistant to cyclosporine.

It appears that cyclosporine has a minimal effect on B lymphocytes. It is postulated that there are two distinct subsets of B lymphocytes that may be stimulated by two different mechanisms, one that may be cyclosporine sensitive while the other is not.[82,83] Cyclosporine has been shown to affect macrophage recruitment and activation; however, it does not directly inhibit macrophage activities such as phagocytosis, migration, and chemotaxis.[84] Cyclosporine does not affect neutrophil response, suggesting that although cyclosporine halts T lymphocyte proliferation, it does not adversely affect important precursor neutrophilic mechanisms.[85]

Pharmacokinetic profile. Cyclosporine is available in an oral and an intravenous solution. After oral administration, cyclosporine absorption is slow and incomplete.[86,87] There is considerable variation in peak cyclosporine concentrations after oral administration in renal, cardiac, bone marrow, and hepatic transplant recipients. Peak concentrations after oral administration vary between 1 and 8 hours, but usually peak levels occur within 4 hours. The absorption half-life ranges between 0.6 and 2.3 hours.[86,88]

Approximately 37% of an oral dose of cyclosporine is absorbed, 27% of which undergoes first-pass metabolism in the liver, leaving an absolute bioavailability of 27%.[88,89] There is marked variability in the extent of cyclosporine absorption in patients after organ transplantation. The absolute bioavailability of cyclosporine may vary from 20% to 50% in bone marrow transplant patients,[87] and from less than 5% to 89% in renal transplant patients.[90] In cardiac transplant patients, the bioavailability of cyclosporine is approximately 35%,[91] and in liver transplant patients, the bioavailability ranges from 8% to 60%.[92] The effects of food on the bioavailability of cyclosporine are equivocal. Early reports suggested that food may delay and alter the absorption of cyclosporine[93]; however, later reports stated that food had no consistent effect on cyclosporine absorption.[94] The effect of food on cyclosporine absorption may be related to the nature of the diet and the temporal relation of food consumption and cyclosporine administration.

The absorption of fat and fat-soluble substances is impaired in patients with liver dysfunction. Because cyclosporine is fat soluble, the bioavailability of cyclosporine is decreased in patients with severe liver dysfunction.[92] Studies have shown that patients with elevated total bilirubin levels have decreased absorption of cyclosporine.[95] This decrease in bioavailability is felt to result from an insufficient amount of bile and bile salts necessary for cyclosporine absorption.

After liver transplantation, the absorption of

cyclosporine is erratic in patients with external bile drainage (e.g., a draining T-tube). There is a significant increase in cyclosporine trough blood concentrations after clamping of the external biliary drain.[96] After the removal of the external biliary drain, there is an increase in the rate and extent of biliary drainage, and there is an increase in the rate and extent of absorption. Whenever external biliary diversion is instituted or discontinued, cyclosporine dosage adjustments will need to be made.

Since cyclosporine is highly lipid soluble, it diffuses readily across biologic membranes and distributes widely in the body. The volume of distribution for cyclosporine has been reported to vary between 4.5 L/kg of body weight after intravenous administration to 13 L/kg of body weight after oral administration.[88] In blood, cyclosporine is primarily bound to red blood cells (approximately 58%). Four percent is bound to granulocytes, 5% to lymphocytes, and the remaining 33% is distributed in the plasma.[97] Approximately 80% of the drug found in the plasma is bound to plasma lipoproteins. Of the different lipoproteins, the high-density lipoprotein fraction binds 57% of drug, the low-density lipoprotein fraction binds 25%, and the very-low-density lipoprotein fraction binds approximately 2%.[98] Lipoprotein profiles may be altered significantly in patients with renal and hepatic dysfunction. Therefore, in these conditions, a change in the binding capacity (increased unbound drug) of cyclosporine may be anticipated.

Because of its lipophilic nature, body fat contains a high concentration of cyclosporine. Therefore, in the obese patient, cyclosporine remains in the body for long periods after discontinuation of the drug. Other tissues such as the liver, pancreas, lungs, kidneys, adrenal glands, spleen, and lymph nodes contain higher concentrations of cyclosporine than the serum.[99-102] Low levels of cyclosporine are found in brain tissue. Early studies demonstrated that cyclosporine was undetectable in cerebrospinal fluid; however, this is inconsistent with the clinical evidence of central nervous system toxicity in some patients receiving cyclosporine therapy.[103-105]

Cyclosporine is eliminated from the body by hepatic metabolism, primarily through the cytochrome P-450–dependent monooxygenase system.[85] The metabolism of cyclosporine yields more than 17 metabolites, all of which retain the cyclic polypeptide structure of the parent compound and are monohydroxylated or dihydroxylated, or N-demethylated derivatives of cyclosporine. Thus far more than nine metabolites have been structurally identified.[106] Cyclosporine is a drug with low to intermediate hepatic extraction. The hepatic clearance of cyclosporine is dependent on the intrinsic ability of the liver to metabolize the drug, liver blood flow, and blood protein binding.

Age also appears to affect the clearance of cyclosporine. Pediatric patients clear cyclosporine more rapidly than adults. This increased clearance of cyclosporine in pediatric patients appears to be caused by a more rapid removal rate from the body.[107] Because of this phenomenon, children require more frequent and higher doses of cyclosporine per kilogram of body weight than do adults.

Several drugs have been reported to alter the metabolism of cyclosporine. Table 4-6 lists those drugs and their effects on cyclosporine metabolism.

Studies in liver transplant patients with biliary drainage tubes indicate that biliary excretion is a major pathway of elimination of cyclosporine and its metabolites in humans.[88,108] The concentration of cyclosporine in the bile is much higher than corresponding plasma concentrations. Renal excretion is a minor pathway of cyclosporine elimination, with approximately 1% of an administered dose of cyclosporine appearing as unchanged drug in the urine.[89]

Therapeutic uses. Cyclosporine is used to prevent acute rejection and to prolong graft survival in renal, cardiac, and hepatic allografts. The first cadaveric renal transplant was treated with cyclosporine in 1978.[109,110] The initial experience with cyclosporine demonstrated the potent immunosuppressive effects; however, nephrotoxicity and lymphoma were observed frequently. Since these initial studies using high doses of cyclosporine, subsequent trials with lower cyclosporine doses have demonstrated the potent

Table 4-6 Drugs that interfere with the metabolism of cyclosporine

Drug	Effect
Erythromycin	Possible inhibition of cyclosporine metabolism by effects on liver enzyme systems leading to *increased* cyclosporine blood levels
Ketaconazole	Inhibition of cyclosporine metabolism, with questionable effects on enzyme systems leading to *increased* cyclosporine blood levels
Methylprednisolone	Questionable impairment of elimination of cyclosporine metabolites, leading to *increased* cyclosporine blood levels as measured by radioimmunoassay
	Possible increase in drug elimination, leading to *decreased* cyclosporine blood levels as measured by high-performance liquid chromatography
Long-term corticosteroids	Possible induction of cyclosporine metabolism, leading to *decreased* cyclosporine blood levels
Phenobarbital	Induction of cyclosporine metabolism by enzyme induction leading to *decreased* cyclosporine blood levels
Phenytoin	Induction of cyclosporine metabolism by enzyme induction, leading to *decreased* cyclosporine blood levels
Rifampin	Induction of cyclosporine metabolism by enzyme induction, leading to *decreased* cyclosporine levels
Isoniazid	Induction of cyclosporine metabolism by enzyme induction, leading to *increased* cyclosporine blood levels
Calcium channel blocker	Induction of cyclosporine metabolism by enzyme induction, leading to *decreased* cyclosporine blood levels

immunosuppressive effects of cyclosporine without a high incidence of irreversible adverse effects.[111-113]

Currently cyclosporine is most frequently administered concomitantly with corticosteroids to prevent acute rejection.[114] Studies have shown 1-year actuarial graft survival ranging from 70% to 90% in patients treated with concomitant cyclosporine-steroid therapy.[115] When compared with conventional therapy (azathioprine, corticosteroids, lymphocyte immune globulin), 1-year patient survival has improved from 76% to approximately 94% in renal transplant patients receiving cyclosporine.[116]

In recent years, conventional immunosuppressive therapy has achieved acceptable results in cardiac transplantation; however, there was substantial morbidity.[117] Cyclosporine has been used to prolong graft and patient survival after cardiac transplantation. Although the use of corticosteroids has not been totally eliminated

from the immunosuppressive regimen, cyclosporine has allowed for a reduction in the amount of corticosteroid needed.[118] The use of cyclosporine and low-dose corticosteroid therapy has been associated with an improved 1- to 2-year patient survival (80%) when compared with patients treated with corticosteroids and azathioprine (58%).[119]

The use of cyclosporine has had a positive effect on the survival of liver transplant patients. One-year hepatic graft survival before the institution of cyclosporine ranged from 20% to 40%.[120,121] The use of cyclosporine and low-dose corticosteroids has achieved a 1-year hepatic graft survival rate of 60% to 80%.[122] With the advent of cyclosporine, there has also been a reduction in the incidence of postoperative infections. Cyclosporine has also been used in the prophylaxis of rejection in pancreatic transplant and for the treatment of graft versus host disease in bone marrow transplantation.[123-125]

Dosage and administration. Cyclosporine is administered orally and by IV infusion. Oral doses of cyclosporine should be measured carefully using the graduated pipette provided by the manufacturer. The oral dose should be drawn up in the graduated pipette and transferred to a glass container to minimize the adherence of cyclosporine to the side of the container. To increase the palatability of the oral solution, the measured dose should be diluted with plain or chocolate milk or orange juice at room temperature. The diluted solution should be administered immediately, not allowing the mixture to stand before administration. After the initial dilution is administered, the container should be rinsed with additional diluent and administered to ensure that the entire dose of the drug has been ingested.

Because of the risk of anaphylaxis and increased risk of nephrotoxicity, the intravenous form of cyclosporine should be reserved for patients with a contraindication or intolerance to oral therapy. Cyclosporine for injection must be diluted before administration. Each milliliter of cyclosporine for injection should be diluted with 20 to 100 ml of diluent (0.9% saline or 5% dextrose). The prescribed dose of intravenous cyclosporine should be infused over 2 to 6 hours.

The dosage of cyclosporine should be individualized according to blood or plasma cyclosporine concentrations and serum creatinine concentrations. For the prevention of allograft rejection in adults and children, the initial oral dose of cyclosporine is 10 to 20 mg/kg of body weight initially administered 4 to 12 hours before transplant. Postoperatively, the maintenance dose is approximately 10 to 20 mg/kg of body weight per day administered once or twice daily. As therapy progresses, the dose of cyclosporine may be tapered, usually at a rate of approximately 5% per week. A stable maintenance dose is achieved when cyclosporine levels remain within the therapeutic range, with the patient manifesting no signs and symptoms of rejection or toxicity.

In patients unable to tolerate oral cyclosporine, the drug may be administered by IV infusion, administering one third of the recommended oral dose. The initial dose of 5 to 6 mg/kg of body weight is administered 4 to 12 hours preoperatively, and the initial postoperative dose is 5 to 6 mg/kg of body weight daily. Again, each IV dose of cyclosporine is administered over 2 to 6 hours. The daily dose can be divided into two or three infusions. The patient should be converted to oral therapy as soon as possible after surgery.

Because of poor bioavailability in liver transplant patients, the IV dose of cyclosporine is usually tapered with the addition of oral cyclosporine. Many times the conversion to oral therapy is extremely difficult, especially in children, and the added effect of IV cyclosporine is needed.

Therapeutic monitoring. The quantitation of drug levels in biologic fluids is an essential part of the clinical management of patients receiving immunosuppressive regimens using cyclosporine. Currently clinicians are faced with a choice of measuring cyclosporine in plasma or whole blood using three different assay procedures: (1) radioimmunoassay (RIA), (2) high-performance liquid chromatography (HPLC), and (3) polarized fluorescence. The analysis of different biologic specimens by any of the available methods produces different results.

Biologic specimen. The purpose of monitoring blood concentrations of cyclosporine is to determine whether a given dose has produced a therapeutic, although not toxic, level. Cyclosporine monitoring has been performed using whole blood, serum, and plasma. Because of the extensive binding of cyclosporine to red blood cells, the concentrations of cyclosporine in whole blood are approximately two times that in plasma.[97,98] The relative distribution of cyclosporine between red blood cells and plasma depends on the temperature of the separation of plasma, the hematocrit, the drug concentration, and the lipoprotein composition of the plasma. Plasma samples separated at room temperature have shown cyclosporine levels to be as much as 50% less than plasma samples separated at 37° C.[126,127] The temperature-dependent concentration of cyclosporine is related to an altered red blood cell and lipoprotein uptake of cyclosporine at different temperatures. The optimal temperature for cyclosporine separation in plasma appears to be 37° C, which simulates in vivo distribution of cyclosporine in the blood. This approach may be impractical in routine clinical monitoring because of the lack of temperature-controlled centrifuges in many clinical laboratories. Because plasma cyclosporine concentrations are lower, there tends to be greater variability in cyclosporine estimations in plasma compared with whole blood.[128] Because of the variabilities in the assay of plasma cyclosporine concentrations, and whole blood concentrations of cyclosporine are more reproducible, whole blood samples are preferred for cyclosporine monitoring.[129]

Assay procedures

RADIOIMMUNOASSAY. An immunoassay method is based on the ability of a given drug to inhibit the reaction between drug-specific antibodies and an appropriately labeled drug. The labeled drug should structurally resemble the true drug and should interact with the antibody as if it were the drug itself. The technique of RIA is best understood in terms of competitive protein binding. A variable quantity of nonradiolabeled drug and a fixed amount of radiolabeled drug compete for a constant quantity of antibody binding site. After equilibrium is reached, the fractions are separated and the radioactivity is measured.

The RIA procedure depends on the production of an antiserum with high affinity for the drug being assayed, the synthesis of a labeled drug or drug derivative, and a convenient separation step. Currently, there are two RIA procedures available for the analysis of cyclosporine: (1) RIA polyclonal antibody procedure, and (2) RIA monoclonal antibody procedure. The polyclonal assay procedure measures the parent cyclosporine compound and has a high cross-reactivity with the metabolites of cyclosporine.[130] The monoclonal assay procedure is sensitive to parent cyclosporine compound only.[131]

Radioimmunoassay is readily available in most clinical laboratories and may be used to analyze cyclosporine in whole blood and plasma. There are various polyclonal and monoclonal procedures kits available that incorporate either ^{125}I or ^3H radiolabeled cyclosporine into the procedure. There are several disadvantages to the use of RIA: (1) the cross-reactivity of the antibody with metabolites in the polyclonal procedure, (2) long sample turn-around times are required, and (3) a high level of technical competence is required. Despite these deficiencies, RIA remains a reliable method for therapeutic monitoring of cyclosporine in the clinical setting.

HIGH-PERFORMANCE LIQUID CHROMATOGRAPHY. Analysis of cyclosporine by HPLC was first introduced in 1980 by Niederberger.[132] Since its introduction, several HPLC methods have been published.[133,134] This technique is designed to specifically measure parent cyclosporine and is much more labor intensive than the RIA technique. Essentially, three steps are necessary in the HPLC technique: (1) lysis of the red cells if whole blood samples are used, (2) extraction of cyclosporine from the blood or plasma matrix, and (3) chromatograph quantification of cyclosporine. The use of HPLC in monitoring cyclosporine concentrations requires a high level of technical competence. Also, because of the various analysis procedures available, results may differ among laboratories, thereby preventing the comparison of data between institutions. Larger sample volumes and long sample turn-around times are also required when this assay method is used. Although HPLC is time consuming and difficult, this is the preferred method of analysis for pharmacologic and clinical research studies of cyclosporine metabolism and disposition.[135-137]

POLARIZED FLUORESCENCE. The principles of polarized fluorescence were first developed in early 1920 by Perrin.[138] Thirty years later, polarized fluorescence was applied to biologic systems, and its application to the antigen-antibody reaction was first described in 1961.[139] The polarized fluorescence immunoassay procedure makes use of competitive-binding assay principles. The tracer material is measured directly without the need for a separation step. The specificity of an immunoassay procedure is thereby combined with the speed and convenience of a homogenous method, which provides a precise and reliable procedure for determining concentrations in biologic fluids. Polarized fluorescence has been applied in the measurement of such compounds as insulin,[140] cortisol,[141] gentamicin,[142,143] and phenytoin.[144,145] Recently, a polarized fluorescence methodology (Abbott TDx Systems, Abbott Diagnostics Laboratories, Irving, Texas) has been introduced for the analysis of cyclosporine and its metabolites. Because this procedure was developed recently, few studies have been conducted comparing polarized fluorescence analysis to RIA for cyclosporine. Several studies, however, have shown a good correlation between the concentrations obtained with polarized fluorescence and RIA in renal and liver transplant patients.[146,147] Because the polarized fluorescence procedure offers a shorter sample turn-around time, requires less technical expertise, and a large sample load may be analyzed, this procedure may develop into a viable alternative to the RIA procedure. The concentrations obtained with the polarized fluorescence procedure are slightly higher (approximately 20% to 25%) than those obtained with RIA because of differences in the specificity or cross-reactivity between the antibody and the various cyclosporine metabolites.[146]

Blood level monitoring. Although no clear correlation has been established between the concentration of cyclosporine in whole blood or plasma and therapeutic outcome, there are three primary reasons for monitoring cyclosporine levels:

1. *Variable bioavailability of cyclosporine.* As mentioned above, the bioavailability of cyclosporine varies among individuals. There appears to be a time window in which cyclosporine is effective. It is important that adequate absorption of cyclosporine occurs and a therapeutic level is achieved within that time span.[148] Initially, IV cyclosporine may be used to achieve therapeutic levels rapidly.
2. *Variable clearance of cyclosporine.* The clearance of cyclosporine from the body is variable and dose dependent. Some investigators have shown a variable clearance of cyclosporine of 1.1 to 4.3 L/min.[88] There is also enterohepatic circulation of the drug, which may have an effect on the elimination of cyclosporine. This may be a function of intestinal motility.

3. *Relationship of cyclosporine concentration and toxicity.* Numerous authors have advocated a relationship between cyclosporine levels and nephrotoxicity.[94,149,150] Although it is difficult to differentiate between renal graft rejection and cyclosporine toxicity, there seems to be a linear correlation between cyclosporine concentrations and acute tubular necrosis.[150] The concentrations required to produce hepatotoxicity are not clearly defined. Although there is no direct relationship between blood concentrations of cyclosporine and therapeutic response, maintenance of concentrations within the recommended ranges appears to minimize both graft rejection and toxicity.

Adverse effects. The use of cyclosporine has been associated with an array of complications, the most common and clinically important being nephrotoxicity. Acute nephrotoxic reactions may occur after rapid administration of an IV dose. Nephrotoxicity may also be chronic, manifested by a slow rise in the serum creatinine. Nephrotoxicity has been shown to occur in 50% to 75% of patients after renal transplantation, and approximately the same incidence has occurred after cardiac and hepatic transplantation.[150-152] The characteristic profile of cyclosporine nephrotoxicity is a reduced creatinine clearance, elevation of serum creatinine, and a disproportionate increase in blood urea nitrogen (BUN), with preserved urine volume and sodium resorption. Hyperkalemia and hypertension are characteristic; hyperuricemia and hyperkalemic hyperchloremic type IV renal tubular acidosis are also often encountered. One study has documented a reduction in plasma renin activity and renal tubular insensitivity to aldosterone as two of the contributing factors to the hyperkalemia.[153] The exact cause of renin suppression is not known but may be secondary to extracellular fluid expansion or inhibition of renal prostaglandin synthesis.

The mechanisms of cyclosporine-induced nephrotoxicity may be threefold: (1) increased intraproximal tubular pressure activating glomerulotubular feedback, (2) decreased filtration coefficient, and (3) vasoconstriction. The initial hypothesis of cyclosporine-induced nephrotoxicity suggested that cyclosporine caused tubular damage, which led to functional impairment because of back pressure along nephrons blocked by damaged cells. This led to a feedback mechanism whereby angiotensin lowered glomerular flow.[154] The mechanism of tubular injury is not clear. One possibility may be a direct effect resulting from increased cyclosporine levels. This is supported by evidence that patients with increased cyclosporine levels tend to have a greater incidence of nephrotoxicity.[155]

Glomerular toxicity is a proposed mechanism of cyclosporine nephrotoxicity.[156] This phenomenon appears to involve a progressive, diffuse tubulointerstitial fibrosis with focal to total glomerulosclerosis reflected either as a direct result of cyclosporine effects on the glomeruli or as a result of compensatory maladaptive changes in nephron hemodynamics. Reduced glomerular filtration rate with low glomerular capillary ultrafiltration results from functional injury to the glomeruli and leads to an altered filtration fraction.

The third proposed mechanism of nephrotoxicity is an alteration in renal hemodynamics.[157] This alteration in renal hemodynamics leads to proximal tubular hypoxia and results in a reduction in the glomerular filtration rate. There are three possible mechanisms of reduction of renal blood flow: (1) stimulation of the renin-angiotensin-aldosterone system, (2) inhibition of the prostaglandin-mediated vasodilator effect, and (3) efferent arteriolar vasoconstriction. Various authors have demonstrated cyclosporine effects on renal hemodynamics by showing reduced total renal blood flow,[158] increased renal vascular resistance and increased plasma renin activity,[156,160] and reduced synthesis of prostacyclin-stimulating factor, which leads to reduced prostacyclin synthesis.[161]

The important step in evaluating cyclosporine nephrotoxicity, particularly in renal transplant patients, is to differentiate allograft rejection from nephrotoxicity. Factors suggesting cyclosporine nephrotoxicity include a serum creatinine rising slowly over a period of weeks, and whole blood cyclosporine (parent compound)

concentrations greater than 300 ng/ml. The management of cyclosporine-induced nephrotoxicity involves a slow taper of the cyclosporine dose with careful assessment for a gradual improvement in the serum creatinine over a period of days to weeks.

Hepatotoxicity is another serious adverse effect of cyclosporine. The initial reports of hepatotoxicity showed a rise in serum bilirubin (greater than 2 mg%) in 13 of 66 renal transplant patients.[162] Several reports followed, again with hyperbilirubinemia being the major characteristic.[163-165] Hepatotoxicity is also characterized by rises in the serum transaminases (SGOT and SGPT), alkaline phosphatase, gamma GT, and total bilirubin. In the liver transplant population, these changes in liver enzymes tend to be a problem, because it is difficult to rule out toxicity or rejection. This reaction is usually dose dependent and tends to reverse with reduction in the cyclosporine dosage.

Cyclosporine has also been associated with several neurologic effects. These include tremors, paresthesias, muscle weakness, enhanced sensitivity to extreme temperature changes, and seizures.[166] The causes of these effects are uncertain. Some authors have associated electrolyte abnormalities, particularly hypomagnesemia, with neurologic effects.[167] Others have suggested the neurologic effects may be caused by an increase in free cyclosporine in patients who are hypocholesterolemic.[168] Reduction in the cyclosporine dose may aid in the alleviation of neurologic symptoms.

Other adverse effects associated with cyclosporine include malignancy (lymphoma), which probably results from oversuppression,[169] hyperkalemia,[170] and hypertension questionably secondary to renal mechanisms, gingival hyperplasia which may require gingivectomy,[171] hirsutism, and anaphylaxis after IV administration.[172] A complex picture of drug interactions is also beginning to appear with the use of cyclosporine. Table 4-6 lists some of these interactions and their sequelae. Hyperlipidemia and abnormalities in plasma electrophoresis may occur in patients receiving intravenous cyclosporine because of the vehicle in the commercial product. The hyperlipidemia and abnormalities in the lipoproteins are reversible with the discontinuance of the drug; however, the presence of these adverse effects during cyclosporine therapy does not require discontinuance of therapy. Table 4-7 summarizes the side effects and nursing implications for cyclosporine therapy.

Combination drug therapies

Early after its introduction, cyclosporine was used as a single agent for immunosuppression in

Table 4-7 Cyclosporine therapy: summary of side effects and nursing implications

Side effects	Assessment parameters	Nursing interventions
Cardiovascular: fluid and electrolytes		
Nephrotoxicity	Cyclosporine levels	Administer diuretics
Systemic arterial hypertension	Serum creatinine, BUN	Administer antihypertensives oral or parenteral
Hyperkalemia	Creatinine clearance	Administer magnesium
Hypomagnesemia	Peripheral edema	Decrease dosage
Anaphylaxis if administered rapidly IV	Blood pressure	Administer IV cyclosporine over 2-6 hours
	Serum magnesium	
	Serum potassium	
Pulmonary		
None	None	None
Gastrointestinal		
Hepatotoxicity	Cyclosporine levels	Decrease dosage
	Serum transaminases, phosphatases, bilirubin	
	Coagulation factors	
Endocrine		
None	None	None
Hematologic		
Lymphocytopenia	Cyclosporine levels	Decrease dosage
Lymphoma	CBC with differential count	Increase attention to infection control measures
Opportunistic infection	Inspect mucous membranes for opportunistic infection	Administer oral antifungal agent
	Bacterial, viral, and fungal cultures	Administer antibiotics
Neurologic		
Tremors	Cyclosporine levels	Assure patient that tremors and paresthesias are dose related
Paresthesias	Neurologic status	
Muscle weakness		Decrease dosage
Increased sensitivity to temperature changes		Provide physical therapy
		Administer analgesics for headaches
		Initiate seizure precautions in susceptible patient
		Instruct patient about side effects

some renal programs. A complication of mono-therapy with cyclosporine was an increased incidence of nephrotoxicity.[110] Corticosteroids were later added in combination with cyclo-sporine. Since 1980 the combination of cyclo-sporine and corticosteroids has been the main-stay of immunosuppression therapy for organ transplantation. The addition of corticosteroids allowed for a slight decrease in the dosage of cyclosporine, thereby decreasing the incidence of nephrotoxicity. Improved graft survival was demonstrated in patients receiving this double-drug therapy.[112]

More recently, triple-drug immunosuppres-sive regimens have been advocated.[173] Triple-drug regimens usually contain low-dose cyclo-sporine (8 mg/kg of body weight per day, orally), azathioprine (1.5 mg/kg of body weight per day, orally), and prednisone (1 to 2 mg/kg of body weight per day, tapered to 0.3 mg/kg of body weight per day, orally). The theoretic basis of triple-drug regimens is to allow lower doses of the agents to be used, thus avoiding toxicity from the individual agents. As with the advent of any new therapy, variable results have been obtained using triple-drug therapy.

Salaman et al[174] demonstrated a higher fre-quency of rejection episodes in renal transplant patients treated with monotherapy than in those treated with triple-drug therapy. However, pa-tients receiving triple-drug therapy had a higher incidence of serious infections (27%) than in patients receiving monotherapy (8%). Frier demonstrated that triple-drug therapy did not significantly modify graft survival in renal trans-plant patients; however, patient survival was significantly increased.[169] The clinical implica-tions from this study of triple-drug therapy versus monotherapy include the following: (1) triple-drug therapy allows for rapid decreases in corticosteroid dosages, thereby reducing the incidence of serious infections and osteoporosis, and (2) easier management of cyclosporine dosage and adverse effects. Other investigators have reported similar results in other organ transplant patient populations.[175] Although more research is needed, triple-drug regimens seem to offer a flexible means of immunosup-pression. Today various centers are evaluating the effect of quadruple-drug (cyclosporine, cor-ticosteroids, azathioprine, and lymphocyte im-mune globulin or muromonab CD-3) immuno-suppressive regimens.

CONCLUSION

The use of immunosuppression is patient spe-cific. Treatment regimens may vary from insti-tution to institution. Most regimens will incor-porate double- or triple-drug regimens. The advantage of using double- or triple-drug ther-apy is that lower dosages of all drugs used are possible. Most institutions restrict the use of lymphocyte immune globulin and muromonab CD-3 to the treatment of severe acute rejection episodes, although some institutions will rou-tinely use quadruple-drug therapy.

The role of immunosuppression is crucial to patient and graft survival. Over the years, immunosuppression has become an area for intensive research, which has led to the avail-ability of newer agents with increasead speci-ficity and usefulness. With the advent of newer immunosuppression methods, the future of transplantation is sure to be promising.

REFERENCES

1. Billingham RE, Brent L, Medawar PB (1956). The antigenic stimulus in transplantation immunology. *Nature, 178,* 514-519.
2. Katz DH (1982). The immune system: an overview. In Sites DP, Stobo JD, Fudenberg HH et al (eds). *Basic and clinical immunology, 4th ed.* (13-20). Los Altos, Ca: Lange Medical Publications.
3. Cohen DJ, Loertscher R, Rubin MF et al (1984). Cyclosporine: a new immunosuppressive agent for organ transplantion. *Annals of Internal Medicine, 101,* 667-682.
4. Wish JB (1986). Immunologic effects of cyclosporine. *Transplantation Proceedings, 18*(3)(Suppl 2), 15-18.
5. Murray JE, Merrill JP, Dammin GJ et al (1962). Kidney transplantation in modified recipients. *Annals of Surgery, 156,* 337-355.
6. Starzl TE, Marchioro TL, Waddell WR (1963). The reversal of rejection in human renal homografts with subsequent development of homograft tolerance. *Surgery Gynecology and Obstetrics, 117,* 385-395.
7. Hume DM, Magee JH, Kauffman HM et al (1963). Renal homotransplantation in man in modified recip-ients. *Annals of Surgery, 158,* 608-644.
8. Woodruff MF, Robson JS, Nolan B et al (1963). Homotransplantation of kidney in patients treated by preoperative local radiation and postoperative admin-istration of an antimetabolite (Imuran). *Lancet, 2,* 675-682.

9. Murray JE, Merrill JP, Harrison JH et al (1963). Prolonged survival of human kidney homografts by immunosuppressive drug therapy. *New England Journal of Medicine, 268,* 1315-1323.

10. Oplez G, Michey MR and Terasaki PI (1977). HLA matching and cadaver kidney transplant survival in North America: influence of center variation and presensitization. *Transplantation, 23,* 490-497.

11. Starzl TE, Porter KA, Iwasaki Y et al (1967). The use of antilymphocyte globulin in human renal homotransplantation. In Wolstenholme GE and O'Connor M (eds). *Antilymphocyte serum.* (pp. 4-34). London: J and A Churchill.

12. Borel JF, Feurer C, Gubler HU and Stahelin H (1976). Biological effects of cyclosporin A: a new antilymphocytic agent. *Agents and Actions, 6,* 468-475.

13. Calne RY, Rolles K, White DJ et al (1979). Cyclosporin A initially as the only immunosuppressant in 34 recipients of cadaveric organs: 32 kidneys, 2 pancreases, and 2 livers. *Lancet, 2,* 1033-1036.

14. Cosimi AB, Burton RC, Colvin RB et al (1981). Treatment of acute renal allograft rejection with OKT3 monoclonal antibody. *Transplantation, 36,* 535-539.

15. Norman DJ, Barry JM, Henell K, et al (1985). Reversal of acute allograft rejection with monoclonal antibody. *Transplantation Proceedings, 17,* 30-41.

16. Goldstein G, Schindler J, Sheahan M et al (1985). Orthoclone OKT3 treatment of acute renal allograft rejection. *Transplantation Proceedings, 17,* 129-131.

17. Elion GB, Hichings GH and Vander Werff H (1951). Antagonist of nucleic acid derivatives VI. Purines. *Journal of Biology and Chemistry, 192* 505-518.

18. Schwartz R and Damashek W (1959). Drug-induced tolerance. *Nature, 183,* 1682-1683.

19. Calne RY and Murray (1966). Inhibition of the rejection of renal homografts in dogs with Burroughs Wellcome 322. *Sugrical Forum, 12,* 118-120.

20. Ahmed A and Mory R (1981). Azathioprine. *International Journal of Dermatology, 20,* 461-467.

21. Bach JF and Dardenne M (1971). The metabolism of azathioprine in renal failure. *Transplantation, 12,* 253-259.

22. Delphin E (1979). Principles of clinical immunosuppression. *Surgical Clinics of North America, 59*(2), 283-298.

23. Sopko J and Anuras S (1978). Liver disease in renal transplant recipients. *American Journal of Medicine, 64,* 139-146.

24. Elion GB (1967). Biochemistry and pharmacology of purine analogues. *Federal Proceedings, 26,* 898-904.

25. Thorn GW (1966). Clinical considerations in the use of corticosteroids. *New England Journal of Medicine, 274,* 775-781.

26. Fauci A, Dale D and Balow J (1976). Glucocorticosteroid therapy: mechanism of action and clinical considerations. *Annals of Internal Medicine, 84,* 304-315.

27. O'Malley BW (1971). Mechanism of action of steroid hormones. *New England Journal of Medicine, 284,* 370-377.

28. Fauci AS and Dale DC (1974). The effect of in vivo hydrocortisone on subpopulations of human lymphocytes. *Journal of Clinical Investigations, 53,* 240-246.

29. Fauci AS and Dale DC (1975). Alternate-day prednisone therapy and human lymphocyte subpopulations. *Journal of Clinical Investigations, 55,* 22-32.

30. Fauci AS and Dale DC (1975). The effect of hydrocortisone on the kinetics of normal human lymphocytes. *Blood, 46* 235-243.

31. Gesner BM and Ginsburg V (1964). Effect of glycosidases on the fate of transfused lymphocytes. *Proceedings of the National Academy of Science, USA, 52,* 750-755.

32. Rinehart JJ, Sagone AL, Balcerzak SP et al (1974). Effects of corticosteroid on monocyte function. *Journal of Clinical Investigations, 54,* 1337-1343.

33. Claman HN (1983). Glucocorticosteroids I: Anti-inflammatory mechanisms. *Hospital Practice, 18*(7), 123-134.

34. Russo-Marie F, Seillan C and Duval D (1981). Glucocorticoids as inhibitors of prostaglandin synthesis. *Bulletin of European Physiopathology and Respiration, 17,* 587-594.

35. Gillis S, Crabtree GR and Smith KA (1979). Glucocorticoid induced inhibition of T cell growth factor production. II. The effect on the in vitro generation of cytolytic T cells. *Journal of Immunology, 123,* 1632-1638.

36. Larsson EL (1980). Cyclosporine A and dexamethasone suppress T cell responses by selectively acting at distinct sites of the trigger process. *Journal of Immunology, 124,* 2828-2833.

37. Claman HM (1983) Glucocorticosteroids II: The clinical responses. *Hospital Practice, 18*(7), 143-151.

38. Woodruff MF and Anderson NA (1963). Effect of lymphocyte depletion by thoracic duct fistula and administration of antilymphocyte serum on the survival of skin homografts in rats. *Nature, 200,* 702-705.

39. Starzl TE, Marchioro TL, Porter KA, Iwasaki Y and Cerilli GJ (1967). The use of heterologous antilymphoid agents in canine renal and liver homotransplantation and in human renal homotransplantation. *Surgery Gynecology and Obstetrics, 124,* 301-318.

40. Birch AG, Carpenter CB, Tilney NL, Hampers CL, Hager FB et al (1971). Controlled clinical trial of antilymphocytic globulin in human renal allografts. *Transplantation Proceedings, 3,* 762-765.

41. Turcotte TG, Feduska NJ and Haines RF (1973). Antilymphocyte globulin in renal transplnat recipients. *Archives of Surgery, 106,* 484.

42. Sheil AG, Mears D, Kelley GE, Stewart JG et al (1972). A controlled clinical trial of antilymphocyte globulin therapy in man. *Transplantation, 4,* 501-505.

43. Starzl TE, Groth CG, Kashiwagi N, Putnam CW, Corman JL et al (1972). Clinical experience with horse antihuman ALG. *Transplantation Proceedings, 4,* 491-495.

44. Najarian JS, Simmons RL, Condie RM, Thomson EJ et al (1976). Seven years experience with antilymphoblast globulin for renal transplantation from cadaveric donors. *Annals of Surgery, 184,* 352-368.

45. Cosimi AB, Wortis HH, Delmonico FL and Russell DS (1976). Randomized clinical trial of ATG in cadaver and allograft recipients: Importance of T-cell monitoring. *Surgery, 80,* 155-163.

46. Kountz SL, Butt KM, Rao TK, Zieluski CM et al (1977). Antilymphocyte globulin (ATG) dosage and graft survival in renal transplantation. *Transplantation Proceedings, 9,* 1023-1025.

47. Pennock JL, Oyer PE, Reitz BA et al (1982). Cardiac transplantation in perspective for the future, survival, complications, rehabilitation and cost. *Journal of Thoracic and Cardiovascular Surgery, 83,* 168-177.

48. Tursi A, Greaves MF, Torrigiano G et al (1969). *Immunology, 17,* 801.

49. Raff MC (1969). Theta isoantigen as a market of thymus-derived lymphocytes in mice. *Nature, 224,* 378-379.

50. Lance EM, Medawar PB and Taub RN (1973). Antilymphocyte serum. *Advances in Immunology, 17,* 1-92.

51. Chanard J, Bach JF, Assailly J, Funck Bretano JL (1972). Hepatic homing of labelled lymphocytes in man. *British Medical Journal, 2,* 502-504.

52. Starzl TE, Seil R and Putnam CW (1977). Kidney transplantation. Modern trends in kidney transplantation. *Transplantation Proceedings, 9(1),* 1-8.

53. Novick AC, Braun WE, Stinmuller D et al (1983). A controlled, randomized, double-blind study of antilymphoblast globulin in cadaveric renal transplantation. *Transplantation, 35(2),* 175-179.

54. Monaco AP (1972). Antilymphocyte serum and other methods of lymphocyte depletion. In Najarian JS and Simmons RL (eds). (pp 222-251). *Transplantation.* Philadelphia: Lea & Febiger.

55. Monaco AP, Campion JL and Kapnick SJ (1977). Clinical use of antilymphocyte globulin. *Transplantation Proceedings, 9,* 1007-1018.

56. Cosimi AB (1981). The clinical value of antilymphocyte antibodies. *Transplantation Proceedings, 13,* 462-468.

57. Barnes BA and Olivier D (1981). Analysis of NIAID kidney transplant histocompatibility study (KTHS): Factors associated with transplant outcomes I. *Transplantation Proceedings, 13,* 65-72.

58. Hardy MA, Nowygrod R, Elberg A et al (1980). Use of ATG in treatment of steroid-resistant rejection. *Transplantation, 29,* 162-164.

59. Nowygrod G, Appel and Hardy MA (1981). Use of ATG for reversal of acute allograft rejection. *Transplantation Proceedings, 13,* 469-472.

60. Cheeseman SH, Rubin RH, Stewart JA et al (1979). Controlled clinical trial of prophylactic human-leukocyte interferon in renal transplantation. *New England Journal of Medicine, 300,* 1345-1349.

61. Chatenoud L, Baudrihaye MF, Schindler J et al (1982). Human in vivo antigenic modulation induced by the anti-T cell OKT3 monoclonal antibody. *European Journal of Immunology, 12,* 979-982.

62. Chatenoud L and Bach JF (1984). Antigenic modulation. *Immunology Today, 5,* 20-25.

63. Cosimi AB, Colvin RC, Burton RB et al (1981). Use of monoclonal antibodies to T-cell subsets for immunologic monitoring and treatment in recipients of renal allografts. *New England Journal of Medicine, 305,* 308-314.

64. Ortho Multicenter Transplant Study Group (1985). A randomized clinical trial of OKT3 monoclonal antibody for acute rejection of cadaveric renal transplants. *New England Journal of Medicine, 313,* 337-342.

65. Thistlewaite JR, Cosimi AB, Delmonico FL et al (1984). Evolving use of OKT3 monoclonal antibody for the treatment of renal allograft rejection. *Transplantation, 38,* 695-700.

66. Cosimi AB, Burton RC, Colvin RB et al (1981). Treatment of acute renal allograft rejection with OKT3 monoclonal antibody. *Transplantation, 32,* 535-539.

67. Starzl TE and Fung JJ (1986). Orthoclone OKT3 in treatment of allografts rejected under cyclosporine-steroid therapy. *Transplantation Proceedings, 18,* 938-941.

68. Bristow MR, Gilbert, EM, Renlund DG, Gay WA and O'Connell JG (1988). Use of OKT-3 monoclonal antibody in cardiac transplantation. *Journal of Heart Transplantation, 7,* 1-11.

69. Bristow MR, Gilbert EM, O'Connell JB et al (1988). OKT3 monoclonal antibody in heart transplantation. *American Journal Kidney Disease, 11,* 135.

70. Norman DS, Shield CF, Barry J et al (1988). Early use of OKT3 monoclonal antibody in renal transplantation to prevent rejection. *American Journal Kidney Disease, 11,* 107.

71. Millis JM, McDiarmid SV, Hiatt JR, Brems JJ et al (1989). Randomized prospective trial of OKT3 for early prophylaxis of rejection after liver transplantation. *Transplantation, 47(1),* 82-88.

72. Hirsch RL and Goldstein G (1986). Orthoclone OKT3 in the treatment of renal allograft rejection. *Dialysis and Transplantation, 15,* 659-662.

73. Emmons C, Smith J and Flanigan M (1986). Cerebrospinal fluid inflammation during OKT3 therapy. *Lancet, 2,* 510-511.

74. Borel JF (1976). Comparative study of in vitro and in vivo drug effects on cell mediate cytotoxicity. *Immunology, 31,* 631-641.

75. Reitz BA, Bieber CP, Raney AA, Pennock JL et al (1981). Orthotopic heart and combined heart lung transplantation with cyclosporin A immune suppression. *Transplantation Proceedings, 13,* 393-396.

76. Bird G and Britton S (1979). A new approach to the study of human B lymphocyte function using an indirect plaque assay and a direct B cell activator. *Immunology Reviews, 45,* 41-67.

77. Morgan DA, Ruscetti A and Gallo R (1976). Selective in vitro growth of T lymphocytes from normal human bone marrow. *Science, 193,* 1007-1008.

78. Smith KA (1980). T cell growth factor. *Immunology Reviews, 51,* 337-357.

79. Palacios R and Moller G (1981). Cyclosporin A blocks receptors for HLA-DR antigen on T cells. *Nature, 290,* 792-794.

80. Palacios R (1981). HLA-DR antigens render interleukin-2 producer T cells sensitive to interleukin-1. *Scandinavian Journal of Immunology, 14,* 321-326.

81. Palacios R (1982). Mechanism of T cell activation. Role and functional relationship of HLA-DR antigen and interleukins. *Immunology Reviews, 63,* 73-110.

82. Dongworth DW and Klaus GG (1982). Effects of cyclosporin A on the immune system of the mouse – I: Evidence for a direct selective effect of cyclosporin A on B cells responding to anti-immunoglobulin antibodies. *European Journal of Immunology, 12,* 1018-1022.

83. Shidani B, Colle J, Motta I et al (1983). Effect of cyclosporin A on induction and activation of B memory cells by thymus-independent antigens in mice. *European Journal of Immunology, 13,* 359-363.

84. Thomson AW, Moon DK and Nelson DS (1983). Suppression of delayed-type hypersensitivity reactions and lymphokine production by cyclosporin A in the mouse. *Clinical Experimental Immunology, 52,* 599-606.

85. Janco RI and English D (1983). Cyclosporine and human neutrophil function. *Transplantation, 35,* 501.

86. Newberger J and Kahan BD (1983). Cyclosporine pharmacokinetics in man. *Transplantation Proceedings, 15,* 2413-2415.

87. Ptachcinski RJ, Venkataramanan R, Rosenthal JT, Burckart GJ et al (1985). *Clinical Pharmacology and Therapeutics, 38,* 296-300.

88. Beveridge T, Gratwohl A, Michot F, Niederberger W et al (1981). Cyclosporin A: pharmacokinetics after a single dose in man and serum levels after multiple dosing in recipients of allogenic bone marrow grafts. *Current Therapeutic Research, 30,* 5-17.

89. Beveridge T (1982). Pharmacokinetics and metabolism of cyclosporin A. In White DJG (ed). *Cyclosporin A.* (5-17). New York: Elsevier Biomedical.

90. Wood AJ, Maurer G, Niederberger W and Beveridge T (1983). Cyclosporine: pharmacokinetics, metabolism, and drug interactions. *Transplantation Proceedings, 15,* 2409-2412.

91. Ptachcinski RJ, Venkataramanan R and Burckart GJ (1986). Clinical pharmacokinetics of cyclosporin. *Transplantation Proceedings, 11,* 107-132.

92. Burckart GJ, Venkataramanan R, Ptachcinski R, Starzl TE et al (1986). Cyclosporine absorption following orthotopic liver transplantation. *Journal of Clinical Pharmacology, 26,* 647-651.

93. Keown PA, Stiller CR, Laupacis AL, Howson W et al (1982). The side effects of cyclosporine: relationship to drug pharmacokinetics. *Transplantation Proceedings, 14,* 659-661.

94. Keown PA, Stiller CR, Sinclair NR, Carruthers G et al (1983). The clinical relevance of cyclosporine blood levels as measured by radioimmunoassay. *Transplantation Proceedings, 15,* 2438-2441.

95. Venkataramanan R, Ptachcinski RJ, Burckart GJ, Gray J et al (1985). Cyclosporine bioavailability in liver disease. *Drug Intelligence and Clinical Pharmacy, 19,* 451.

96. Andrews W, Iwatsuki S and Starzl TE (1985). Correspondence. *Transplantation, 39,* 338.

97. LeMaire M and Tillement JP (1982). Role of lipoproteins and erythrocytes in the in vitro binding and distribution of cyclosporin A in the blood. *Journal of Pharmaceutics and Pharmacology, 34,* 715-718.

98. Niederberger W, LeMaire M, Maurer G, Nussbaumer K et al (1983). Distribution and binding of cyclosporine in blood and tissues. *Transplantation Proceedings, 15,* 2419-2421.

99. Atkinson K, Boland J, Britton K and Boggs J (1983). Blood and tissue distribution of cyclosporine in humans and mice. *Transplantation Proceedings, 15, 2430-2449.*

100. Kahan BD, Van Buren CT, Boileau M, Reid M et al (1983). Levels in a cadaveric renal allograft recipient. *Transplantation, 35,* 96-99.

101. Niderberger W and Wiscott E (1982). Circular letter to users of RIA or HPLC to measure cyclosporin A in blood.

102. Reid M, Gibbons S, Kwok D, Van Buren CT et al (1983). Cyclosporine levels in human tissue of patients treated for one week to one year. *Transplantation Proceedings, 15,* 2434-2437.

103. Beaman M, Parvin S, Veitch PS and Walls J (1985). Convulsions associated with cyclosporin A in renal transplant recipients. *British Medical Journal, 290,* 139-140.

104. Boogaerts MA, Zachee P and Verwilghen RL (1982). Cyclosporine, methylprednisolone, and convulsions. *Lancet, 2,* 1216-1217.

105. Shah D, Rylance PB, Rogerson ME, Bewick M et al (1984). Generalized epileptic fits in renal transplant recipients given cyclosporine A. *British Medical Journal, 289,* 1347-1338.

106. Maurer G, Loosli HR, Schreier E and Keller B (1984). Disposition of cyclosporine in several animal species and man. Structural elucidation of its metabolites. *Drug Metabolism and Disposition, 12,* 120-126.

107. Burckart GJ, Starzl TE, Williams L, Sanghvi A et al (1985). Cyclosporine monitoring and pharmacokinetics in pediatric liver transplant patients. *Transplantation Proceedings, 17,* 1172-1175.

108. Venkataramanan R, Starzl TE, Yang S, Bruckart GJ et al (1985). Biliary excretion of cyclosporine in liver transplant patients. *Transplantation Proceedings, 17,* 286-289.

109. Calne RY, White DJG, Pentlow BD et al (1979). Cyclosporin A: preliminary observations in dogs with pancreatic duodenal allografts and patients with cadaveric renal transplants. *Transplantation Proceedings, 11,* 860-864.

110. Calne RY, White DJG, Thiru S et al (1978). Cyclosporin A in patients receiving renal allografts from cadaveric donors. *Lancet, 2,* 1323-1327.

111. Calne RY, White DJG, Evans DB et al (1981). Cyclosporin A in cadaveric organ transplantation. *British Medical Journal, 282,* 934-936.

112. Starzl TE, Weil R, Iwatsuki S et al (1980). The use of cyclosporin A and prednisone in cadaveric kidney transplantation. *Surgery Gynecology and Obstetrics, 151,* 17-25.

113. Starzl TE, Klintmalm GBG, Weil R et al (1981). Cyclosporin A and steroid therapy in sixty-six cadaver kidney recipients. *Surgery Gynecology and Obstetrics, 153,* 486-494.

114. Ferguson RM, Tynasiewicz JJ, Sutherland DER et al (1982). Cyclosporin A in renal transplantation: a prospective randomized trial. *Surgery,* 175-182.

115. Milford EL, Kirkman RL, Tilney NL et al (1985). Clinical experience with cyclosporine and azathioprine at Brigham and Women's Hospital. *American Journal of Kidney Diseases, 5,* 313-317.

116. Kahan BD, Flencher SM, Lorber MI et al (1987). Complications of cyclosporine-prednisone immunosuppression in 402 renal allograft recipients exclusively followed at a single center for from one to five years. *Transplantation, 43,* 197-204.

117. Pennock JL, Oyer PE, Reitz BA et al (1982). Cardiac transplantation in perspective for the future. *Journal of Thoracic and Cardiovascular Surgery, 83,* 168-177.

118. Griffith BP, Hardesty RL, Deeb GM et al (1982). Cardiac transplantation with cyclosporin A and prednisone. *Annals of Surgery, 196,* 324-329.

119. Oyer PE, Jamieson SW, Stinson EB et al (1983). Heart and heart-lung transplantation at Stanford. Paper presented to the First International Congress on Cyclosporine. Houston, Texas, May 16.

120. Starzl TE, Koep LJ, Halgrimson CG et al (1979). Fifteen years of clinical liver transplantation. *Gastroenterology, 77,* 375-388.

121. Calne RY and William R (1979). Liver transplantation. *Current Problems in Surgery, 16,* 3-44.

122. Starzl TE, Iwatsuki S, Van Thiel DH et al (1982). Evolution of liver transplantation. *Hepatology, 2,* 614-644.

123. Sutherland DER, Goetz FC, Elick BA et al (1982). Experience with 49 segmental pancreas transplants in 45 diabetic patients. *Transplantation, 34,* 330-338.

124. Powles RL, Barrett AJ, Clink H et al (1978). Cyclosporin A for the treatment of graft-versus-host disease in man. *Lancet, 2,* 1327-1331.

125. Hows JM, Palmar S and Gordon-Smith EC (1982). Use of cyclosporin A in allogeneic bone marrow transplantation for severe aplastic anemia. *Transplantation, 33,* 382-386.

126. Diepernick H (1983). Temperature dependency of cyclosporin plasma levels. *Lancet, 1,* 416.

127. Smith J, Hows J and Gordon-Smith EC (1983). In vitro stability and storage of cyclosporine in human serum and plasma. *Transplantation Proceedings, 15,* 2422-2425.

128. Johnston A, Marsden JT and Holt DW (1986). The UK cyclosporine quality assessment scheme. *Therapeutic Drug Monitoring, 8,* 200-204.

129. Wenk M and Follath F (1983). Temperature dependency of apparent cyclosporin A concentrations in plasma. *Clinical Chemistry, 29,* 1965.

130. Donatsch P, Abisch E, Homberger M, Trabar R et al (1981). A radioimmunoassay to measure cyclosporin A in plasma and serum samples. *Journal of Immunology, 2,* 19-32.

131. Ball PE, Munzer H, Keller HP, Abisch E et al (1988). Specific ^{3}H radioimmunoassay with a monoclonal antibody for monitoring cyclosporine in blood. *Clinical Chemistry, 34*(2), 257-260.

132. Niederberger W, Schaub P and Beveridge T (1980). High-perforamnce liquid chromatographic determination of cyclosporin A in plasma and urine. *Journal of Chromatography, 182,* 454-458.

133. Sawcuck RJ and Cartier LL (1981). Liquid chromatographic determination of cyclosporin A in blood and plasma. *Clinical Chemistry, 27*(8), 1368-1371.

134. Carruthers SG, Freeman DJ, Koegler JC, Howson W et al (1983). Simplified liquid chromatographic analysis for cyclosporine A, and comparison with radioimmunoassay. *Clinical Chemistry, 29*(1), 180-183.

135. Rosano TG, Freed BM, Cerilli J and Lampert N (1986). Immunosuppressive metabolites of cyclosporine in the blood of renal allograft recipients. *Transplantation, 42,* 262-266.

136. Freeman DJ, Laupacis A, Keown PA et al (1984). Evaluation of cyclosporine-phenytoin interaction with observations on cyclosporine metabolites. *British Journal of Clinical Pharmacology, 18,* 886-893.

137. Bowers LD and Singh J (1987). A gradient elution HPLC assay for cyclosporine and its metabolites in blood and bile. *Journal of Liquid Chromatography, 10,* 411-420.

138. Perrin F (1926). Polarization de la lumièr de fluorescence. Vie moyenne des molécules dans l'ete excité. *Journal of Physiology Radium, 7,* 390-401.

139. Dandliker WB and Feigen GA (1961). Quantification of the antigen-antibody reaction by the polarization of fluorescence. *Biochemistry and Biophysiology Research Communication, 5,* 299-304.

140. Spencer R, Toledo F, Williams B and Yoss N (1973). Design, construction and two applications for an automatic flow cell polarization fluorometer with digital read-out: enzyme-inhibitor (antitrypsin) assay and antigen-antibody (insulin-insulin antiserum) assay. *Clinical Chemistry, 19,* 838-844.

141. Kobayashi Y, Amitani K, Watanabe F and Miyai K (1976). Fluorescence polarization immunoassay for cortisol. *Clinica Chimica Acta, 92,* 241-247.

142. Watson RAA, Landon J, Shaw EJ and Smith DS (1976). Polarization fluoroimmunoassay of gentamicin. *Clinica Chimica Acta, 73,* 51-55.

143. Jolley ME, Stroupe SD, Wang CJ et al (1981). Fluorescence polarization immunoassay. I. Monitoring aminoglycoside antibiotics in serum and plasma. *Clinical Chemistry, 27,* 1190-1197.

144. McGregor AR, Crookall-Greening JO, Landon J and Smith DS (1978). Polarization fluoroimmunoassay of phenytoin. *Clinica Chimica Acta, 83,* 161-166.

145. Lu Steffes M, Jolley M, Pittluck G et al (1981). Fluorescence polarization immunoassay of phenytoin and phenobarbital. (Abstract). *Clinical Chemistry, 27,* 1093.

146. Schroeder TJ, Pesce AJ, Hasan FM, Wermeling JR et al (1988). Comparison of Abbot TDx fluorescence polarization immunoassay, Sandoz radioimmunoassay,

and high-performance liquid chromatography methods for the assay of serum cyclosporine. *Transplantation Proceedings, 20*(2, Suppl 2), 345-347.

147. Hooks MA, Millikan WJ, Henderson JM, Mullins R et al (1989). Comparison of whole-blood cyclosporine levels measured by radioimmunoassay and fluorescence polarization in patients post orthotopic liver transplant. *Therapeutic Drug Monitoring, 11,* 304-309.

148. Borel JF, Feuer C, Mangee C et al (1977). Effects of new antilympohcytic peptide cyclosporin A in animals. *Immunology, 32,* 1017-1025.

149. Klintmalm G, Rigden O and Groth GG (1983). Clinical and laboratory signs of nephrotoxicity and rejection in cyclosporine-treated renal allowgraft recipients. *Transplantation Proceedings, 15,* 2815-2820.

150. Klintmalm G, Iwatsuki S and Starzl TE (1981). Nephrotoxicity of cyclosporin A in liver and kidney transplant patients. *Lancet, 1,* 470-471.

151. Hamilton DV, Calne RY, Evans DB et al (1981). Effect of long-term cyclosporin A on renal function. *Lancet, 1,* 1218-1219.

152. Shulman H, Striker G, Deeg HJ et al (1981). Nephrotoxicity of cyclosporin A after allogenic marrow transplantation. *New England Journal of Medicine, 305,* 1392-1395.

153. Bantel JP, Nath KA, Sutherland DE et al (1985). Effects of cyclosporine on the renin-angiotensin, aldosterone system and potassium excretion in renal transplant recipients. *Archives of Internal Medicine, 145,* 505-508.

154. Whiting PH, Thomson AW, Blair JT et al (1982). Experimental cyclosporine A nephrotoxicity. *British Journal of Experimental Pathology, 63,* 88-92.

155. Kahan BD, Van Buren CT, Lin S et al (1982). Immunopharmacologic monitoring of cyclosporin A treated recipients of cadaveric kidney allografts. *Transplantation, 34,* 330-337.

156. Myers BD, Ross J, Newton L et al (1984). Cyclosporine-associated chronic nephrotoxicity. *New England Journal of Medicine, 311,* 699-703.

157. Baxter CR, Duggin GG, Willis NS et al (1982). Cyclosporin A-induced increased in renin storage and release. *Research Communication Chemistry Pathology and Pharmacology, 37,* 305-309.

158. Humes HD, Jackson NM, O'Connor RP et al (1985). Pathogenic mechanisms of nephrotoxicity: insights into cyclosporine nephrotoxicity. *Transplantation Proceedings, 17,* 51-61.

159. Paller MS and Murray BM (1985). Renal dysfunction in animal models of cyclosporine toxicity. *Transplantation Proceedings, 17,* 155-159.

160. Sullivan BA, Hak LJ and Finn WF (1985). Cyclosporine nephrotoxicity: studies in laboratory animals. *Transplantation Proceedings, 17,* 145-154.

161. Neild GH, Ivory K and Williams DG (1983). Glomerular thrombi and infarction in rabbits with serum sickness following cyclosporine therapy. *Transplantation Proceedings, 15,* 2782-2786.

162. Klintmalm GB, Iwatsuki S and Starzl TE (1981). Cyclosporin A hepatoxicity in 66 renal allograft recipients. *Transplantation, 32,* 488-489.

163. Rodger RS, Turney JH, Haines I et al (1983). Cyclosporine and liver function in renal allograft patients. *Transplantation Proceedings, 15*(4, Suppl 1), 2754-2756.

164. Schade RR, Gugliemi DH, Van Thiel DH et al (1983). Cholestasis in heart transplant recipients treated with cyclosporine. *Transplantation Proceedings, 15*(4, Suppl 1), 2757-2756.

165. Atkinson K, Biggs J, Dodds A et al (1983). Cyclosporine-associated hepatoxicity after allogenic marrow transplantation in man: differentiation from other causes of posttransplant liver disease. *Transplantation Proceedings, 15*(4, Suppl 1), 2761-1767.

166. European Multicenter Trial (1982). Cyclosporin A as sole immunosuppressive agent in recipients of kidney allografts from cadaveric donors. *Lancet, 2,* 57-60.

167. Thompson CB, Sullivan KM, June CH and Thomas ED (1984). Association between cyclosporin neurotoxicity and hypomagnesemia. *Lancet, 2,* 1116-1120.

168. de Groen PC, Wiesner RH and Krom RA (1988). Cyclosporine A-induced side effects related to a low serum cholesterol level: an indication for a free cyclosporine A assay? *Transplantation Proceedings, 20*(2, Suppl 2), 374-376.

169. Matter BE, Donatsch P, Racine R et al (1982) Genotoxicity evaluation of cyclosporin A, a new immunosuppressive agent. *Mutation Research, 105,* 257-264.

170. Adu D, Turney J, Michael J et al (1983). Hyperkalemia in cyclosporine treated renal allograft recipients. *Lancet, 2,* 370-371.

171. Wysocki GP, Gretzinger HA, Laupacis A et al (1983). Fibrous hyperplasia of the gingiva; side effect of cyclosporin A therapy. *Oral Surgery, 55,* 274-278.

172. Kahan BD, Widemann CA, Flechner S et al (1984). Anaphylactic reaction to intravenous cyclosporine. *Lancet, 1,* 52.

173. Fries D, Hiesse C, Santelli G, Gardin JP et al (1988). Triple therapy with low-dose cyclosporine, azathioprine, and steroids: long-term results of a randomized study in cadaver donor renal transplantation. *Transplantation Proceedings, 20*(3, Suppl 3), 130-135.

174. Salaman J (1988). Cyclosporine mono-drug therapy. *Transplantation Proceedings, 20*(3, Suppl 3), 117-120.

175. Andreone PA, Olivari MT, Elick B, Arentzen CE et al (1986). Reduction of infectious complications following heart transplantation with triple-drug immunotherapy. *Journal of Heart Transplantation, 5*(1), 13-19.

PART TWO

The Issues

5

Tissue and Organ Donation and Recovery

Danny Hawke, James Kraft, and Susan L. Smith

The field of tissue and organ transplantation has expanded tremendously in both its purpose and scope over the past 35 years. What began not so long ago in a few animal laboratories as experimental surgery has become a major biomedical thrust in the United States. Tissue and organ transplantation has been added to the armamentarium of therapies that can now snatch terminally ill victims from the clutches of death. Evidence of the industrialization of transplantation abounds in many large tertiary care facilities. The infrastructures of these hospitals have changed to accommodate transplant programs; special operating rooms and intensive care units are equipped solely to handle transplant recipients. Medical residency programs in transplantation now exist, and the specialty of transplantation psychiatry has evolved.

PUBLIC AND PROFESSIONAL ATTITUDES
Public attitudes

Despite the technologic feasibility of performing an unlimited number of tissue and organ transplant procedures, thousands of persons with end-stage organ disease continue to wait for a lifesaving procedure. The donor pool necessary to meet transplant needs is projected at 10,000 to 15,000 per year.[1-3] The major limiting factor in organ transplantation continues to be a shortage of donor organs. According to the United Network of Organ Sharing

(UNOS), in the 15-month period ending December 1988, organ donation for all types of organs in the United States increased.[4] However, of the 12,500 to 27,000[1,5] potential organ donors and 50,000 potential tissue donors[6] in the United States each year, only 15% to 20% are recovered.[6] Contributing factors to this problem include reluctance by the general public to donate organs and medical professionals to initiate the donation process.

Public and professional attitudes about organ donation are crucial to organ and tissue transplantation. Several public opinion polls on attitudes toward organ donation were taken in the 1980s. In 1981, a poll indicated that between 50% and 70% would donate organs of their loved ones.[7] A 1985 Gallup poll revealed that 93% knew about organ transplantation and donation, 75% approved, and 27% stated they would donate organs, but only 17% had signed donor cards.[8] More than 70% of those polled would not donate and gave the following reasons: (1) fear that their death would be hastened for the purpose of taking organs, (2) fear of being mutilated, (3) not understanding "brain death," and (4) having to face their own mortality.

Public attitude polls of Americans were also conducted in 1984, 1986, and 1987.[8] These polls revealed that 98% of Americans were aware of organ transplantation, indicating an increased level of awareness in recent years. This in-

Table 5-1 Religious considerations in tissue and organ donation and transplantation

Amish	Organ donation and transplantation are acceptable, but the Amish are reluctant to donate their organs if the transplant outcome is known to be questionable.
Assemblies of God	There is no position.
Baptist	Organ donation is encouraged.
Buddhist	Organ donation is an individual decision. Those who donate their bodies and organs to the advancement of medical science are honored.
Catholic	Organ donation and transplantation are acceptable. Catholics view organ donation as an act of charity, fraternal love, and self-sacrifice.
Christian Church (Disciples of Christ)	Organ donation is an individual decision.
Christian and Missionary Alliance Church	Organ donation and transplantation are acceptable.
Christian Reformed (Reformed Church of America)	Members are urged to support the Anatomical Gift Act.
Church of the Brethren	Organ donation is encouraged.
Church of Christ	Organ donation is an individual decision.
The Church of Christ Scientist	Christian Scientists normally rely on spiritual, rather than medical, means for healing. However, organ donation is an individual decision.
Church of Jesus Christ of Latter Day Saints (Mormons)	Organ donation is an individual decision.
Episcopal Church	The Church does not object to donation as long as it is done reverently.
Evangelical Covenant Church of America	There is no position.
Evangelical United Brethren	Organ donation is encouraged.
Greek Orthodox Church	Donation is not consistent with traditional Orthodox practice and belief.
Gypsies	Gypsies are opposed to organ donation. Although they have no formal resolution, their opposition is associated with their belief about the afterlife. Gypsies believe that for 1 year after a person dies, the soul retraces its steps. All of the body parts must be intact because the soul maintains a physical shape.
Hindu	Organ donation is an individual decision.
Islam	In 1983, the Moslem Religious Council initially rejected organ donation by followers of Islam, but it has reversed its position, provided donors consent in writing prior to their death. The organs of Moslem donors must be transplanted immediately and should not be stored in organ banks.
Jehovah's Witnesses	Organ donation is an individual decision. All organs and tissue must be completely drained of blood before transplantation.
Jewish	Judaism teaches that saving a human life takes precedence over maintaining the sanctity of the human body.
Lutheran Church	Organ donation is an individual decision.
Mennonite Church	Organ donation and transplantation are acceptable.
Methodist Church	Organ donation is encouraged.
Presbyterian Church	There is no position.
Protestant	Protestants encourage and endorse organ donation. The Protestant faith respects an individual's conscience and a person's right to make decisions regarding his or her own body.
Quaker Religious Society (Friends)	Organ donation is an individual decision.
Reformed Church in America	Members are urged to support the Anatomical Gift Act.
Seventh-Day Adventists	Organ donation and transplantation are acceptable.

creased awareness was attributed primarily to media coverage of organ transplantation. Nine percent of those surveyed indicated that their increased awareness was as a result of personal experience, and 7% credited public education. Lowest levels of awareness were identified in blacks and individuals from lower educational and income groups.

One person in five in the United States carries a donor card.[9] This number has remained fairly constant over the past 4 years. The public attitude polls cited also indicate that Americans are more likely to consent to donate another family member's organs and tissues than their own.[10] Of those surveyed, 66% stated that they would probably donate a loved one's organs. In contrast, only 30% stated that they would probably donate their own organs. Individuals least likely to donate are individuals over the age of 55, blacks, persons with less than a high school education, and individuals with a household income of less than $15,000.[9] Forty-three percent of persons signing donor cards did not realize that in most cases, their next-of-kin's consent is necessary for donation. Only two out of three persons who considered themselves potential organ donors had shared their intentions with a family member. These surveys indicate the need for further education regarding organ donation and transplantation, especially in minority and lower income populations.[10]

Religious considerations

The clerical, ethical, and moral leaders of our country support tissue and organ donation and transplantation.[10-12] The national Episcopal, Lutheran, and Presbyterian churches have passed resolutions encouraging their members, as a part of their Christian ministry, to become organ donors. Religious views and practices related to organ donation and transplantation are presented in Table 5-1.

Professional attitudes

The donation process in the majority of cases is initiated by a medical professional. Ninety-eight percent of actual organ donors die in a critical care unit.[13] Approximately 20% die within 6 hours of admission and approximately 50% die within 24 hours.[14] Therefore critical care nurses

play a key role in the donation process. Critical care nurses spend the greatest amount of time with potential organ donors, donor families, and organ procurement organization (OPO) personnel. If critical care nurses are uncomfortable with the concept of donation, their attitudes will have a negative impact on the donation process when they interact with families. Initiating and facilitating organ donation must be incorporated as a natural component of the medical and nursing care of potential donors for it to be successful.

The attitudes of critical care nurses and physicians regarding organ donation changed positively in the 1980s.[9] This could be the result of the increased frequency and success of organ transplantation and/or supportive federal legislation that now requires hospitals to develop policies and procedures for organ donor identification and referral. Before these developments, nurses and physicians often did not refer potential donors for various reasons: They were not educated about recognizing potential donors, which reflected a lack of institutional support; nurses were unlikely to refer potential donors unless they were confident of the physician's support; there is a very real emotional strain involved in the process; and there are legal considerations that may have caused physicians and nurses to be hesitant to initiate the process.[15] Many physicians did not wish to become involved in donation because they feared a lawsuit. Responsibility for the potential donor is not always clear, and physicians may be reluctant to certify brain death, because it may result in additional responsibility for maintaining the donor until organs are recovered. It is the responsibility of hospital administrators to ensure that their staff are informed and educated about organ donation.

In addition to volunteerism, various solutions—presumed consent, required request, financial incentives, primates as donors, and anencephalic donors—to the shortage of cadaver donor organs have been proposed over the past several years. All but one, required request, are laden with ethical issues. *Required request* or routine inquiry policies require that the families of prospective donors be approached at the time of death about the possibility of organ donation. In October 1987, required request policies became a condition of a hospital's eligibility for Medicare reimbursement.

Presumed consent, or presuming that an individual desired to donate his or her organs unless otherwise formally specified, is law in several European countries. In countries in which presumed consent is law, organs are routinely harvested from cadavers as long as the option to refuse donation was presented to the family and they waived that option. Presumed consent is based on the concept of utility. And in the United States, 12 states have presumed consent legislation for cornea donation.[16] Presumed consent, however, has not been effective in increasing organ donation in those countries where it is practiced.

Several financial incentives to donate have been proposed, including cash, tax credits, and payment for funeral expenses. The Senate Committee on Labor and Human Resources responded to these proposals by stating that "individuals should not profit by the sale of human organs for transplantation and the human body should not be viewed as a commodity."[16] The House Committee on Energy and Commerce concurred, further stating that permitting the sale of organs might cause the system of volunteerism to collapse.[16] Marketing organs in the United States is now a federal crime punishable by a $50,000.00 fine and/or 5 years in prison.

Transplantation of primate organs into humans (xenografting) is highly experimental, has met with little success when attempted, and is highly controversial from an ethical perspective. It is highly unlikely that xenografting will be accepted by society as a partial solution to the problem.

Anencephalic infants are born with a neural tube defect in which most or all of the cerebral hemispheres are absent. The anencephalic infant has no cognitive capabilities and will die soon after birth. However, because the brainstem is functional at birth, the infant is not considered brain dead and technically cannot be considered an organ donor. For anencephalics to be considered organ donors, one of two changes in brain death legislation would have to occur: (1) the definition of death would have to be amended to include anencephaly as a qualifying condition, or (2) the current definition of death would be maintained, with the legal exception that organs can be taken from non-brain-dead anencephalic infants.[17]

NATIONAL LEGISLATION
The Uniform Anatomical Gift Act

The shortage of organs and tissues for transplantation is a national problem. The initial effort to address the many complex issues impeding donation was the passage of the Uniform Anatomical Gift Act (UAGA) in 1968.[18] The UAGA established a legal framework for cadaveric organ donation. The purpose of the UAGA was to prevent presumed consent legislation from being enacted and to ensure respect for individual autonomy and dignity. The act grants authority to competent persons over 18 years of age to donate their organs for transplantation. An individual may specify his or her wishes regarding organ donation through a will or Uniform Donor Card. The Act also recognizes the authority of next of kin to donate organs of the deceased. The UAGA has been adopted in all 50 states and the District of Columbia.

An individual's decision to donate after his or her death may be formally documented on a donor card, driver's license, living will, or other document witnessed by at least two individuals. The Uniform Donor Card is a method developed to encourage the voluntary donation of one's organs and tissues. Donor cards have been incorporated onto the back of driver's licenses in 45 states.[8] A telephone survey of transplant coordinators and hospital administrators in 50 states revealed that only in Louisiana is there a written policy requiring the state police department to look for donor cards at the scene of an accident and to alert hospital personnel if one is found.[19] In most cases of vehicular trauma, the driver's license never makes it to the hospital where the potential donor is taken; therefore the medical staff is frequently unaware of the trauma victim's wishes regarding organ and tissue donation.

Even when an individual has signed a donor card expressing his or her wish to donate and the medical staff is made aware of this, the donor card is not considered a legal document in the majority of states. Most states, for legal and moral reasons, require permission from the next of kin before organs can be recovered. However, at the 1987 National Conference of Commissioners on Uniform State Laws, a recommendation was made for revising the Uniform Anatomical Gift Act. Section 2-H states, "An anatomical gift that is not revoked by the donor before death is irrevocable and does not require the consent or concurrence of any person after the donor's death."[20]

As stated earlier, relatively few Americans carry signed donor cards,[6] which leads experts to question the effectiveness of the system of "volunteerism" in organ recovery. The UAGA, now in existence for over 20 years, has not alleviated the shortage of organs and tissues for transplantation.

The National Organ Transplant Act

In 1984 Congress passed the National Organ Transplant Act (PL 98-507), which established a 25-member multidisciplinary task force on organ transplantation. The task force was charged with conducting comprehensive examinations of the medical, legal, ethical, social, and economic issues presented by human organ recovery and transplantation.[21] The task force concluded that the serious gap that existed between the need for organs and the supply of donors resulted in part from a lack of uniform standards of accountability and quality assurance in organ and tissue procurement. Recommendations from the task force to alleviate this problem included (1) development of uniform standards for organ procurement, (2) implementation of the Uniform Determination of Death Act in all states, and (3) implementation of routine inquiry or required request policies in all states.

Recommendations were also made regarding public and professional education related to organ donation, recovery and transplantation. It was recommended that the American Council on Transplantation (ACT) serve as the umbrella organization for facilitation of public programming to community and minority groups, and the distribution of educational materials. ACT is a private organization founded in 1983 that represents more than 1000 community members, physicians, nurses, scientists, organiza-

tions, hospitals and insurers. The goal of ACT is to promote donor identification and referral, multiple organ and tissue donation, and equitable distribution of organs. A further recommendation was that a national educational program on organ transplantation, similar to other national health-related programs, be instituted. To increase medical professionals' awareness, recommendations to incorporate content on organ transplantation into medical and nursing school curricula, to make continuing education on organ transplantation for medical professionals mandatory, and to include content on organ transplantation in specialty certification examinations were made.

Furthermore, the National Organ Transplant Act of 1984 prohibited the purchase of organs for transplantation, established grants to OPOs, and established a national organ sharing system, the National Organ Procurement and Transplant Network (OPTN). The OPTN provides for a unified national system of organ sharing that encompasses a patient registry and coordinates organ allocation and distribution.

The Omnibus Reconciliation Act of 1986

In 1986 Congress incorporated the Organ Transplantation Task Force recommendations into the Omnibus Reconciliation Act. Specifically, the following provisions were tied to Medicaid or Medicare reimbursement in an effort to strengthen the organ recovery system and impose quality control in organ recovery and transplant programs. First, required request policies must be implemented by hospitals participating in Medicaid or Medicare programs. Second, transplant centers must be members of the OPTN. Third, OPOs must be members of the OPTN to participate in Medicaid or Medicare programs. And fourth, renal transplantation would be reimbursed by Medicare only when performed at centers that conform to federal regulations, and who are members of the OPTN. The Omnibus Reconciliation Act of 1986 also required OPOs to meet certification requirements, and allowed for Medicare reimbursement of the cost of immunosuppressive drugs.[9]

The first required request laws were enacted in 1985 in Oregon and New York. By 1988, 43 states had passed legislation either to require hospitals to request donation from next of kin of potential donors or to notify local OPOs of potential donors.[22] Again, failure of the voluntary donor process has necessitated this recent legislation. Unfortunately, however, after implementation of these laws, an initial decrease in organ donation occurred, suggesting a negative influence. Another possible explanation is that the temporary decline was related to the usual confusion and uncertainty associated with major change.

ORGAN PROCUREMENT ORGANIZATIONS

Organ recovery services in the United States are provided by nonprofit OPOs. They are an integral link in the acceptance of organ transplantation as an appropriate treatment option. There are two types of OPOs: hospital-based and independent. The earliest "hospital-based" programs were established for the sole purpose of providing kidneys for transplantation and were funded by the Social Security Amendment of 1972.[23] As more hospitals began performing transplants, the need to regionalize OPOs became clear. "Independent" OPOs were formed to provide services to donor hospitals and transplant centers within a given geographic area.

The task force established by the National Organ Transplant Act of 1984 examined organ recovery in the United States. This task force found that the organ recovery system in effect at that time was ineffective and that in some metropolitan areas there were too many OPOs. In 1986, as part of the Omnibus Reconciliation Act, the Health Care Finance Administration (HCFA) was charged with responsibility for the certification of OPOs.[24] HCFA developed a certification process. To be certified, an OPO must (1) demonstrate a working relationship with 75% of the hospitals within its service area and provide organ recovery, organ sharing, and professional education services, (2) arrange for appropriate tissue typing of donated organs, (3) discuss its accounting procedures and make available the name and address of its accounting firm, (4) explain its method of transportation of donated organs to transplant centers, (5) submit quantifiable data about the service area, population base, and number of donors yielded per year, (6) arrange to cooperate with tissue banks

for the retrieval, processing, preservation, storage and distribution of tissue, (7) have a board of directors or board of advisors consisting of members who represent hospital administrators, intensive care or emergency room personnel, tissue banks, voluntary health associations, members of the community, a physician skilled in the field of histocompatibility, a neuroscience physician, and a transplant surgeon from each center within the service area. HCFA also required that OPOs define their service areas.

Seventy-two OPOs were designated by HCFA as of March 31, 1988. HCFA established service areas and determined that there would be only one OPO per service area. However, a hospital within a given service area is free to use an OPO from another service area.[25]

OPOs provide a wide range of services, including public and professional education, 24-hour assistance to hospitals in the evaluation of potential donors, and, when suitable potential donors are identified, the coordination of organ recovery. When requested, an organ transplant coordinator will determine the suitability of organs and tissues for transplantation.

Organ transplant coordinators

The responsibilities of the organ transplant coordinator are critical and include (1) assisting in donor management, including the coordination of necessary laboratory tests, (2) arranging necessary transportation of the transplant center's recovery teams to and from the donor hospital, and (3) assisting surgeons in surgical recovery procedures. After organ recovery, the organ transplant coordinator provides verbal and written feedback about disposition of donated organs and tissues to the physicians and hospital staff directly involved in the organ recovery. The donor family is also contacted and informed of the age, sex, and postoperative status of the recipients. By learning of the benefit that comes from their tragic loss, the donor family is helped through the grieving process. Anonymity, if possible, of the donor, recipient, and their respective families is maintained both before and after donation.

The critical care nurse's role in the recovery process does not end with contacting the OPO. His or her skills are needed to assist in the evaluation and management of organ and tissue donors. The critical care nurse is not only crucial in donor management; he or she also acts as a liaison to the donor family.

An often overlooked factor is the emotional strain experienced by nurses caring for patients who die. Nurses are asked to look beyond the tragedy and proceed with the care and management of the brain-dead patient. Many OPOs are now introducing recipients of organs to nurses in donor hospitals so that they can experience first-hand the results of their efforts. This approach to providing positive feedback to critical care nurses involved in organ donation is both innovative and successful.

THE NATIONAL ORGAN SHARING SYSTEM

In 1972 the Kidney Disease and Control Agency of the Public Health Service began providing funding for the development of a kidney-sharing system for potential recipients. This agency also began investigating methods for preserving cadaveric kidneys as well as for developing a mechanism for establishing the cost of organ recovery. The first group of transplant centers to receive this funding included the Medical College of Virginia, Duke University, the University of North Carolina, Georgetown University, Johns Hopkins University, the University of Maryland, the University of Virginia, Emory University, and Danville Memorial Hospital. This group came to be known as the Southeastern Regional Organ Procurement Agency.

To appropriate funding for organ recovery and sharing, organ acquisition charges were developed that are billed to the transplant centers. Charges were also established for listing potential recipients on the national recipient computer program. Funding for this contract expired in June 1973; in July 1973, renewed financial support for kidney recovery costs was provided through amendments to existing Medicare legislation. The Southeastern Regional Organ Procurement Program expanded to include many new members, which resulted in its incorporation as a nonprofit organization, the Southeastern Regional Organ Procurement Foundation (SEOPF), on January 14, 1975.[22]

An important outcome of SEOPF was the development of a system for listing of recipients and cross-matching capabilities. This included the establishment of recipient serum sample trays, which enabled any donor to be cross-matched against any potential recipient in the computer match sharing program. Each participating transplant center submitted a serum specimen from each of its potential kidney recipients to a central laboratory, which then prepared the cross-match trays and returned them to the transplant centers' tissue typing labs. Thus any donor organ, regardless of location, could be cross-matched against any potential recipient listed with SEOPF.

In May 1977, responding to a request from the Medical College of Virginia's heart transplantation program, SEOPF coordinated the first long-distance recovery of a heart.[26] The organ was successfully transplanted, and thus began the long distance recovery of organs other than kidneys. From that point on, the SEOPF computer became the repository for data pertinent to all types of solid organ transplantation.

In 1982 SEOPF, in conjunction with the American Kidney Fund, established the Kidney Center to facilitate organ sharing. The objective of this center was to decrease organ wastage by serving as a central clearinghouse for referral and donation. This pilot project was successful, and funding was approved by HCFA on March 15, 1984.[7] Because of a growing demand for multiorgan listings by the Kidney Center, the Center's name was changed to The Organ Center.

The National Organ Transplant Act of 1984 created the OPTN. According to the Act, the OPTN was to develop a national system for the recovery and distribution of donor organs for transplantation. The OPTN was to be administered by the U.S. Department of Health and Human Services through a contract with a private, nonprofit organization. In September 1986 the contract to operate the OPTN was awarded to UNOS. UNOS policy requires that transplant centers list all potential recipients in the UNOS computer system.

UNOS operates 24 hours a day in Richmond, Virginia. The following scenario explains the relationship between UNOS and OPOs. An OPO with a kidney donor notifies UNOS of the donor availability and provides donor information to the UNOS computer. The UNOS computer will then provide a list of potential recipients based on match and need. Matching is based on ABO compatibility, HLA compatibility, presensitization, recipient's medical status, and organ size.

Since its inception, UNOS has established (1) a national waiting list for individuals in need of organ transplantation, (2) a national system for computerized matching of potential recipients with available organs, (3) a 24-hour central office to ensure access to the recipient list, (4) methods to assist OPOs in distribution of organs to transplant centers, and (5) standards for organ recovery and transplantation. UNOS also provides professional education programs nationwide and collects, analyzes, and publishes national data on donation and transplantation. UNOS operates a toll-free telephone number (800-666-1884) to provide the public with information on organ donation.

ROLE OF THE CRITICAL CARE NURSE IN TISSUE AND ORGAN DONATION AND RECOVERY

Despite the widespread distribution of information regarding organ donation and the adoption of state and national legislation to facilitate the donation of transplantable organs, a major discrepancy between the number of potential organ donors and the number of actual organ donors continues to exist. A major factor in increasing organ recovery is the identification of potential donors in critical care units and the ability of health care professionals to obtain family consent for donation. The role of the critical care nurse in addressing these problems is essential to increasing the availability of organs for transplantation. This fact has been recognized by the American Association of Critical Care Nurses (AACN), and addressed in two position statements[27,28] supporting this critical step in the organ donation process (see Appendixes A and B).

The ideal organ donor candidate is an individual who has suffered a fatal injury to the brain, has previously been healthy, and is free of contagious disease. Severe head injury is the cause of death in 56% to 77% of cases.[14,29-31] Other causes include brain tumors, cerebrovascular accidents, cardiac arrest, and drug overdose. By virtue of the nature of their injuries, these individuals are normally cared for in critical care units. The critical care nurse, therefore, becomes a key individual in the process of organ donation through early identification of potential organ donors, referral of potential donors to an OPO, and in understanding family dynamics during the organ recovery process.

The family should be assured that every effort has been made to save their loved one's life; however, when brain death does occur, they may find solace in the option of donation. If the sensitive and emotional nature of organ donation is understood, these issues can be addressed in a timely and compassionate manner. Early identification of donor candidates by the critical care nurse is essential to the success of this process.

Brain death

Brain death is an absolute criterion for vascular organ donation, although not for tissue or cornea donation. Therefore understanding the concept of brain death is essential to the successful recovery of organs. The declaration of death in a mechanically supported individual allows for surgical removal of viable organs for donation. Without mechanical support of ventilation, vital organs would become irreversibly damaged and unsuitable for transplantation. Brain death most frequently results from open and closed head injuries, cerebrovascular accidents, primary brain tumors, and cerebral anoxia. Patients who are brain dead as a result of these conditions should be considered as potential multiorgan donors.

Evolution of the concept of brain death. Before the 1950s, the commonlaw definition of death was "total stoppage of circulation of the blood and a cessation of vital functions."[32] During the 1950s and 1960s, cardiopulmonary resuscitation (CPR) techniques were perfected, and CPR became a standard of care for the cardiopulmonary arrest victim. However, it became evident that cardiopulmonary function could be revived while brain function could not in cases where respirations were absent for prolonged periods. As a result of this knowledge, decisions were made not to resuscitate in such cases.

Biomedical technologic advances made it necessary to reexamine the definition of death.

In 1968 the Ad Hoc Committee of the Harvard Medical School to Examine the Definition of Death issued a landmark report, stating criteria to determine brain death. The Committee defined brain death in terms of the entire brain when they said, "a person is dead if the brain is dead."[33] This simple definition remains a standard for determination of death despite biomedical advances. With biomedical advances in the 1960s, including surgical techniques for organ transplantation, there evolved a clear need for criteria for the legal recognition of brain death. These criteria began to be spelled out with considerable variation in state statutes.

In 1974 the American Medical Association (AMA) recognized brain death as one criterion for making the medical diagnosis of death by resolving that "death shall be determined by the clinical judgment of a physician using the necessary available and currently accepted criteria," and "that permanent and irreversible cessation of the function of the brain constitutes one of various criteria which can be used in the medical diagnosis of brain death."[34] In 1975, the American Bar Association (ABA) House of Delegates adopted the following definition of death: "For all legal purposes, a human body with irreversible cessation of total brain function, according to usual and customary standards of medical practice, shall be considered dead."[2]

In 1980 the Uniform Law Commissioners adopted the Uniform Determination of Death Act (UDODA). According to the Act, "An individual who has sustained either (1) irreversible cessation of circulatory and respiratory functions, or (2) irreversible cessation of all functions of the entire brain, including the brainstem, is dead."[1] The UDODA has been endorsed by the AMA, the ABA, the President's Commission for the Study of Ethical Problems in Medicine and Biomedical and Behavioral Research, the American Academy of Neurology, and the American Electroencephalographic Society.[11] By 1987, 39 states and the District of Columbia had enacted brain death legislation.[11]

Younger et al surveyed 195 health professionals about their knowledge of brain death and organ retrieval.[35] Their concepts of death varied widely, and only 35% correctly identified legal

---

BRAIN DEATH CRITERIA

Apnea despite adequate carbon dioxide stimulus
Total unresponsiveness:
    No response to noxious stimuli
    No reflex activity except of spinal cord origin
    Fixed, dilated pupils
    Absent corneal reflex
    Absent gag, cough reflex
Known cause of condition

---

and medical criteria for determining death. This lack of conceptual clarity about brain death is troublesome, because a correct understanding of brain death is a necessary prerequisite to the success of organ donation and transplantation.

The role of the critical care nurse. Although the pronouncement of death and the determination of the medical diagnosis of brain death are the responsibility of the physician, the critical care nurse plays several important roles, including early recognition of impending brain death, open communication with the physician, peer support to nurses caring for brain dead patients, assistance in testing for brain death criteria (see the box above), and care of the family.[32] The critical care nurse is in an ideal position to provide the family with and reinforce information about brain death. Only through an understanding and acceptance of the concept of brain death will the potential donor family consent to organ donation.

Donor identification

General criteria for the donation of vascular organs are outlined in the box below. Criteria

---

GENERAL DONOR CRITERIA FOR VASCULAR ORGANS

Age: Newborn to 65 years
Negative history of active systemic infections
Negative history of carcinoma, except tumors of
    CNS
Hemodynamically salvageable
Relatively normal organ function

from the U.S. Public Health Service for exclusion of high-risk donors are listed in the box at right. The suitable organ donor has suffered brain death yet has intact cardiovascular function. Mechanisms of injury that may lead to brain death include, but are not limited to, trauma, cerebrovascular accidents, anoxic encephalopathy, and primary brain tumors. Although the typical organ donor is in a surgical intensive care unit, suitable donors may also be identified in emergency departments, medical intensive care units and, occasionally, on general care floors. Despite the location of the potential donor, all candidates who are to be considered as potential donors must (1) meet brain death and general age criteria, (2) be free of infection, (3) have no history of carcinoma (except primary tumors of the central nervous system), (4) be hemodynamically salvageable, and (5) have relatively normal organ function. Organ-specific criteria are listed in Table 5-2.

CURRENT CRITERIA FOR EXCLUSION OF HIGH-RISK DONORS

Clinical or laboratory evidence of HIV infection
Men who have had sex with another man one or more times since 1977
Past or present intravenous drug abuse
Persons immigrating since 1977 from countries where heterosexual activity is thought to play a major role in the transmission of HIV (e.g., Haiti, central Africa)
Persons with hemophilia who have received clotting factor concentrates
Sexual partners of any of the above
Men and women who have engaged in prostitution since 1977 and persons who have been their heterosexual partners within the past 6 months

From American Federation of Clinical Tissue Banks (1989). *Operational Standards*, p. 9. Richmond, Va: The Federation.

Table 5-2 Donor criteria

Organ or tissue	Age	Cause of death	Specific criteria	General criteria
Organ				
Kidney	6 mo-65 yr	Brain death	No preexisting renal disease or injury	No sepsis, transmittable diseases, extracranial malignancy, IV drug abuse, or death of unknown etiology
Heart	Term newborn to 55 yr	Brain death	No preexisting cardiac disease or injury	No sepsis, transmittable diseases, extracranial malignancy, IV drug abuse, or death of unknown etiology
Liver	Term newborn to 55 yr	Brain death	No preexisting hepatic disease or injury	No sepsis, transmittable diseases, extracranial malignancy, IV drug abuse, or death of unknown etiology
Pancreas	1-60 yr	Brain death	No preexisting pancreatic disease or injury	No sepsis, transmittable diseases, extracranial malignancy, IV drug abuse, or death of unknown etiology

Adapted from LifeLink of Georgia, Atlanta, Ga, 1989.

Age criteria. The age of the potential donor can range from term newborn to over 65 years, depending on the organ considered for donation and the recipient need. Several programs across the country have active neonatal transplant programs and use hearts, livers, and kidneys from infants. At this time the anencephalic program at Loma Linda University in California has been discontinued; however, new technologies and changing philosophies could reactivate this and other similar programs in the future. In general, procurement agencies will evaluate the newborn donor on an individual basis, assess the need for the respective organs offered in donation by accessing the national computer, and make recommendations based on those identified needs.

As the transplantable population ages, the upper limit for age of the organ donor becomes more liberal. It is not unusual for organs to be recovered from donors who are older than 60 years of age. Age criteria are evaluated relative

Table 5-2 Donor criteria—cont'd

Organ or tissue	Age	Cause of death	Specific criteria	General criteria
Lung	12-55 yr	Brain death	No preexisting pulmonary disease or injury, no smoking history, no chest tubes	No sepsis, transmittable diseases, extracranial malignancy, IV drug abuse, or death of unknown etiology
Heart-lung	Term newborn to 65 yr	Brain death	No preexisting cardiac or pulmonary disease or injury, no smoking history, no chest tubes	No sepsis, transmittable diseases, extracranial malignancy, IV drug abuse, or death of unknown etiology
Tissue				
Bone Facia Connective tissues Bone marrow Heart valves	15-65 yr	Brain death or cardiac death	Documented time of death	No malignancy No uncontrolled infections No deaths of unknown etiology No tissue radiation No transmittable diseases No chronic steroid therapy No IV drug abuse No history of homosexuality
	Term newborn-55 yr			
Eye	No age limit	Brain death or cardiac death		No active hepatitis, AIDS No viral encephalitis No Creutzfelt-Jakob disease No rabies No death of unknown etiology

to the function of the organs rather than chronologic absolutes.

Absence of infection. The organ donor must be free of active infection. Donors with a recent history of infection documented by positive blood, sputum, or urine culture must receive appropriate antibiotic coverage and have negative culture results to be considered for donation. Of prime concern is prevention of the transmission of active pathogens into a patient who is immunosuppressed and the subsequent development of a fatal infection. Regardless of the length of hospital stay or the use of antibiotics, all potential organ donors have blood cultures drawn before organ recovery.

Of prime concern today is the presence of sexually transmitted disease in the organ donor. Thus, before organ recovery, serologic tests for syphilis, hepatitis B, and HIV are performed. Organ donation cannot proceed without negative results to serologic tests for all three infections.

Absence of severe systemic disease. The ideal organ donor is a relatively young individual who is free of and has no history of end-organ disease. As a general rule, no one disease, other than carcinoma (except a primary CNS tumor), should be considered a contraindication to evaluation for organ donation.

Each organ system is evaluated individually. Clearly, if an individual has been diagnosed as having primary renal hypertension, he or she could not be considered a renal donor. However, if that individual is diagnosed as having essential hypertension with normal renal function, then the history of hypertension would not necessarily exclude that individual as a renal donor. In summary, all organ donors must be considered on an individual basis, and no single systemic disease process should exclude a donor from consideration.

Initiation of organ donation

The initiation of organ donation occurs at the time the health care professional recognizes the potential organ donor and makes a referral to the OPO. Referral of a potential organ donor does not commit the physician, nurse, or family to donation. It does allow the OPO to assess the particular situation and determine an appropriate course of action. Without referral, the family cannot be offered the option of donation. To be offered the option to donate a loved one's organs is a family's right; failure to offer this option to families is a violation of their rights.

Initiation of donation should proceed according to hospital policy, which should reflect a positive institutional commitment toward the donation process. The policy should be written in clear and concise terms, and all potentially involved personnel should not only understand the policy but also be capable of implementing it.

Regardless of the policy developed by an individual hospital, certain basic information is needed by the OPO to assess the suitability of the potential donor. This includes the potential donor's name, age, sex, race, diagnosis, cause of death, date of admission, availability of next of kin, the attending physician's name, and a brief summary of vital signs and pertinent laboratory values.

The role of the organ recovery team is varied; however, a team member should be available to coordinate the donation process, manage the organ donor and/or make recommendations for donor management to the local physician, and be available to answer questions of the donor family.

Family consent. Perhaps nowhere is the role of the critical care nurse more important than when supporting the family who are considering organ donation. When families are asked to make a decision about organ donation, they do so at a time of crisis, the time of a loved one's death. For donation to have been considered and presented to the family means the death came unexpectedly. Feelings of disbelief, grief, helplessness, and guilt are commonly expressed. At this time the family requires much emotional support. The critical care nurse is in an ideal position to offer this support.

At first thought, to make a decision about organ donation in the face of this tragedy seems too much to ask of a grieving family. However, in a recent study, 82% of families were willing to donate their loved ones' organs when given the option.[36] Family members report that they find solace in being given the opportunity to enhance the lives of others through the gift of organ donation.

A key concept of organ donation is that it is

PRIORITY OF NEXT-OF-KIN CONSENT

Donors over 18 years of age

Spouse
Adult son or daughter
Either parent
Adult brother or sister
Legal guardian
Any person authorized or under obligation to dispose of the body

Donors under 18 years of age

Both parents
If both parents are not readily available, and no contrary indications of the absent parent are known, one parent
If the parents are divorced or legally separated, the custodial parent
In the absence of the custodial parent, when no contrary indications of the absent parent are known, the noncustodial parent
If there are no parents, the legal guardian
Any other person authorized or obligated to dispose of the body

---

Data from Caplan AL (1988). Beg, borrow or steal: the ethics of solid organ procurement. In Mathieu D (ed). *Organ substitution technology. Ethical, legal and public policy issues.* Boulder: Westview Press (59-68).

offered as an option to the family. It is the family's right to accept or refuse this option, and either decision must be respected and supported. It is the joint responsibility of nurses, physicians, and the OPO to offer this option, prepare the family to make an informed consent, and provide an environment that is supportive to this process.

Before offering the option of organ donation, the potential donor's next of kin must be identified. Consent by the next of kin as defined by the UAGA is shown in the box above.

Donor management

After the diagnosis of brain death, the focus of clinical care shifts from interventions aimed at saving the life of the patient to interventions aimed at maintaining the viability of potentially transplanted organs. The main goal of organ

donor management is the maintenance of optimal conditions that will ensure functional, intact, and infection-free organs.[11] The function of organs to be recovered is preserved by optimal management of the following parameters: hydration and perfusion, oxygenation, diuresis, avoidance of infection, and temperature control. Multiple organ recovery has become commonplace in the past several years; consequently, it can take up to 12 hours to coordinate the activities of several organ recovery teams with the donor institution. It is during this extended period of time that donor management becomes critical to the recovery of viable organs.

Invasive monitoring for the purpose of providing clinical parameters of organ function is considered essential to donor stabilization and maintenance. Direct arterial blood pressure monitoring via a peripheral arterial catheter allows for continuous monitoring of blood pressure and immediate recognition of hypotension (and hypertension). Central venous pressure (CVP) monitoring is critical to balanced hydration. The triple-lumen catheter is ideal for this purpose in that it has additional ports for administration of fluids, blood products, and pharmacologic agents. Brainstem herniation leads to disruption in thermoregulation, which can cause hypothermia, ventricular dysrhythmias, and cardiac arrest; therefore temperature monitoring via a rectal or esophageal probe is desirable.

Clinical parameters considered pertinent to the management of the vascular organ donor include systolic blood pressure, mean arterial blood pressure, CVP, urine output, heart rate, and body temperature. Ideal parameters for potential donors are listed in Table 5-3. Vital signs are monitored every 15 minutes until the donor is stable, then hourly if the donor remains stable. A baseline laboratory series including CBC, blood cultures, serum electrolytes, arterial blood gases, and urinalysis is obtained to determine the course of subsequent therapeutic management. Additional laboratory studies and/or procedures that may be ordered for organ specific donation are found in Table 5-4. With aggressive fluid resuscitation, electrolytes and blood gases are monitored about every 4 hours. In cases of suspected hemorrhage, he-

Table 5-3 Ideal clinical parameters for potential organ donors

Parameter	Optimal value
Systolic blood pressure	90-160 mm Hg
Mean arterial blood pressure	Greater than 70 mm Hg
Central venous pressure	6-12 cm H_2O
Urine output	Greater than 1.0 ml/kg/hr
Heart rate	60-120 beats/min
Arterial blood gases	$pao_2 \geq 80$ torr
	$paco_2$ 35-45 torr
	pH 7.35-7.45
	$Sao_2 \geq 90\%$
Body temperature	36.1°-38.9° C

moglobin and hematocrit values are monitored about every 4 hours until stable. Several conditions that threaten organ viability may be present in the potential organ donor that warrant immediate attention. A discussion of these conditions and interventions to preserve organ viability follows.

Table 5-4 Laboratory studies and procedures for organ-specific donation

Organ	Laboratory study/procedure
Kidney	Creatinine clearance
Heart	Cardiology consultation
	12-lead ECG
	Cardiac enzymes and iso- enzymes
	Chest x-ray examination
Liver	Bilirubin (total and direct)
	SGOT
	SGPT
	LDH
	PT, PTT
	Platelet count
Single lung	Sputum culture and Gram stain, chest x-ray examination
Heart/lung	Sputum culture and Gram stain, chest x-ray examination, 100% oxygen challenge
Pancreas	Amylase
	Lipase

Hypotension and shock

Hypotension is the most frequently encountered problem in the potential organ donor. The following conditions contribute to hypotension in this setting: brainstem herniation, collapse of peripheral vascular resistance, customary dehydration in head injured patients, blood loss, and excessive urine output secondary to diabetes insipidus.[7]

Shock is a clinical syndrome defined by tissue perfusion that is inadequate to meet the metabolic demands of the body. Various cardiovascular and neuroendocrine compensatory mechanisms are activated to maintain perfusion to the heart and brain, but ultimately at the expense of unprotected organs (kidneys, liver, and pancreas) and peripheral tissues. If shock is acutely severe or untreated, compensatory mechanisms will fail and hypotension will result. In the organ donor, there are two major causes of hypotension and shock: a major neurogenic insult and hypovolemia.

"Neurogenic shock" results from herniation of the brainstem, with subsequent loss of vasomotor function and vascular tone. "Hypovolemic shock" can result from internal or external hemorrhage, decreased circulating plasma volume during the treatment of cerebral edema with diuretics, and diabetes insipidus that results from pressure on the pituitary gland during brainsteam herniation. Neurogenic shock and hypovolemic shock require the same primary intervention: immediate restoration of effective circulating plasma volume.

Interventions for hypotension secondary to neurogenic shock. Acute hypotension resulting from brainstem herniation is treated by fluid resuscitation and administration of inotropic agents. If serum electrolyte values are normal, the rapid intravenous (IV) infusion of several liters (1 to 3) of lactated Ringer's solution is indicated. The endpoints of therapy are a systolic blood pressure greater than 90 mm Hg and a CVP of 6 to 10 mm Hg. If the patient is hypernatremic, crystalloid solutions such as $D_5.2NS$ or D_5W are used.

Frequently, rehydration alone is insufficient to maintain blood pressure at levels adequate to ensure organ perfusion. In this case, inotropic agents are administered in the lowest possible dosages and weaned as soon as tolerated by the patient. Dopamine and dobutamine are most commonly used for this purpose. Other inotropic agents that are also potent vasoconstrictors, such as metaraminol bitartrate (Aramine), norepinephrine bitartrate (Levophed), methoxamine hydrochloride (Vasoxyl), epinephrine, and phenylephrin hydrochloride (neo-Synephrine), are avoided.

Dopamine. Dopamine (Inotropin) is administered as a continuous IV infusion, beginning at a rate of 5 µg/kg/min and not exceeding 15 µg/kg/min. The endpoint of therapy is a systolic blood pressure greater than 90 mm Hg. When dopamine is given in dosages higher than 15 µg/kg/min, renal and mesenteric vasculature is constricted, which can jeopardize perfusion to the kidneys, liver, and pancreas.

Dobutamine. Dobutamine (Dobutrex) is administered as a continuous IV infusion, beginning at a rate of 5 µg/kg/min and titrated to maintain a systolic blood pressure greater than 90 mm Hg.

Interventions for hypotension secondary to hemorrhage. Hypotension resulting from hemorrhage is treated with the aggressive infusion of packed red blood cells and volume expanders such as hespan. Hemoglobin and hematocrit values are obtained about every 2 hours until stabilized, then about every 4 hours. Concomitant crystalloid therapy is instituted based on serum electrolyte values and vital signs. The endpoints of therapy are the same as those stated above.

Interventions for hypotension secondary to therapeutic dehydration for cerebral edema. A primary intervention for the patient with a closed head injury is the promotion of osmotic diuresis to decrease cerebral edema and intracranial hypertension. The pharmacologic agents most commonly used are mannitol and furosemide. Osmotic diuresis, in combination with other cardiovascular effects of a severe CNS insult, can result in significant depletion of intravascular volume and hypotension. Crystalloid fluid administration sufficient to maintain the CVP at 6 to 12 cm H_2O pressure is the appropriate preventive and therapeutic intervention.

Interventions for hypotension secondary to diabetes insipidus. Diabetes insipidus (DI) is a condition that occurs when intracranial hypertension is sufficient to compress the pituitary gland, which lies over the brainstem. Compression of the pituitary gland prevents the action of antidiuretic hormone, resulting in massive diuresis. It is characterized by urine output greater than 7 ml/kg/min, urine specific gravity less than 1.005, serum osmolarity greater than 300 mOsm, and serum sodium greater than 150 mEq/L. Interventions for DI include replacement of urine output milliliter for milliliter with D_5W and intravenous aqueous vasopressin tannate (Pitressin). The normal concentration of aqueous vasopressin tannate used is 50 units in 500 ml D_5W, and it is infused at 1 to 2 units/hr. Desmopressin (DDAVP), a potent derivative of vasopressin tannate, may also be used, particularly if Pitressin is ineffective.

Electrolyte imbalances. Various abnormalities in the serum electrolyte balance occur as a result of brain death. The mechanism of injury and treatment modalities discussed contribute to this problem. The most common electrolyte imbalances complicating donor management are hypernatremia, hypokalemia, and hyperkalemia. Management of these imbalances depends on an understanding of the altered physiology of the donor. The goal of electrolyte management in the organ donor is restoration of serum electrolytes to normal values.

Hypernatremia. Hypernatremia is defined as a serum sodium greater than 145 mEq/L. In the organ donor, hypernatremia results from dehydration secondary to therapeutic diuresis and DI. Clinical manifestations include elevated serum sodium, serum chloride, BUN, and serum creatinine; decreased urine output; and elevated urine specific gravity (except in DI). Interventions begin with resuscitation with sodium-poor fluids and later the administration of furosemide to promote normal diuresis. In extreme cases, correction of hypernatremia should take place over 8 to 12 hours to prevent extracellular fluid overload.

Hypokalemia. Hypokalemia is defined as a serum potassium level of less than 3.5 mEq/L. In the organ donor, hypokalemia results from excessive therapeutic diuresis and DI. The most serious complication is the development of ventricular dysrhythmias secondary to ventricular irritability. Correction of hypokalemia is accomplished by adding potassium chloride to maintenance IV fluids (e.g., 20 mEq potassium chloride per liter) or, in more serious cases, by administration of potassium chloride boluses (e.g., 10 mEq potassium chloride in 50 ml D_5W over 1 hour).

Hyperkalemia. Hyperkalemia is defined as a serum potassium level greater than 5.5 mEq/L. Although hyperkalemia is rare in the organ donor, it can occur in the oliguric multiple-trauma victim or as a result of excessive potassium supplementation. Life-threatening dysrhythmias, hypotension, and cardiac arrest can occur in extreme cases.

Mild cases of hyperkalemia are treated by removing any potassium from IV fluids and forced diuresis. More severe cases are treated with the administration of IV sodium bicarbonate; 50% dextrose and insulin (5 to 10 units of regular insulin per ampule of 50% dextrose); or the combination of 10% dextrose, sodium bicarbonate, and insulin.

Oliguria. Oliguria is defined as a urine output of less than 0.5 ml/kg/min for 2 consecutive hours. The maintenance of optimal renal function is critical in the organ donor. To prevent oliguria, urine output is replaced milliliter for milliliter on an hourly basis. When oliguria occurs, interventions include fluid resuscitation in the form of fluid boluses, followed by diuretics such as furosemide and mannitol.

Hyperosmolar diuresis. Hyperglycemic hyperosmolar diuresis is not uncommon in the organ donor as a result of the administration of large volumes of dextrose-containing solutions. Clinical manifestations include a serum glucose greater than 500 mg/dl, serum osmolarity greater than 350 mOsm, and increased urine output. Interventions include removal of dextrose from IV solutions, discontinuation of vasopressin tannate (Pitressin), and administration of insulin.

Pulmonary compromise. The brain-dead organ donor loses function of the respiratory center in the brainstem and requires mechanical ventilatory assistance and oxygenation. Without this support, hypoxemia and cellular death would occur. Optimal donor management includes close monitoring of pulmonary function, including arterial blood gas (ABG) monitoring and pulmonary hygiene. The endpoints of therapy are pao_2 greater than 80 to 90 torr, a $paco_2$ between 35 and 45 torr, and Sao_2 greater than 90%. Mechanical ventilatory parameters are manipulated frequently to maintain ABGs within these limits.

Several conditions can compromise pulmonary function in the organ donor. These include pulmonary edema, pneumonia, and pneumothorax.

Pulmonary edema. Pulmonary edema can occur as a result of aggressive fluid resuscitation. Manifestations include elevated CVP, distended neck veins, pulmonary crackles and, eventually, a decreased pao_2. Interventions include diuresis, the addition of positive end-expiratory pressure (PEEP), and increasing the FIo_2.

Pneumonia. Pneumonia is defined as an inflammatory condition in the lungs caused by bacterial, viral, fungal, or protozoal infection. In the organ donor, etiologic factors include the presence of an endotracheal tube, poor pulmonary hygiene, immobility, weakened resistance to infection, and aspiration. Interventions include preventive pulmonary hygiene, administration of antibiotics, and manipulation of mechanical ventilatory parameters to optimize oxygenation and ventilation.

Pneumothorax. Pneumothorax is defined as free air in the pleural space resulting in collapse of the lung. In the organ donor, pneumothorax can be the result of initial trauma, trauma sustained during central venous catheter placement, or high levels of PEEP. Pneumothorax is manifested by a sudden decrease in the pao_2, an increase in the $Paco_2$, decreased breath sounds over the affected lung, increased ventilatory pressures, and tracheal deviation away from the affected lung. The immediate intervention is placement of a chest tube in the affected pleural space.

Loss of thermoregulation

Brain-dead individuals lose the ability to regulate body temperature and thus have a tendency to become hypothermic after brainstem herniation. It is necessary to monitor temperature constantly by use of a rectal or esophageal probe, and it is desirable to maintain a core temperature of at least 34.4° C. Temperatures below 36.1° C can lead to decreased glomerular filtration, decreased heart rate, and increased serum glucose. Temperatures of 33.8° C and below can lead to ventricular fibrillation and cardiac arrest. Therapy consists of use of a hyperthermia blanket, radiant warmers, wrapping of head and extremities, and administration of warmed IV fluids and blood products.

Infection

Because of the nature of injuries (many are traumatic) and the need for intensive care and invasive interventions, the development of infection is a potential problem in all potential organ donors. Avoidance of infection is accomplished with the same precautions used for any patient. Blood and sometimes sputum cultures are routinely obtained, and broad-spectrum antibiotics are routinely ordered for potential organ donors.

ORGAN RECOVERY

Organ recovery is undertaken in the operating room of the donor hospital only after an important series of events takes place: timely recognition of a potential donor, notification of an OPO, diagnosis of brain death, family consent, and optimal donor management throughout this process. The organs recovered vary from situation to situation and depend on the family's consent, condition of the donor, height and weight of the donor, and proximity of the donor to other transplant centers. The operating room at the donor hospital customarily has at least several hours to prepare for organ recovery because of the time involved in coordinating multiple surgical teams, many times geographically distant in many directions. Recovery and preservation times for recovered organs and tissues are shown in Table 5-5. It is during this process that the invaluable role of the organ recovery coordinator is most realized.

It is also during this time that the psychosocial support skills of the critical care nursing team are called on. Careful consideration of the family's special needs at this time are of paramount importance to the effort of increasing organ donation. There is, of course, no one description of a family's response to this crisis,

Table 5-5 Tissue and organ recovery chart (after cessation of vital signs)

Organ/ tissue	Maximum recovery time	Maximum preservation time	Preservation medium
Bone	24 hr	2 hr/indefinite	Fresh frozen, sterilized in ethylene oxide or irradiated
Bone Marrow	6 hr	Indefinite	Frozen in liquid nitrogen
Cornea	6 hr	7 days	Cold gentamicin with pH buffer
Heart	Immediate	3-5 hr	Cold normal saline
Kidney	Immediate	48 hr	Cold Euro-Collins, Viaspan
Liver	Immediate	24 hr	Cold Euro-Collins, Viaspan
Pancreas	Immediate	8 hr	Cold Euro-Collins, Viaspan

Adapted from LifeLink of Georgia, Atlanta, Ga, 1979.

and interventions are therefore highly individualized. In addition to obvious crisis interventions, the family may need pastoral support and assistance with making funeral arrangements. A family may have difficulty saying goodbye and leaving the hospital for the final time. Sensitivity to this issue by the critical care nursing team can assist the family in coping with their loss.

And let us not forget about each other, because caring for a critically injured patient is stressful in its own right. Caring for the brain-dead patient and family is a special situation with its own unique set of stressors. Tremendous personal resources are expended during the donor management phase, and then as quickly as it all began, it is over—the patient is taken to the operating room, not to return. The primary nurse needs the same sensitivity from her or his nurse colleagues that she or he gives to the family in this situation. This is, unfortunately, too often overlooked. There is often little or no time to debrief, because the next situation requiring the nurse's full attention is minutes away.

Transport of the donor

Donor management continues until the aorta is clamped in the operating room to begin the actual removal of organs. Transport of the donor from the intensive care unit to the operating room is a critical time in the organ recovery process. Considering the tenuous condition of the patient, necessitating the presence of multiple intravenous catheters, the use of inotropic drugs, the need for continuous ventilatory support, and the number of personnel involved, numerous avenues for error can present during this time. Extreme care is taken not to interrupt any of these interventions vital to organ viability.

Multiple organ recovery

With the current status of renal and extrarenal organ transplantation and the proliferation of transplant centers, multiple organ recovery has become commonplace. Multiple organ recovery can be done effectively in any hospital capable of performing routine major surgical proce-

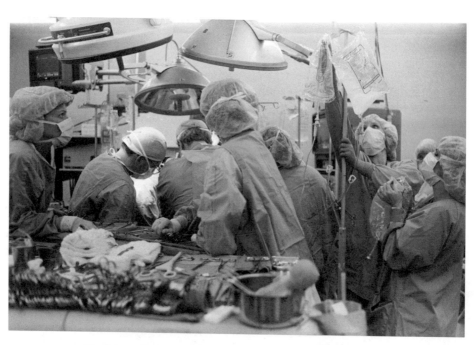

Fig. 5-1 Multiple-organ recovery team in the operating room.

dures. However, each recovery team must provide its own special equipment.

During multiple organ recovery, as many as four separate surgical teams may be operating in the same surgical field (Fig. 5-1). At no time is collaboration more important in the operating room. The future viability of all recovered organs is dependent on this cooperative effort. Regardless of the organs to be recovered, a standard midline incision is made from the suprasternal notch to the pubis.

Organ preservation

Successul preservation of cadaver kidney grafts by continuous hypothermic pulsatile perfusion or simple cold storage was demonstrated almost 20 years ago by Belzer and Collins.[37,38] The three principles of cold storage are (1) vascular flushing with rapid cooling, (2) prevention of cellular swelling with establishment of equilibrium between the graft tissue and preservation solution, and (3) prevention of excessive cellular acidosis.

Until recently, the only commercially available preservation solution was Euro-Collins solution, essentially a balanced electrolyte solution. Euro-Collins solution provides a simple means of short-term organ preservation. However, problems with delayed kidney graft function and the need for posttransplant dialysis, prompted investigations for a superior preservation solution.[39] The University of Wisconsin developed a solution that contains hydroxylethyl starch, which provides better metabolic substrate for organ metabolism. Using this solution, canine liver, pancreas, and kidney have been effectively preserved for as long as 30 hours,[40] 72 hours,[41] and 5 days,[42] respectively. Preservation times of human organs have greatly increased, also. Human liver preservation times now exceed 10 hours.[43] The Wisconsin solution is commercially available as Viaspan.

SUMMARY

"Successful organ procurement requires sincerity and sensitivity, dedication and determination, statesmanship and citizenship, honesty and integrity."[44] The technology of organ and tissue transplantation has evolved into a multidimensional effort to assist those facing a sure death from various forms of end-stage organ disease. However, the major rate-limiting factor continues to be a shortage of donor organs. The effort to increase organ recovery for transplantation begins with each of us and extends to all levels of the nursing and medical professions.

REFERENCES

1. President's Commission for the Study of Ethical Problems in Medicine and Biomedical and Behavioral Research (1981). *Defining death: medical, legal and ethical issues in the determination of death.* Washington, DC: US Government Printing Office.
2. Guidelines for the determination of death: report of the medical consultants on the diagnosis of death to the President's Commission for the Study of Ethical Problems in Medical and Biomedical and Behavioral Research (1981). *Journal of the American Medical Association, 246,* 2184-2186.
3. Black PMcL (1978). Brain death. *New England Journal of Medicine, 299,* 338-344.
4. United Network for Organ Sharing (1989). *UNOS Update, 5,* Issue 2, Richmond, VA.
5. Black PMcL (1978). Brain death. *New England Journal of Medicine, 299,* 393-401.
6. Younger SJ, Allen M, Bartlett ET, Cascorbi HF, Han T, Jackson DL, Mahowald MB and Martin BJ (1985). Psychosocial and ethical complications of organ retrieval. *New England Journal of Medicine, 313,* 321-324.
7. Council on Scientific Affairs of the American Medical Association (1981). Organ donor recruitment. *Journal of the American Medical Association, 246,* 2157-2158.
8. The Gallup Organization (April 1987). *The U.S. Public's attitudes toward organ transplants/organ donation: 1987.* Survey conducted for the Dow Chemical Company. Princeton, N.J., The Gallup Organization.
9. Office of Organ Transplantation (1987). *The status of organ donation and coordination services: Report to the Congress for fiscal year 1987,* U.S. Department of Health and Human Services.
10. The Catholic Hospital Association (1975). *Religious aspects of medical care.* St. Louis: The Catholic Hospital Association.
11. LifeLink of Georgia (1987). *Organ and tissue donor manual.* Atlanta, Ga.
12. Pittsburgh Transplant Foundation. *Statement of major faiths regarding anatomical gifts.* Pittsburgh: Pittsburgh Transplant Foundation.
13. Bart KJ, Macon EJ and Humphries AL (1981). Increasing the supply of cadaveric kidneys for transplantation. *Transplantation, 31,* 383-387.
14. Bart KJ, Macon EJ and Humphries AL (1979). A response to the shortage of cadaveric kidneys for transplantation. *Transplantation Proceedings, 11,* 455-458.

15. Corlett S (1985). Professional and system barriers to organ donation. *Transplantation Proceedings, 17*(753), 111-119.

16. Caplan AL (1988). Beg, borrow or steal: the ethics of solid organ procurement. In Mathieu D (ed). *Organ substitution technology. Ethical, legal and public policy issues.* Boulder: Westview Press (59-68).

17. Robertson JA (1988). Relaxing the death standard for organ donation in pediatric situations. In Mathieu D (ed). *Organ substitution technology. Ethical, legal and public policy issues.* Boulder: Westview Press, pp. 69-76.

18. Sadler AM, Sadler BL and Stason EB (1968). The Uniform Anatomical Gift Act: a model for reform. *Journal of the American Medical Association, 206,* 2501-2506.

19. Overcast TD, Evans RW, Bower LE, Hoe MM and Lirak CL (1984). Problems in the identification of potential organ donors: misconceptions and fallacies associated with donor cards. *Journal of the American Medical Association, 251,* 1559-1562.

20. Commissioners on Uniform State Laws (July 1987). *Uniform Anatomical Gift Act of 1987.* National Conference of Commissioners on Uniform State Laws. Newport Beach, Calif.

21. Task Force on Organ Transplantation (April 1986). *Organ transplantation: issues and recommendations.* Rockville, Md: Health Resources and Services Administration. (NTIS No. HRP-0906976).

22. Harrel AE. Director of Professional and Public Affairs, American Council on Transplantation. Personal communication. April 1988.

23. DeChesser AD (1986). Organ donation: the supply-demand discrepancy. *Heart and Lung, 15,* 547-551.

24. Metz RA (1988). Organ procurement and transplantation, a view from the front lines. *Contemporary Dialysis and Nephrology,* July, 38-39.

25. Prottas JM (1985). The structure and effectiveness of the U.S. organ procurement system. *Inquiry, 22,* 365-376.

26. Personal communication: Southeastern Organ Procurement Foundation. July 1988.

27. American Association of Critical-Care Nurses (1986). *Position statement: roles and responsibilities of the critical care nurse in organ and tissue transplantation.* American Association of Critical-Care Nurses.

28. American Association of Critical-Care Nurses (1986). *Position statement: required request and routine inquiry: methods to improve the organ and tissues donation processes.* American Association of Critical-Care Nurses.

29. Davis FD (1987). Coordination of cardiac transplantation: patient processing and donor organ procurement. *Circulation, 75,* 29-39.

30. Cecka JM (1987). In Terasaki PI (ed). *Clinical transplants 1987.* (423-434). Los Angeles, Calif: UCLA Tissue Typing Laboratory.

31. Kormos RL, Donato W, Hardesty RL, Griffith BP, Kiernan J and Trento A (1988). The influence of donor organ stability and ischemia time on subsequent cardiac recipient survival. *Transplantation Proceedings, 20* (Suppl 1), 980-983.

32. Rudy E (1982). Brain death. *Dimensions of Critical Care Nursing, 1*(3), 178-184.

33. Beecher HKA (1968). Definitions of irreversible coma. Report of the Ad Hoc Committee of the Harvard Medical School to examine the definition of brain death. *Journal of the American Medical Association, 205,* 337-340.

34. American Medical Association House of Delegates (1974). Definition of death. *Journal of the American Medical Association, 227,* 728.

35. Younger SJ, Landefeld CS, Coulton CJ and Juknialis BW (1989). Brain death and organ retrieval. A cross-sectional survey of knowledge and concepts among health professions. *Journal of the American Medical Association, 261,* 2205-2210.

36. Van Thiel DH, Shade RR, Hakala TR and Starzite DD (1984). Liver procurement for orthotopic transplantation: an analysis of the Pittsburgh experience. *Hepatology, 4,* 66S-71S.

37. Belzer FO, Ashby BS and Dumphy JE (1967). 24- and 72-hour preservation of canine kidneys. *Lancet, 2,* 536-539.

38. Collins GH, Bravo-Shugarman MB and Terasaki PI (1969). Kidney preservation for transplantation: initial perfusion and 30 hour ice storage. *Lancet, 2,* 1219.

39. Sanfilippo F, Vaughn WK, Spees EK and Lucas BA (1984). The detrimental effects of delayed graft function in cadaver donor renal transplantation. *Transplantation, 38,* 643.

40. Jamieson NV, Sandberg R, Lindell S, Southard JH and Belzer FO (1988). Successful 24- and 30-hour preservation of the canine liver: a preliminary report. *Transplantation Proceedings, 20,* 945-947.

41. Wallberg JA, Love R, Landegaard L, Southard JH and Belzer FO (1987). 72-hour preservation of the canine pancreas. *Transplantation, 43,* 5-8.

42. McAnulty JF, Ploeg RJ, Southard JH and Belzer FO (1989). Successful five-day perfusion preservation of the canine kidney. *Transplantation, 47,* 37-41.

43. Kalayoglu M, Sollinger HW, Stratta RJ, D'Alessandro AM, Hoffman RM, Pirsch JD, and Belzer FO (1988). Extended preservation of the liver for clinical transplantation. *Lancet, 1,* 617-619.

6

Ethical Issues

Anna Omery

This chapter examines the moral and ethical issues that surround transplantation. Successes in transplantation have led to an ever-increasing number of transplants. In 1987, there were 1400 cardiac transplants performed in nine centers.[1,2] And in 1986, in slightly less than a 2-year period, one liver transplant center performed its one-hundredth transplant.[3]

Not only are the number of transplants increasing, the transplantation of an increasing number of organs or tissues, such as the pancreas, is occurring.

Before their transplant surgeries, the individual patients whom these numbers represent may be significantly dependent on the health care system. This dependency may be dramatic. It may mean that their very lives depend on multiple trips to medical centers in just 1 week's time to maintain life. Patients often are critically ill.

After the transplant, the nurse sees a completely different individual from that pretransplant patient: The successful transplant patient may return to full participation in life, to the great satisfaction of health care providers. The fact that the health care team cannot only perform transplants, but also perform them successfully, results in the transplant procedure's taking on a positive value orientation for many, including the nurse.

At the same time that transplantation is taking on its positive orientation, it often becomes obligatory; that is, the nurse comes to believe that not only is it good to do transplants, it is required of the health care system to do so.

Isn't this the purpose of the health care system? Isn't it required that doctors and nurses deliver this course of treatment to the best of their ability and to the greatest extent possible? When the value associated with a medical intervention or treatment such as transplantation moves from being a singular good to being a good that the nurse must, or ought to, actualize, the nurse moves into the moral domain. It is in this domain that ethics exist.

THE ETHICAL RESPONSE

Ethics has been described as the way of teaching one how to live with another.[4] It reflects the critical normative analysis of how one ought to live with another. As a result, it distinguishes the "ought" or "should" of our daily existence.

Much like nursing, ethics can be defined as an art and science. Ethics is an art in that it involves an intuitive sense of association with the world in which we live. As with any art, it can only be actualized in the lived experience of our day-to-day world. It is a science in that it weighs, assesses, analyzes, and studies relationships of empirical data. This art/science seeks to bring sensitivity and method to the discernment of moral values, that is, values of right or wrong, ought or ought not.[5]

The ethical response then becomes that deliberate and critically analyzed response that is both prescriptive and normative. It is prescriptive in that it prescribes or defines for the critical care nurse the appropriate course of action. It is normative in that it establishes the norms or standards for that issue.

Ethics can be divided into at least two classifications, normative and descriptive ethics. Normative ethics is the analysis of how the individual moral agent ought to live or behave. It examines both the possible alternatives for any ethical dilemma and the ethical implications or foundations for those alternatives. Descriptive ethics is the appraisal of the actual thoughts and behaviors of the individual in any given moral-ethical situation. The focus in this chapter is on normative ethics.

When faced with an ethical dilemma in practice, some nurses believe that being ethical is to consult the last court case or law related to that issue. If they abide by that societal directive, they will then have adequately addressed the ethical dilemma.

Certainly ethics has a relationship to the legal system. The content of any legal system consists of codified standards of behavior regarding right or wrong for any group of society. Ethics is not, however, the same as the legal system. What is legal (i.e., accepted and codified) is not necessarily ethical. Consequently, when one is faced with the decision-making process that is the result of an ethical dilemma, one may be concerned with (or even advised to be concerned with) legal standards. The nurse should realize that these standards (i.e., laws) will not necessarily give the definitive answer for that dilemma. To truly be a moral-ethical agent, it may become necessary to challenge the societal standard of what is right or wrong for the individuals in that particular ethical dilemma.

Any response to an ethical dilemma should be assessed, analyzed, and studied. This analysis should include a clarification of the ethical principles used to support or justify the final decision. Ethical principles are the relevant generalizations about what befits or does not befit the behavior of human beings.[6] The box above, right lists the ethical principles considered in this chapter.

Identifying the foundation of ethical principles may enable one to become aware of her or his value system. Personal value systems play a significant role in the decisions of the health care provider. Enhanced awareness will not necessarily make the resolution of an ethical dilemma easier. It can, however, result in more

---

ETHICAL PRINCIPLES

Autonomy
Beneficence
Justice
Nonmaleficence
Respect for persons
Utility
Veracity

---

effective communication for the nurse with her or his peers, fellow professionals, and patients. It can also give her or him a perspective of self that would otherwise be missing. This increased sense of self can support the nurse so that she or he feels more competent in the day-to-day moral decisions inherent in clinical practice.

Many of the ethical issues that critical care nurses face occur under emergent conditions. Frequently, then, a nurse may have to go with a "gut" response initially. While this type of response may be effective for the short term, the inconsistencies that accompany the continued use of such intuitive strategies can lead to frustration and even burnout. As a result, it is much more effective to identify the issues of concern that will be ongoing and address them in a systematic and rigorous way, or as an ethical response.

ETHICAL ISSUES SURROUNDING TRANSPLANTATION

The ethical issues that result from transplantation exist at the macro, or societal, level and at the micro, or institutional or individual, level. This is not to say that macro and micro issues have no relationship to each other. Almost all ethical issues have implications for both levels. However, those issues at the macro level are best addressed through public policy. Specific macro issues related to transplantation are allocation of scarce resources, and the expansion of transplantation technology. Micro issues are more likely to be addressed at the institutional level through the interpretation of already established policies or at the individual level through moral standards. Micro issues related to transplantation include the meaning of death and its relationship to the transplant process, and transplantation as a cure versus chronic disease.

Macro ethical issues

There are few in this country who believe adequate resources exist to meet all the health care needs of each individual citizen. The issue then becomes "who shall receive the available health care?"[7] And for many patients, including most transplant recipients, the question becomes "who shall live?"

Organ allocation. There have always been more potential organ recipients than available organs. What, then, are the moral obligations of a society to make such organs and tissues available? What moral authority does the society have to ensure or assist in organ recovery and donation?

Most societies that have the resources to perform transplants are peaceable, pluralistic ones that have renounced the use of force to impose a particular ideology or view of the good life. These societies usually include numerous communities with both convergent and divergent views on how their citizens should live and use their resources. In such societies morality, as opposed to force, is the basis for resolution of disputes related to distribution of a limited resource. The focus in resolving any dispute is on mutual respect of persons and autonomy.[8-10] Autonomy is the ethical principle that supports the right of the individual to determine his or her own course of action and act on it. Any possible resolution to procurement and distribution of a limited resource, such as an organ or tissue, will reflect this focus of respect for persons and autonomy. Any force or coercion in the strategies will therefore be unacceptable.

In the United States, the first national effort directed toward organ donation and recovery was a form of encouraged volunteerism. This ideal of voluntarily donating organs reflects those values of respect and personal autonomy. This first effort was the Uniform Anatomical Gift Act, drafted in 1968 and adopted by all states by 1971. The purpose of the Act was to increase organ recovery and donation through (1) the authorization of persons 18 years or older to donate all or part of their bodies after death for medical purposes, (2) giving the next of kin of any potential donor the authority to donate (if the individual who was to be the donor had not indicated prior opposition), and (3) specifying mechanisms for donation, such as carrying a donor card.

Although the Act standardized state laws pertaining to organ donation, it provided little direction for the mechanism of making a request for an organ. It also gave little direction on how, and to what extent, consent should be sought. As a result, health care providers continued to feel uneasy about requesting organ donation and sought consent from immediate family members even when a donor card was signed and available.[12]

Given these constraints, the Uniform Anatomical Gift Act has not resulted in the desired, increased availability of donor organs. There is still a dramatic need, with approximately one third of patients accepted for transplantation dying while awaiting a donor organ.[13]

Given the lack of success, other options or alternatives for increasing organ donation have been suggested.[14-17] These options are required request,[18] presumed consent,[19] and the marketing and selling of organs.[20,21]

Required request is the recovery option that has been most readily implemented to increase the number of donor organs available in the United States. Under this alternative, the option of organ donation must be presented to individuals and/or their families.[22] The Report of the U.S. Department of Health and Human Services Task Force on Organ Transplantation[23] strongly recommended required request over other alternatives for increasing the availability of transplantable organs. This report urged the adoption of required request legislation by all state governments.

Mechanisms vary for the implementation of required request. The least intrusive of these mechanisms includes the use of check-off boxes on government documents such as driver's licenses or social security cards. Childress[24] noted, however, that the public has expressed concerns about donor cards. Those laypersons surveyed felt that if they signed a donor card, they would not be aggressively treated. The respondents expressed their belief that they would be treated as potential donors, from whom organs could be recovered, rather than as possible survivors. Given this perspective, it is unlikely that the use of noncompulsory check-off boxes will meet with any more success than the carrying of voluntary donor cards. If our society continues to operate from the values of respect and personal autonomy, there will be little impetus to encourage participation. The probable result is, then, that this mechanism will have little impact on future organ availability.

Another mechanism for required request includes the mandatory requirement by the state government that hospitals develop some policy that will ensure that families of potential donors are given the option to donate. The result of this mechanism is usually a policy whereby physicians and nurses are required to complete an educational program on early identification of potential donors. They are then obligated to offer the option of donation to family members of dying or dead patients.

Supporters of required request cite polls in which eight of ten families in the United States responded that if approached they would donate. The supporters also argue that the mechanism is consistent with the values of respect for person and autonomy. Consequently, supporters feel that this mechanism has the greatest chance of increasing the number of donor organs available without violating these ethical principles.

This mechanism is not, however, without difficulties. As previously indicated, respect and autonomy are the normative principles that prescribe the actions surrounding organ recovery in our society. Do these principles have any less relevance when the individual is not the potential recipient or donor, but is the physician or nurse? Does an individual lose her or his right of autonomy when she or he takes on the role of a health care provider? Should nurses and physicians be constrained into making a required request for potential donor organs? Whether autonomy is valued can be critically debated if there is legal constraint or coercion for any participant in the recovery process.

What about those clinical situations in which to request would be, in the health care provid-

er's best judgment, harmful to the potential donor's family? A possible scenario includes the family of an accident victim who has a massive head injury. The severity and the suddenness of the illness may have left the family in extreme distress, possibly in psychologic crisis. An important and legitimate question is: Should the health care provider be required to make a request under these circumstances? The reality is that this represents the most common scenario involving potential organ donors.

Under certain required consent statutes, such as those in Oregon, the health care provider has the option not to make the request if such a request would be of significant harm to the family. Under these statutes, the health care provider retains her or his right to autonomous clinical judgment. She or he may, however, open a door for not requesting organs, thereby defeating the purpose of increasing the supply of donor organs.

Indeed, supporters of the second strategy, presumed consent, point out that with the failure of encouraged volunteerism–based strategies, there is no reason to expect any substantial increase in the number of organs resulting from required request. Presumed consent gives authority to physicians to remove organs for the purpose of transplantation without the explicit consent of the individual or family. Families, if approached, would not be asked whether they consent to the donation but rather whether they have any objections. Unless the individual has placed her or his name on a central computer registry indicating an objection to transplantation, or families have raised an explicit objection, the organ would be recovered.

Thirteen, mostly European, countries have presumed consent laws.[19] In about half of those countries (Finland, Greece, Italy, Norway, Spain, and Sweden), physicians still consult the family of the donor to make sure there is no objection on their part. In Austria, Czechoslovakia, Denmark, France, Israel, Poland, and Switzerland, physicians proceed with retrieval of organs without asking, unless an objection is raised by the family.

Supporters of the presumed consent argue that not only will the strategy increase the supply of organs, it also has ethical advantages.

They argue that there would be more respect for person using this strategy. The individuals involved would understand that organ donation was routine and would not have to make a difficult decision while experiencing a tragic and unexpected loss. Proponents also maintain that any loss in autonomy could be minimized through the establishment and use of a registry.

Opponents of presumed consent raise the counter point that presumed consent has not resulted in meeting the organ needs in the countries where it has been implemented. Critics note that presumed consent may violate the relationship of trust and/or the promise of fidelity that are important, perhaps even essential, constituents of the nurse-patient or physician-patient relationships.[25,26] They also question whether the potential donor and/or donor family's autonomy (as well as the respect for their persons) might be more easily abused under a strategy in which health care providers are not required to meet with or talk to the individual or the family.

The final strategy to increase the availability of donor organs is the market approach. Under the market approach, bodies and body parts are considered property for possible sale. Marketing approaches range from financial inducements to the selling of organs by the individual or family to the person or group willing to pay the best price.

Supporters of the market approach contend that society would benefit from such a strategy and that the financial inducement could greatly increase the availability of organs. Strategies for protecting the donor under the market approach include development of standards that would (1) require donor consent for use of organs in research, (2) protect the donor from coercion, and (3) ensure reimbursement for donations.

Opponents focus on potential harms to the donor and to society, especially some of its most vulnerable members—the poor and children. Critics note that while autonomy might be maximized under this strategy, in that there is freedom for the individual or family to proceed as they and/or the market wishes, there is certainly a danger to respect for person. It may become possible for persons to be treated as a means to an end, as a potential organ donor, rather than being respected in and for themselves, as a valuable human being.

In addition, this strategy would very likely violate the principle of justice. Rather than being distributed equitably, organs would go to the persons who could best afford them. There would be no assurance that the purchaser would also be the individual who could benefit most from the organ in terms of the potential for return to a full and productive life.

The nurse's role. There is no certainty that any of these potential or actual strategies will definitively increase the supply of donor organs or tissues. In addition, there are moral advantages and disadvantages to each of these strategies. How then should the critical care nurse address the ethical issues surrounding the recovery and donation of the scarce resource that is the donor organ?

Good ethics depends on valid and reliable facts and on open dialogue. Critical care nurses need to share their knowledge and values at public hearings where these issues are addressed. Nurses should also take note of witnesses to closed hearings and membership on government task forces addressing transplant issues to determine whether nurses are actively participating. When nursing is not represented, nurses should notify both their government representatives and their professional organizations. For it is only when nursing representatives share nursing facts and values in these dialogues that nursing's ethical voice will be heard.

The American Association of Critical-Care Nurses (AACN) has authored two position papers related to organ transplantation. These papers are "Roles and Responsibilities of Critical Care Nurses in Organ and Tissue Donation"[27] and "Required Request and Routine Inquiry: Methods to Improve Organ and Tissue Donation."[28] The presence of position statements, however, does not ensure active involvement. What is incumbent on the profession is the enabling of each nurse in the practice setting. Conditions must be created in each setting that will enable the nurse to act on her or his autonomy.

Allocation of nursing care. Currently there is a substantial worldwide shortage of nurses. Although there has been some increase in enrollments in schools of nursing recently, it will be several years before these nurses will be practicing at the bedside, let alone able to provide the complex and comprehensive care that the transplant patient requires.

In the interim, nurse managers are faced with the question of how to adequately distribute an increasingly precious resource: quality nursing care. Competent nursing care determines, in many cases, the difference between success and failure for many procedures, including organ transplantation.

Often, ethical discussions about the allocation of a scarce resource, such as the nurse, rely on the principle of justice (fairness) to defend decisions regarding distribution of that resource. Considerations of equity and impartiality are requirements of the principle of justice. Justice, in this context, implies that patients have equal right to consideration for health care, and the right to a similar standard of care.[29,30]

Although the application of the principle of justice may be appropriate in many circumstances, the use of this principle to defend any allocation of nursing care may be inadequate to support a totally comprehensive moral response. Consideration of equity may raise more dilemmas than it solves. Is nursing care to be distributed equitably according to expertise? What if the nurse who would best meet that requirement is also the nurse who has worked the most overtime in the last month and is about to burn out? To whom is the charge nurse or nurse manager obligated to be fair—the patient or the nurse?

Nurses may have difficulty in fulfilling the consideration of impartiality when making decisions regarding the distribution of nursing care to some transplant recipients. Nurses may feel that some transplant patients, especially certain liver or cardiac transplant patients, are culpable or responsible for their condition. It may be difficult for the nurse to impartially distribute care when perceiving that the patient is to blame and would not have needed a transplant if she or he had made different life-style choices.

Given these inadequacies of the principles of justice in this context, is there any other ethical standard, theory, or principle that the critical care nurse might use to guide the distribution of her or his resources? Perhaps use of the principle of beneficence would serve the nurse more effectively.

Beneficence, the moral imperative to do good, has always been a consideration in ethical decision-making in health care. Concerns about unrestricted beneficence, however, have made this principle secondary to other principles such as justice and autonomy. For beneficience run amok denies autonomy and becomes paternalism. Despite these legitimate concerns, beneficence remains, for many, the primary principle that should guide the ethics of health professionals.[31] Indeed, the application of this principle to allocation decisions concerning the nurse may have advantages.

Maguire has noted that a necessary component to ethical decision-making is creative imagination.[5] This creative imagination breaks the moral reasoner out of the bondage of the current state of things. Although application of the principle of justice may not deny the use of creative imagination, it may, with its emphasis on impartiality and equity, restrict it. The use of beneficence, of acting in the best interest of another to do good, may free the nurse to rationally perceive the actual, yet artfully perceive the possible. It may open her or his moral options to new and unique strategies.

Such strategies might include use of the media to exploit its potential for making others aware of the special role that nurses play in the care of transplant patients. It might include the development of new societal supported models for delivery of nursing care, such as the development of corporations, owned by the public and run by nurses, which lease their services back (under the corporation's control) to the health care institution.[32] Perhaps as we struggle to actualize beneficence in our care of patients there will also be another benefit. Perhaps we will also begin to feel more comfortable in actualizing greater beneficence in our orientation toward each other.

Allocation of resources. There are still other ethical concerns about allocation of resources related to transplantation that need to be addressed. Just because we can do transplants, should we?

Transplantation is an expensive procedure.[16] Renal transplantation is the least expensive, with an average cost of $25,000 to $30,000. The cost of a heart transplant may range from $57,000 to $110,000. The cost of a liver transplant may range from $135,000 to $238,000. These dollar amounts are averages. Although they do not reflect the case that proceeds very well and costs less, they also do not reflect the more complicated case that may cost substantially more. In addition, these numbers do not reflect the ongoing costs associated with transplantation. Immunosuppressive drugs can cost a patient $10,000 per year. The cost of ongoing medical care to monitor the posttransplant progress of the patient has yet to be comprehensively calculated.

More and more often, society is asking, "Is the survival of the one worth the cost to many?" The National Commission for the Study of Ethical Problems in Medicine and Biomedical and Behavioral Research examined this issue in a three-volume report.[33] In its summary, the Commission concluded that society has an ethical obligation to ensure equitable access to health care for all.

At least two states, Massachusetts and Oregon, have interpreted this statement to mean that just because a technology or procedure is available this does not mean that society is obligated to provide it. For the availability of a new or costly technology or procedure that is likely to save the lives of a few individuals should not jeopardize the access of all citizens to an adequate level of health care.[38] However, for the patient in need of a transplant residing in one of these states, this position is viewed as an unfair solution to an unfair problem.[34]

There is no clear consensus in this country on the definition of an adequate level of health care. A national social policy is needed that identifies for the citizen values and obligations related to transplantation. Such a policy might mean that fewer transplants would be performed. Yet, if interpreted equitably, it may be the closest that society can come to guaranteeing equal access to transplant resources.

Recipient selection. Most health care providers and ethicists who work with transplant patients would prefer that the recipient selection process for transplantation be based on criteria that are rational, objective, and scientific. These criteria should be data based and clearly associated with positive patient outcomes, such as survival.[35] Yet to date there is little empirical evidence to provide the basis for such criteria. Given that fact, transplant teams struggle, using current selection critera, to make the best choices.

Patient selection criteria. In the developmental stages of transplant technologies, the criteria for recipient selection were limiting. In 1969 a survey of renal transplant programs in the United States revealed that the most common criteria for selection were (1) willingness of the patient to cooperate, (2) medical suitability, (3) absence of other disabling disease, (4) ability to understand the treatment, (5) the likelihood for vocational rehabilitation, and (6) psychiatric stability. Selection criteria for hepatic and cardiac transplantation are usually a variation of the renal survey criteria. Liver transplant programs may add abstinence from alcohol or drug abuse for longer than 1 year. Cardiac transplant programs may add New York Heart Association class IV disability, or life expectancy of less than 6 months.

Patient selection criteria usually become more flexible as the procedures become more successful. As the transplant team becomes more expert, it is usually positively motivated by its successes. The positive motivators include the desire to increase research knowledge and to demonstrate expertise in what may be a difficult procedure. The team is also motivated by a desire to do good and to distribute its expertise justly. The result is that fewer patients with end-stage organ disease are denied candidacy for transplantation.

However, given the scarcity of resources such as donor organs and skilled nursing care, decisions still have to be made as to who will receive the organs and care that are available. Some argue that given the lack of definitive patient outcome criteria, determination of greatest medical need be used as a criterion for patient selection. The question then becomes, "How does one determine medical need?" Is it based on acuity? What determines acuity? Even if acuity can be determined, how does one select among several individuals if their acuity is comparable?

The Massachusetts Organ Donation Task Force advised that recipient selection criteria be just, fair, and equitable. This recommendation supports the selection of those individuals who could benefit most from the transplant in terms of long-term survival and potential for rehabilitation.[36] The Task Force specified, however, that in making this recommendation it was not endorsing age-specific criteria or social worth criteria.

Indeed, the question of age is one that has remained problematic. In the early years of transplantation, age was often a criterion. Many programs, for instance, used an upper age limit of 55. However, as selection criteria became less stringent and older individuals received organ transplants, it became evident that denying transplant based on age is not necessarily sound.

One issue related to transplant recipient selection that is not commonly discussed in the ethics literature is performing transplants for individuals who are not U.S. citizens. Currently some foreign residents, particularly if they have personal financial resources, are receiving transplants. Those who support performing transplants for such individuals note that the purpose of health care is to do good. Given that the resources in the donating country may be more plentiful than those in the recipient's country, is it not beneficent and just to do the transplant? Is it not maleficent not to do the transplant?

Persons who oppose performing transplants for individuals who are not citizens ask several cogent questions. Are health care providers truly doing good for these foreign citizens? Is it assuredly beneficent to send the recipient back to his or her home country if the recipient's home country does not have the resources to do the transplant surgery or provide the necessary immunosuppressants and follow-up care? If the answers are no to these questions, is the responsibility to give organs to those with the greatest chance for success being ignored? Is the selection of such patients really doing harm rather than good to the patient?

In an effort to move beyond these current debates, the suggestion has been made that all medically acceptable individuals be placed in a national transplant pool.[37] Once in the pool, each individual would receive a transplant on a first come, first served basis. Supporters of such a strategy believe it is the only way to truly be just or fair in selecting transplant recipients.

Until there are objective, reliable criteria (and one can question whether there ever will be), Caplan[38] suggests that strategies at the national level might best resolve the issue of transplant selection criteria. He contends that any transplant system that relies on public donation of organs must accept public regulation. Caplan proposes that there be (1) standardized selection criteria, (2) statements to candidates from transplant centers outlining their priorities (education, research and/or patient care), (3) a consensus that the second or greater transplant in the same individual be treated as experimental and given lower priority over other first transplants, (4) a national organ allocation network to which all transplant centers must belong, and (5) regulation of the number and quality of transplant centers.

Transplantation and technology. The allocation of scarce resources and related issues are not the only macro issues of concern for nurses. Issues also relate to the expansion of transplant technology. As with the other issues, it is necessary to understand their ethical foundations for an adequate ethical response to be drafted. Those issues related to the expansion of transplant technology are the use of xenografts and assistive devices.

Use of xenografts. Xenografting is a highly experimental procedure in organ transplantation. There is little scientific information to guide a transplant team caring for a xenograft recipient. The transplant of a 7-month-old baboon's heart into the infant Baby Fae at Loma Linda University in 1984 resulted in dramatic dialogs about the ethics of xenografting. It raised to the forefront questions about the human-animal relationship. It also forced many health care providers who work in transplantation to examine their own values related to the use of animals in medical research.

Baby Fae's baboon heart was not the first attempt to transplant an animal's organ into a human recipient. There have been at least seven other documented attempts.[39] Most took place in the 1960s, and all failed within 2 months. The use of xenografts raises at least two ethical issues. The first involves the justification of such a highly experimental procedure, and the second, the foundation for killing animals for organs.

Given that there is so little information available, is the ethical risk worth the potential cost? Is the unknown risk justifiable? Is it worth whatever life is offered? Does the need for organs justify the use of xenografts?

The second concern related to the use of xenografts involves the killing of animals. Do animals have equal rights to life? Do the rights of humans outweigh the rights of animals? When we begin to use animals as a means to an end, are we beginning an uncertain utilitarian process? Will the use of animals as organ donors be the beginning of use of others of our own species (such as the severely mentally retarded) as donors, rather than as valued members of the species?

These are but a few of the moral questions that need to be addressed if our health care system and society are to justify the use of xenografts. At present the past lack of success with xenografting has decreased the intensity of the debates surrounding this concern. As other attempts at xenografting are made, the debate will no doubt be heightened.

Use of assistive devices. The lack of available organs for transplant has led to the development of many new technologic devices related to organ and life support. The purpose of these devices is to temporarily or permanently assist an individual in survival, despite organ failure. Examples of such assistive devices include the hemodialysis machine, the extraventricular assist device, and the total artifical heart. These devices are not merely aids to human activities, but are powerful forces acting to reshape human activities and their meanings.[40] Before the development of assistive devices, providing health care to the patient with a failing organ meant giving comfort and treatment to maintain dignity until death. Now it may mean bridging the gap between life and death.

Commitment to a device should not overshadow the moral effort to do good through the use of technology. The use of an assistive device is most often a last life-prolonging effort. Concentration on the perfection or mainte-

nance of such devices, however, can result in losing sight of the human, with her or his associated rights of autonomy, connected to the device.

The use of such devices also raises, once more, the issue of allocation of a scarce resource, because access to the more sophisticated assistive devices is limited to patients at certain major medical centers. Once more, how is the choice of the patient to receive the device to be made? What recipient criteria are appropriate? Once more the question becomes, "How can we be fair to all?"

Macro issues summary. The macro issues of concern to nurses are (1) allocation of scarce resources (both the organ and the nurse), with the resulting issues of competition for the use of resources and patient selection criteria, and (2) the expansion of transplant technologies, to include xenografts and assistive devices. These issues will also be of concern to other members of the transplant community. However, the resolution of these issues will reflect nursing's perspective, values, and moral agency only when the nurse participates in the decision-making process.

Several recurring themes have surfaced in the discussion. The first of these is the requisite that nursing clarify its ethical response to these issues. A majority of the ethics-focused transplant literature reflects the traditional principles of justice, autonomy, beneficence, and respect for persons. The ethical principles underlying nursing's ethical response may be the same, but they may also include the principle of veracity—to tell the truth, and not to lie to deceive others.[41] There cannot be any certainty which principles are foundational to the ethical responses of nurses and nursing until those principles are identified and examined.

Mechanisms for the identification and examination of the principles that underlie the ethical response to issues related to transplantation include the literature and open forums. Nurses need to contribute to the general bioethics literature so that nursing's normative ethical responses are included in the total ethical response to transplantation. In addition, open forums at local, regional, and national professional conferences can provide opportunities for nurses to reflect their values in regards to transplantation and the allocation of resources.

The second recurring theme is the individual nurse's, and the nursing profession's, participation. Individual nurses and the nursing profession need to be involved in the discussion and resolution of issues related to transplantation. One way that this can happen is for nurses to participate on committees and task forces addressing these issues. Widespread participation, however, is necessary. If it is not, nursing ethics, as perceived by society and the rest of the transplant community, runs the danger of reflecting the ethics of only a few.

It may be difficult, after working an entire shift, to gather the energy to participate, especially when the second shift of spousehood and parenthood begins. The nurse may consider, however, that not to participate may mean being obligated to function under an ethical response that is inconsistent with that held personally.

Collectively, nursing's professional organizations can make a difference by making their positions known to the public and participating in health policy decision-making. Not to take a position on these issues, and failure to participate, is to take a position of laissez-faire and ambiguity.

Micro ethical issues: the nurse, the individual patient, and the transplant experience

Each of the macro issues previously discussed touches on each individual transplant experience. Yet there are certain ethical issues that impact and seek resolution at the bedside more frequently than at societal forums. Some of these issues began as societal issues but are now implemented at the bedside. On the other hand, there are also micro issues now evident at the bedside that will, with time, become broader, societal issues. The micro issues to be discussed are (1) the necessity of death for life through transplantation and (2) transplantation as a perceived cure.

The necessity of death for life through transplantation. Currently each organ or tissue donation requires a gift from another human being. In most cases, death is necessary for that gift to be actualized. For families and critical care nurses, it is often difficult to give up the

effort at life support and allow death. Because the potential organ donor is frequently aggressively resuscitated to maintain the viability of organs to be recovered, there may be a sense that life is not over for the donor. The death of the potential donor may also be perceived as a defeat, especially after many hours of complex care and hard work.

Although death may be perceived as a defeat, the idea of recovering organs without death is totally incompatible with any sense of morality. In fact, it was the public's fear that their vital organs might be taken from them that resulted in the first public debates regarding the advances in transplant technology. Before 1968, the generally accepted criteria for death were the absence of spontaneous heartbeats and/or respirations. In 1968, the now famous Ad Hoc Committee of the Harvard Medical School for the Definition of Death proposed that the absence of discernible central nervous system (CNS) activity be recognized as an acceptable criterion for defining death.

The eventual outcome was the Uniform National Determination of Death Act. Recommended by the President's Commission for the Study of Ethical Problems in Medicine and Biomedical and Behavioral Research,[42] this Act not only broadens the definition of death but also provides guidelines for identifying a condition that will sooner or later lead to cardiopulmonary cessation. The Act reads as follows:

An individual who has sustained either (1) irreversible cessation of circulatory and respiratory functions, or (2) irreversible cessation of all functions of the entire brain, including the brainstem, is dead. A determination of death must be made in accordance with accepted medical standards.

Much of the ethical debate surrounding death subsided after this act. After meeting the condition in the Act and gaining permission from the family, organs for donation can be recovered; however, the scarcity of organs for transplantation in infants prompted the identification of a potential donor source for organs. This potential source was the anencephalic infant.

Proponents of the use of anencephalic infants as organ donors began to reexamine the Uniform National Determination of Death Act, realizing that anencephalic infants did not meet the criteria of the Act and were therefore necessarily excluded as potential organ donors. The provisions of the Act do not provide criteria for death in infants under 7 days of age,[43] and vital organs of the anencephalic can become nonviable during that time period. Proponents argued that if death is a social construct, could society not redefine it once again using higher brain function criteria? Wouldn't the increased numbers of organs available, and the survival of increased numbers of children through transplantation of those organs, outweigh any social consequence of redefining death?[44] The ethical basis of this argument lies in the principle of utility. Utility justifies any moral decision that results in maximizing good to many (the recipients), as opposed to doing harm to a few (the anencephalic donor).

Opponents argued that such a revision of the Act might open a Pandora's box of redefinition of death. They pointed out that use of higher brain criteria for death would not only be applicable to anencephalic infants, use of such criteria would also be applicable to children or adults locked in a chronic vegetative state. Would allowing this redefinition, with its prevailing ethic of utility, result in an ever-changing definition of death? Would more and more persons with brain "abnormalities" be labeled dead, therefore available as potential donors? Once so labeled, would these individuals be denied their human status or personhood?

Opponents further base their objections on prima facie obligations of respect for the vulnerable life of the anencephalic infant. In other words, the anencephalic infant has the right to be treated as a person and not as a means to an end. If that means the loss of organs, that loss is not as tragic as it might be when it is weighed against the loss of sensitivity to humanity that might occur if the death criteria are changed.[45]

There is nothing inherently wrong with either position related to the proposed redefinition of death. There are cogent arguments for both sides. For most critical care nurses the debates surrounding the possible redefinition of death have heightened already existing concerns about death and organ donation.

It may be neither more important, nor more proper, for an individual nurse to operate from an ethical foundation of utility than it is to operate from a perspective of respect for individual autonomy. What may be more important is that the individual critical care nurse have insight into the implications of any decision that she or he might make based on one or more of these principles. This insight into the foundation of one's ethical response has the potential to enable the nurse to feel comfortable with her or his decision and, perhaps as a result, to feel less powerless and less frustrated with the ethical response.

To gain insight into one's ethical response, the nurse may need support from his or her colleagues. This support may not come freely; the nurse may have to request it. It may mean asking one's colleagues for a few minutes' time to think. And it may mean nurses caring for nurses. Recognizing that critical care nursing interventions may mean the difference between life and death and that their delay may have critical consequences, nurses may find it difficult to implement the nursing process with each other at the same time. Given, however, that caring for each other in stressful situations may mean better patient care in the long run, or perhaps preventing the loss of a nurse from the profession, can we afford not to care for each other?

Transplantation as a perceived cure. The public view of transplantation is often as a magical cure. Indeed, patients themselves may, if their experience is consistently positive, perceive themselves as "cured." This perception has, in the past, resulted in patients making the decision to stop taking their required immunosuppressive medications. In actuality most transplant recipients trade one set of problems related to end-stage organ disease for another set of problems related to necessary posttransplant care. The ethical issues raised as a result of the conflict between the perceptions that transplantation is a cure, as opposed to a disease syndrome related to chronic immunosuppression, are issues of informed consent and quality of life.

Informed consent. Informed consent is a process of shared decision-making between the patient (or the patient's surrogate) and the transplant team. The principles of respect for person and autonomy of the individual provide the ethical basis for the process.

The informed consent process for the transplant patient should include details about the surgical procedure, including all potential outcomes. There should also be a discussion of the expectations by the transplant team of the patient and family after surgery, including the necessity of complying with a lifetime immunnosuppression regimen and regular follow-up visits to the clinic or hospital. The reality, including the financial reality, of life after transplant is what the patient and family need to understand for a truly informed consent.

Obtaining informed consent may be difficult when the patient and family are attempting to comprehend a terminal disease or condition and, at the same time, a second chance at life. It is even more difficult when the transplant is recommended under emergency conditions, such as when a liver transplant is recommended for a patient with acute hepatic necrosis. However, to withhold information that is part of informed consent because of the already stressful nature of the situation, or to make a decision for the patient or family, is to respond from the ethical perspective of paternalism. Paternalism is in conflict with respect for the right of autonomy.

Moral distress can result when the nurse perceives that the patient or family has not been adequately informed, or does not understand the information that is fundamental to the consent. Strategies for dealing with this moral distress include discussion of this concern with the transplant team, particularly the attending physician, or an ethicist, if available. Unit-based ethics rounds, where the focus is the identification of moral-ethical issues active in a particular situation and development of individual strategies for dealing with these issues, are also valuable in relieving moral distress.

Quality of life. It is not uncommon for critical care nurses to cite quality of life as a moral construct that is foundational to her or his ethical decision-making. Yet when pressed few are able to define quality of life.

When quality of life is defined from a limited scope, it may refer to survival rates. That is, if the patient lives, regardless of his or her condition, he or she is considered to have quality of life. In this view the emphasis is on "life." The moral principle supporting this interpretation may be beneficence; that is, the continued preservation of all life in any form is good.

Quality of life can also be defined as the experience of the transplant recipient, the sense of value that life has for her or him. In this view, the emphasis is on the word "quality." The moral principle supporting this interpretation may be nonmaleficence, to do no harm. That is, the continued aggressive support of life without perceived value is not doing good, but rather is doing harm.

When the interpretation, by the patient or a family, of quality of life conflicts with the interpretation by the transplant team, an ethical dilemma exists and moral distress may result. Distress usually stems from the decision to continue, withdraw or withhold life-saving therapies.

Again, a resource to consult to address moral conflict is the clinical ethicist, if available. The clinical ethicist may be a nurse, a philosopher, a physician, or a member of the clergy. The nature of an ethical dilemma, however, is that there is no right or wrong answer. So this should not be the expectation when making such a consult. The ethicist can, however, clarify the principles at work for the parties involved and, in some cases, make recommendations for outcomes.

Another resource for addressing moral-ethical dilemmas is the institutional or nursing ethics committee. Ethics committees usually have two purposes. The first is education of the health care team. The second is case review, usually for the purpose of clarifying the issues and the underlying ethical principles.

Micro issues summary. The micro issues surrounding transplantation include the need for some to die so that others can live and the perception of transplantation as a magical cure. The scarcity of organs has resulted in continuing debate over criteria for defining death. The issues surrounding the use of the anencephalic infant as an organ source have fueled this debate. When transplantation is perceived as a cure, the informed consent process and quality of life's relationship to the posttransplant course raises moral concerns.

Nursing's ethical response to transplantation

In caring for the transplant recipient, physicians and nurses establish a special relationship — a covenential relationship.[46] A convenential relationship does not exist without the presence of three essential elements. The first of these elements is the gift. In transplantation, the gift is the donation of an organ or tissue, a gift of the physical self. The second element is the promise to strive to achieve the outcome that is most consistent with the values of the recipient. The final element is the set of obligations that are necessary to meet the promise. These obligations involve the ethical principles of respect for persons, autonomy, justice, beneficence, nonmaleficence, and sometimes utility.

Nursing's ethical response, though, runs deeper than these elements. Foundational to nursing's ethical response are the knowledge and ethics of caring. Caring cannot exist in a direct and cold relationship with these principles. It requires the additional requisites of knowing the facts, honesty with ourselves, our patients, and our peers, hope for the best, and courage to continue with the ethical struggles that accompany even a wondrous, modern miracle like the new life that may follow a successful transplant.

REFERENCES

1. Futterman L (1988). Cardiac transplantation: a comprehensive nursing perspective, Part 1. *Heart and Lung,* *17*(5), 499-509.
2. Futterman L (1988). Cardiac transplantation: a comprehensive nursing perspective, Part 2. *Heart and Lung,* *17*(6), 631-640.
3. Busuttil R, Colona J, Hiatt J, Brems JJ, Khoury G, Goldstein LI, Quinones-Baldrich WJ, Abdul-Rasool IH and Rammings KP. (1987). The first 100 liver transplants at UCLA. *Annals of Surgery, 206*(4), 387-402.
4. Campbell J (1988). *The power of myth.* New York: Doubleday.
5. Maguire D (1978). *The moral choice.* New York: Winston Press.
6. Maguire D (1984). *Death by choice.* New York: Doubleday.
7. Fuchs V (1974). *Who shall live? Health, economics, and social choice.* New York: Basic Books.
8. Engelhardt T (1984). Allocating scarce medical resources and the availability of organ transplantation. *New England Journal of Medicine, 311*(1), 66-71.
9. Engelhardt T (1986). *The foundations of bioethics.* Oxford, England: Oxford University Press.
10. Macklin R (1987). *Mortal choices.* Boston: Houghton-Mifflin.
11. Bouressa G and O'Mara RJ (1987). Ethical dilemmas in organ procurement and donation. *Critical Care Nursing Quarterly, 10*(2), 37-47.
12. Sophie L, Salloway J, Sorock G, Volek P and Merkel F (1983). Intensive care nurses' perception of cadaver organ procurement. *Heart and Lung, 12*(3), 261-267.
13. Kozlowski L (1988). Case study in identification and maintenance of an organ donor. *Heart and Lung, 17*(4), 366-371.
14. Boyd KM (1983). The ethics of resource allocation. *Journal of Medical Ethics, 9*(1), 25-27.
15. Caplan A (1983). Organ procurement: it's not in the cards. *Hastings Center Report, 13,* 23-32.
16. Cowan D, Kantorowitz J, Moskowitz J and Rheinstein P (eds). (1987). *Human organ transplantation: societal, medical-legal, regulatory, and reimbursement issues.* Ann Arbor: Health Administration Press.
17. Irwin BC (1986). Ethical problems in organ procurement. *ANNA Journal, 13*(6), 305-310.
18. Ingelhart J (1983). Transplantation: the problem of limited resources. *New England Journal of Medicine, 309*(2), 123-128.
19. Caplan A (1983). Organ transplantation: the costs of success. *Hastings Center Report, 13,* 23-32.
20. Andrews L (1986). My body, my property. *Hastings Center Report, 16*(5), 28-38.
21. Moore FD (1988). Three ethical revolutions: ancient assumptions remodeled under pressure of transplantation. *Transplant Proceedings, 20*(1, Supp.1), 1061-1067.
22. Wright R and Clark L (1988). Required request for organ donation: moral, clinical, and legal problems. *Hastings Center Report, 18*(2), 27-34.
23. Report of the Task Force on Organ Transplantation. Organ transplantation: issues and recommendations. Washington, DC: US Department of Health and Human Services, 1986.
24. Childress J (1988). Organ transplants return to center of ethical debate. *Kennedy Center Institute of Ethics Newsletter, 2*(6), 1-2.
25. Marsden C (1988a). Ethical issues in cardiac transplantation. *Journal of Cardiovascular Nursing, 2*(2), 23-30.
26. Marsden D (1988b). Care giver fidelity in a pediatric bone marrow transplant team. *Heart and Lung, 17*(6), 617-625.
27. American Association of Critical-Care Nurses (1986). *Position statement: role and responsibility of critical care nurses in organ and tissues transplantation.* Newport Beach: American Nurses Association.
28. American Association of Critical-Care Nurses (1986). *Position statement: required request and routine inquiry: methods to improve the organ and tissues donation processes.* Newport Beach: American Nurses Association.

29. Bandman B (1978). The human rights of patients, nurses, and other health professionals. In Bandman EL and Bandman B (eds). *Bioethics and human rights.* New York: McGraw-Hill Book Co.

30. Thompson J and Thompson H (1985). *Bioethical decision making for nurses.* Connecticut: Appleton-Century-Crofts.

31. Pellegrine E and Thomasma D (1988). *For the patient's good: the restoration of beneficence in health care.* Oxford, England: Oxford University Press.

32. Omery A and Caswell D (1988). A nursing perspective of the ethical issues surrounding liver transplantation. *Heart and Lung, 17*(6), 626-630.

33. President's Commission for the Study of Ethical Problems in Medicine and Biomedical and Behavioral Research (1986). *Securing access to health care.* Vols 1-3. Washington, DC: US Government Printing Office.

34. Jonsen A (1987). Organ transplants and the principle of fairness. In Cowan D, Kantorowitz J, Moskowitz J and Rheinstein P (eds). *Human organ transplantation: societal, medical-legal, regulatory, and reimbursement issues.* Ann Arbor: Health Administration Press.

35. Evans R and Yagi J (1987). Social and medical considerations affecting selection of transplant recipients: the case of heart transplantation. In Cowan D, Kantorowitz J, Moskowitz J and Rheinstein P (eds). *Human organ transplantation: societal, medical-legal, regulatory, and reimbursement issues.* Ann Arbor: Health Administration Press.

36. Annas G (1985). Regulating the introduction of heart and liver transplantation. *AJPH Journal, 75,* 93-95.

37. Childress J (1970). Who shall live, when not all shall live? *Soundings, 53,* 339-355.

38. Caplan A (1987). Equity in the selection of recipients for cardiac transplants. *Circulation, 75,* 10-19.

39. Caplan A (1985). Ethical issues raised by research involving xenografts. *Journal of the American Medical Association, 254*(23), 3339-3343.

40. Winner L (1986). *The whale and the reactor: a search for limits in an age of high technology.* Chicago: University of Chicago Press.

41. Beauchamp T and Childress J (1979). *Principles of bioethics.* New York: Oxford University Press.

42. President's Commission for the Study of Ethical Problems in Medicine and Biomedical and Behavioral Research (1981). *Defining death.* Washington, DC: US Government Printing Office.

43. Task Force on Brain Death in Children (1987). Guidelines for the determination of brain death in children. *Pediatrics Journal, 18,* 11-19.

44. Walters J and Ashwal S (1988). Organ prolongation in anencephalic infants: ethical and medical issues. *Hastings Center Report, 18*(5), 19-27.

45. Fost N (1988). Organs from anencephalic infants: an idea whose time has not yet come. *Hastings Center Report, 18*(5), 5-11.

46. Gadow S (1988). Covenant without cure: letting go and holding on in chronic illness. In Watson J and Ray M (eds). *The ethics of care and the ethics of cure: synthesis in chronicity.* New York: NLN Publications.

7

Psychiatric Aspects of Transplantation

Anne Marie Riether

GENERAL PSYCHOLOGIC CONCERNS OF ORGAN TRANSPLANT PATIENTS

During the past 30 years, organ transplantation has become an accepted treatment for organ failure. Only in the past several years, with the development of antirejection drugs such as cyclosporine and OKT-3 and improved surgical techniques, have the long-term survival rates increased significantly.

Kidney transplants, performed since the 1950s, are today considered almost routine. More recently, other types of transplants have been the subject of media coverage and ethical concerns. In 1986 alone, 1368 heart transplants and 924 liver transplants were performed in the United States.[1] In the cyclosporine era, the majority of patients survive the first postoperative year and are doing well at 5 years.[1]

As transplantation becomes an option for more patients, the technical aspects are becoming less challenging. We are just beginning, however, to address the psychiatric morbidity associated with organ transplantation. To date much of the literature in this area has been anecdotal, and many of the psychiatric complications from this surgery have been ignored in the hope that they will "go away" when the patient recovers and leaves the hospital with "a new lease on life."

Patients facing transplantation share many concerns, regardless of the organ transplanted. Most are quite frightened when they realize that a vital organ is failing and that they will need a transplant (or, in the case of renal failure,

dialysis) to survive. The psychologic difficulties of transplant patients include anxiety and fear about the transplant, guilt about being a burden to their families, differing levels of depression, behavioral problems, loss of self-esteem, changes in body image, sexual dysfunction, marital conflicts, and a sense of isolation.[2] They may experience hopelessness or helplessness, dependency and regression, financial stresses, organic brain dysfunction, psychotic states, cognitive changes, and, occasionally, have suicidal ideations.[3,4]

Fears that patients have reported seem fairly consistent, regardless of the organ transplanted, and include fear of the unknown, not getting a donor, the pain of surgery, rejection, and long-term health problems.[2,5]

Traditionally psychologic concerns have been addressed by social workers, chaplains, or nurses, or sometimes through a brief psychiatric consultation. Only recently has a new area of consultation psychiatry come to the forefront: the liaison psychiatrist for the transplant service.

Psychiatric intervention that begins in the evaluation period can help address these problems, lessening the difficulty for many patients and perhaps helping some of them avoid significant difficulty altogether. It can also help to identify high-risk patients so that they may receive additional treatment to optimize their chances for successful transplantation.

Although some patients seem to adjust fairly well, others seem to need to work through a

117

psychologic integration, in which the organ from the donor is accepted physically as well as psychologically into a stable internal body image.[6] This integration has been called the *psychologic transplant,*[7] during which the patient assimilates the new organ as part of his or her own body. It is said to be dependent on the real, as well as the fantasized, qualities of the donor, and the relationship (if any) between the donor and the recipient.[5]

In the initial stage, the patient reacts to the transplanted organ as a "foreign body," reporting that the organ "feels funny." They may worry that the organ might "fall out" or "get loose." During the next stage the patient is less preoccupied with the foreignness of the organ. And finally, when the patient begins to psychologically accept the organ as part of her or his body during the complete incorporation stage, the organ is completely assimilated.[7]

Although all transplant surgeries have in common the replacement of a healthy organ for a diseased one, distinct psychologic features characterize patients who receive each kind of transplant.[5]

Kidney transplantation

Kidney transplantation is generally "less stressful" than long-term dialysis[5]; however, it has its own set of complex problems, which are discussed in Chapter 11.

Kidney transplantation, unlike heart or liver transplantation, does not engender the same urgency in the transplant team or the recipient. Dialysis may be used to optimize patient conditions before surgery and sustain them while waiting. However, waiting for a compatible kidney donor is difficult and has been referred to as *dialysis stress.*[8]

Living organ donation, until recently, has been limited to kidney transplantation, although patients receiving heart-lung transplants may donate a heart to a cardiomyopathy patient, and there have been some attempts at transplanting partial pancreas grafts from living donors.[9] Unlike heart and liver transplants, in which only minimal donor-recipient histocompatibility testing is necessary, extensive histocompatibility testing is necessary to identify a compatible kidney donor. A family member may

volunteer to be tested for compatibility but, once determined to be a good "match," may feel ambivalent about donating.[5] They may fear renal failure themselves later in life or may wonder whether another family member, to whom they are closer, might need that kidney later.[3] They may fear the pain of surgery and wonder whether the risk of graft rejection is worth their donation.

Unlike the anonymity of a cadaver donor, living-related donors are known to the patient. There is usually a relationship between the potential donor and recipient, and once the transplant has been completed, the patient must adjust to life with the new organ, just as the donor must adjust to the organ's loss.[5] Although no studies have been done comparing experiences of recipients of living-related donor kidneys with those of recipients of cadaver donor kidneys, the patient who receives a relative's kidney may have difficulty incorporating the kidney into his or her body image if the donor continues to see the kidney as his own, even though it is residing in another's body.

The recipient of a living-related donor kidney may also have difficulty psychologically integrating the organ because of the fear of acquiring the donor's characteristics.[5] For example, one woman feared that she would acquire her mother's "mean streak," and a young boy demanded that his kidney graft be removed after his brother (who had donated his kidney 18 months earlier) announced that he was homosexual.

Although most patients do not have a great deal of difficulty with incorporation of the transplant, preoperative psychiatric screening of potential donors and recipients is helpful in determining which patients may have more difficulty with this process. In studying kidney transplant recipients, Kemph[10] found that although the recipients might deny any feelings toward the donors, their responses on the Thematic Apperception Test (TAT) were preoccupied with theft, robbing, and punishment. This suggests that the conflicts associated with the transplant have become unconscious through repression and may be undetected if projective testing is not done.

Patients with kidney failure may feel guilt

about accepting a donor organ and may express a feeling of undeservedness.[11] Dysphoria (depressed mood) and other disturbances of affect are common among renal failure patients,[11-13] and many report that coping with end-stage renal disease is the most difficult emotional problem of their lives.[14]

Using DSM-III-R criteria[15] for major depression, there is a high prevalence of major depression in patients who have end-stage renal disease.[16,17] It has been estimated that 47% of the patients who have a major depression concurrent with their renal disease before transplant continue to be depressed after transplant.[14]

According to one study, the suicide rate for dialysis patients is 100 times that of the general population and 400 times as high if deaths caused by noncompliance with treatment recommendations are included.[13] In a series of 292 kidney transplants, 55 patients developed severe depression, and seven attempted suicide.[18] In this study preoperative psychiatric problems were linked to postoperative psychiatric complications. Other researchers have found no link between psychiatric disorders and survival but have found that hospital readmissions after transplant and the duration of those admissions are related to psychosocial problems detected during the first interview.[19]

In addition to emotional distress, dialysis patients and potential kidney transplant patients may suffer cognitive changes as a result of uremia.[20] These changes may affect incorporation of the transplanted kidney and the quality of life after transplant. However, at least one longitudinal study of 237 kidney transplant patients has shown that despite some early adjustment problems or dysphoric mood states, most kidney transplant patients report increased self-esteem and independence and say that they feel more in control of their destiny.[21]

Heart transplantation

The psychologic symptoms encountered in heart transplant patients are different in some cases from those in patients receiving other types of transplants. Unlike the kidney or liver, the heart is not a silent organ—its beat can be felt by the patient and can be heard by the physician.

Unlike kidney patients, patients awaiting heart transplants cannot be maintained indefinitely on artificial life support.

The heart is the most symbolic of our internal organs. We talk of having a tender heart, the heart of a child, or cold-heartedness, as if this organ had emotions of its own. When we cry our hearts out or are brokenhearted, we convey a picture of one who is very depressed and distraught. We worry when someone we know has a change of heart and wonder whether it was caused by something we did. Conversely, when we give our hearts to others or give heartfelt thanks, we evoke an image of a very loving, grateful person. The heart is the symbol of love, romance, and life in our literature and in our everyday speech. The lay press marvels at heart transplants, and people speculate on how the person will be "changed" by this operation.

Like patients with other forms of organ failure, patients with end-stage cardiac disease have a decreased quality of life and may show varying amounts of depression, anxiety, and cognitive changes. In addition, they may have psychotic reactions after surgery that are related to sensory deprivation, metabolic disturbances, medications, or emotional events.[22] Heart transplantation is associated with a high incidence of postoperative psychiatric complications, ranging from acute brain syndromes to major mood disorders and psychosis.

Patients who have had previous cardiac problems, such as myocardial infarction or coronary artery bypass surgery, seem to have less difficulty than patients who, until the need for transplant was discussed, were unaware of any problems with their heart. This may result from the fact that in the former group, their identity as a "heart patient" is already present and therefore they experience less of a shock when they hear that their heart is failing and that they will need surgery.

Psychiatric symptoms may herald the onset of neurologic or infectious complications. In a retrospective study of 83 cardiac transplant patients, 54% had at least one neurologic complication, 16% had more than one, and 20% died of neurologic complications.[23] Because of the high doses of corticosteroids, transplant patients are at risk for viral and fungal infections such as candidosis and aspergillosis, which are associated with metastatic brain abscesses and meningeal involvement. Many patients with early infections have mild signs of cognitive impairment. If these mental status changes are blamed on metabolic encephalopathy or "ICU psychosis," diagnosis and treatment of a life-threatening infection may be delayed.

Liver transplantation

Unlike other patients with end-stage organ disease, patients in need of a liver transplant often bear a social stigma. Patients with liver disease are often assumed to be alcoholics or drug addicts. Family and friends may be ignorant of the causes of liver failure, and when patients talk about their need for a liver transplant they may be judged harshly for having "brought the disease on themselves."

Liver failure cannot be hidden. The body image changes are obvious. These patients frequently become jaundiced and may, as one patient put it, "glow in the dark." The body image changes are obvious. They may get "liver spots," and brawny skin changes. Their hair loses its luster, and they bruise easily. Their bones may break spontaneously or from minor trauma resulting from liver disease and steroid-induced metabolic bone disease. Ascites may elicit questions about when the baby is due, and the patient who is tired of explaining may reply, "soon." As is true of patients with uremia or cardiomyopathy, the liver-failure patient may show cognitive changes from hepatic encephalopathy and may exhibit organic brain syndromes such as delirium or dementia.

DEFENSE MECHANISMS

Many patients awaiting transplant use defense mechanisms to help them cope. These may include denial, displacement, minimization, rationalization, isolation of affect, projection, and reaction formation.[24]

According to Vaillant's longitudinal study of life-style and psychologic adaptation,[25] defensive and coping mechanisms are hierarchic. Persons who use primarily lower-level mechanisms such as projection and denial have generally unsatisfying, unsuccessful, even psychotic, lives. However, those using higher-order mech-

anisms, such as sublimation, report rewarding, successful lives.

Denial

Denial is the most common defense seen early in the patient's illness or in the evaluation for transplantation. Denial may be a way of dealing with unconscious ambivalent feelings about transplant. Since depression often results when denial totally breaks down, a certain amount of denial may actually be adaptive and may help patients cope with their life-threatening situation. Excessive denial of the severity of the situation, however, may lead to noncompliance or refusal to accept the current medical situation and the treatment team's recommendations. Patients being evaluated for transplant may need additional time to absorb the results of their diagnostic tests and to intellectually and emotionally understand and accept what is happening to their bodies. It is essential that the patient accept that she or he has a terminal disease. Once this is accepted, the patient should be able to accept the need for a transplant.

Displacement

Displacement is a defense mechanism in which emotions, ideas, or wishes are transferred from one individual to another. This mechanism is often used to allay anxiety or to avoid unpleasant feelings. Patients may find it difficult to become angry at their physician for fear that they will not get a new organ, and so instead "displace" their feelings onto a "safer" individual. An example of displacement is when patients are really angry at their surgeon for not spending enough time talking to them, but instead they bitterly complain that their nurse, who has spent the last 8 hours with them, is never available.

Minimization

Patients may also minimize their disease as a coping mechanism. Not wanting to accept the severity of their illness, they may forget to mention important signs and symptoms to caregivers, an omission that may produce a very distorted account of their illness. Despite realistic explanations of their disease and the transplant procedure, patients may continue to believe that they will not need a transplant or that their surgery will not be as complicated as most. They may minimize the potential complications or limitations associated with the transplant, focusing instead on the transplant team's success stories.

Patients who continue to minimize their disease despite repeated explanations from the medical team may be having difficulty coping with their illness. For these patients, supportive therapy or family sessions may prove helpful. If the patient's minimization results from not fully comprehending the severity of the illness, additional education for the patient and the family is indicated.

Rationalization

Rationalization is used as a defense mechanism when patients attempt to justify their actions, beliefs, or behaviors based on faulty reasoning. Patients who attempt to convince their nurse that they do not need to stop smoking, because their father lived to be 90 and smoked three packs of cigarettes a day, are rationalizing.

Isolation of affect

Isolation of affect is frequently seen in the obsessive person who deals only with the facts. Finding it hard to deal with the highly charged emotions of the situation, they tend to intellectualize the illness. They may quote endless statistics and facts about the operation but be baffled when asked how they are feeling about having the surgery. These patients tend to see the operation as mechanistic and the surgeon as an unemotional carpenter tacking in spare parts. They want details about the technical aspects of the surgery but deny having any feelings about losing the organ or having it replaced by someone else's.

A typical response by a patient who exhibits isolation of affect is "I just don't think about it" (the surgery). As is true of most defense mechanisms, being unemotional can be helpful to some degree, but patients who rigidly refuse to acknowledge any emotions associated with the transplant may become overwhelmed by anxiety when their defenses break down. When obsessive patients who use this kind of defense

mechanism are no longer in control, or when the surgery or the postoperative course is no longer by the book, they may become overwhelmed by anxiety and fear.

Projection

Projection occurs when patients attribute their own unacknowledged feelings, thoughts, and impulses that are personally undesirable or unacceptable to others. Transplant patients who are racially prejudiced, but find this trait socially unacceptable, may bitterly complain that they are not being transplanted because the hospital staff is discriminating against them. This defense mechanism protects the person from anxiety arising from inner conflict.

Reaction formation

Reaction formation is sometimes seen in transplant candidates and recipients who are in psychologic conflict. This often-confusing defense mechanism causes the patient to do the opposite of what he or she is feeling. For example, a patient may be very angry at the transplant surgeon because of the long wait for a donor organ, but because he or she fears that showing anger may jeopardize her or his position on the waiting list, the patient may be overly solicitous, showering the surgeon with compliments or gifts.

Another example of reaction formation is the patient who is in conflict from an unconscious wish for others to die (so that a donor organ will become available). This person may joke about drinking and driving fatalities, refer to motorcyclists as "mobile kidney donors" and then volunteer to work in a motor vehicle campaign against drunk driving. If this psychologic conflict remains unconscious, the patient may have unexplained guilt or anxiety.

PSYCHOLOGIC RITES OF PASSAGE

For most patients and families, the psychologic stresses of organ failure culminate after months or years of living with a chronic illness. When a patient finally comes to terms with the recommendation for transplant, very predictable psychologic stages or psychologic rites of passage occur: denial, anger, accentuation of personality characteristics, magical expectations, idealization, and acceptance. These stages are experienced on the patient's own timetable. More than one stage may be experienced at the same time, and regression to a previously experienced stage can occur. Psychiatric intervention can be helpful to a patient who is stuck in a particularly difficult emotional stage.

Denial

The first stage is denial, an unconscious defense mechanism that may allow the patient to cope successfully with a stressful situation. Denial in patients with organ failure frequently takes the form of not believing that they are sick enough to need a transplant. Despite their serious limitations, medical complications, and frequent hospitalizations, they may minimize their symptoms. This denial enables a jaundiced patient to believe he has a suntan, a patient with ascites to believe she is simply gaining weight, and a patient with increasing shortness of breath and angina to blame it on anxiety or stress.

Anger

Once a patient's denial has been replaced with realism, anger, depression, and grief may follow. Patients with end-stage organ disease may be angry about their physical limitations, inability to work, changing family roles, sexual dysfunction, or a host of other limitations that accompany their illness. Anger at their illness is often displaced onto the family or the nursing staff. Patients rarely displace this anger onto the transplant team, since it is this team that will decide whether they are placed on a donor waiting list.

Patients in this stage may be difficult to care for. They may be demanding and sullen and never satisfied with their care. They may argue about thier diet, medications, or seemingly minor incidents. They may become hostile and sarcastic when they hear about another patient's successful operation, and their anger may seem to increase proportionally with their perceived stress.

When anger is not openly expressed, these patients become depressed and withdrawn. Supportive or insight-oriented psychotherapy may be needed to help them express their internal anger. Their depression may be reactionary, because they are dealing with the immediate losses and changes in their lives, or it may be preparatory, which is common in patients with terminal illnesses.[26]

As patients deal with the reality of their situations and begin working through their anger, they also begin grieving. Transplant patients grieve for the loss of their health, independence, privacy, fantasies of immortality, and body image. Placed on medical disability and no longer able to enjoy their hobbies and recreational activities, these patients may lose their image of themselves as productive individuals. Finally, as patients become more disabled, they may lose relationships that are important to them.

The onset or exacerbation of disease is commonly preceded by affective states variously designated as despair, depression, or grief.[27] In a study of the role of grief and fear in the death of kidney transplant patients, 8 of 11 patients who died following renal transplantation had suffered a sense of abandonment by their families. These patients had also shown extreme anxiety that was not observed in other patients who survived the procedure. It may be that after experiencing the loss of the supportive relationship, these patients gave up.[27]

When looking specifically at grief, we find well-substantiated reports that grief negatively affects mortality. The death rate among bereaved relatives has been reported as seven times higher than among a control group of nongrieving persons.[28] In conversations, transplant patients may reveal that they clearly feel not only their loss and disability, but also the grief and sorrow of others around them.

Some patients find it difficult to work through the grieving stage and continue to be angry, refusing to accept their losses. They may continue to ask "why me," never moving on to accepting the reality of the present.

Accentuation of personality characteristics

In this stage, patients' individual personality characteristics are accentuated. Coming closer to transplantation, each potential recipient reacts differently, according to his or her own personality style. Obsessive, paranoid, borderline antisocial, and dependent personality traits may become apparent.

Obsessive individuals will absorb themselves in a flurry of activity, researching the statisitics on transplantation, writing to members of Congress, and doing public relations work for organ donation. These patients channel their anxiety by organizing projects. One potential heart transplant patient wanted to redecorate the transplant wing of a hospital while waiting, so that he and other patients would have a "psychologically more pleasing" environment after transplant. Other obsessive patients may write books about their experiences or keep extensive logs with minute details of their illness. These individuals are sometimes difficult to manage because they want to be in control of their illness and treatment and find it difficult not to know when the transplant will take place, let alone the outcome.

Persons with paranoid personality traits become more suspicious and more paranoid during the waiting period. They may be extremely sensitive to any hint of partiality or special privileges given to another waiting patient. They may accuse the transplant team of favoritism or sometimes even unethical practices in "choosing" the order of transplanted patients. They tend to see themselves as victims and seem ready to fight at the slightest provocation. Needless to say, they find it difficult to establish trust relationships with their physicians and other caregivers.

Because paranoid patients are difficult to care for, they may be ignored or given less time by the transplant team, which further compounds the problem. Supportive therapy to help these patients build a trusting relationship is often effective. Frequent short contacts by the transplant team, combined with honest communication about their status, helps to reassure these patients that they are not forgotten or being ignored.

Patients with borderline personality traits can also be very difficult to care for. They are often demanding and may be considered "ungrateful" by the staff. They can be very rigid, only seeing situations as either black or white, and individuals as either all good or all bad. These patients have difficulties with interpersonal relationships and, like paranoid patients, may see themselves as victims. They may attempt to split the transplant team by pitting one member against another. They frequently ask for special favors and become angry if they are not granted. Firm, consistent limiting setting is an imperative component of the care plan for this type of patient.

In the more severe borderline personality cases, resorting to drugs or alcohol as a coping mechanism is common. They may have a history of self-destructive acts and noncompliance. They typically blame their troubles on others, and few continue in therapy long enough to benefit from it. During extreme periods of stress, such as is encountered during the waiting period for transplant, transient breaks with reality may occur and the patient may become psychotic, necessitating a psychiatric hospitalization.

Patients with antisocial traits may have a history of illegal activities, drug dependence, alcoholism, or promiscuity. They tend to disregard rules and authority and are quite manipulative. Although they may be on good behavior while being evaluated for a transplant, their personality style will come to the forefront while they wait to be transplanted. They may attempt to con their way into a transplant and can be quite seductive, offering special favors and gifts to the nurses and other members of the transplant team. These patients tend to be noncompliant once the crisis has passed.

Patients with dependent personality features tend to become more passive while waiting for the transplant. They may become quite regressed and childlike, not assuming responsibility for even their most basic care. They may lie in bed all day, being fed and cared for by family members. In the most severe cases, patients with marked dependent personality features may be unable to make any decisions regarding their treatment; instead, they delegate total responsibility for their care to others. After transplant these patients have difficulty giving up this dependent role and may actually have more of a fear of life than a fear of death.

Magical expectations

During the stage of magical expectations, patients accept their illness and the need for a transplant, but with unrealistic expectations. As they eagerly look forward to the transplant, they minimize the time it will take to find a compatible donor, the complexity of the surgery, and potential complications. They have unrealistic expectations and may make elaborate plans to travel soon after their surgery. They are sure they will get the perfect donor match and be a "star patient."

Patients in this stage tend to see the transplant as a panacea for life's problems, as if a new organ can fix their health, marriage, and financial problems. They view the organ as making them new persons. Although this stage can help patients move toward ultimate acceptance of the transplant, patients may need help in assessing their situations realistically, without destroying their dreams and goals.

Idealization

Idealization is similar to magical expectations. In this stage patients tend to attribute more to a situation or a person than reality warrants. Patients may idealize the surgeon and the hospital; they may dream about their physicians, and boast to family and friends about their physician's training and list of accomplishments. Patients may worry about their surgeon and tend to see him or her as a person with an *"M Deity"* rather than an M.D. Some patients become preoccupied with members of the transplant team and, in a peculiar reversal of dynamics, begin taking care of them. One patient was heard asking members of the team whether the surgeon was getting enough rest, because he looked awfully tired. Another patient asked the transplant psychiatrist to "counsel" the surgeon because he "looked depressed."

The physicians and nursing staff should be aware of the dynamics of this stage, because patients may become disillusioned with these idealized persons when this stage ends. A physician who was "perfect" one week may be the target of an angry tirade over some minor disappointment the following week.

Acceptance

The final psychologic stage of the waiting period is acceptance. During this period, patients realistically acknowledge their illness and await their transplant. They are aware of the risks and potential benefits but have made an informed decision to proceed with the surgery. They have some anxiety and fear but are generally able to cope effectively as they live their lives one day at a time.

Not every patient goes through each stage described. Some patients never get past the denial stage, and others may experience them out of order. Patients who do accept their organ failure and who work through the related emotions make the best psychologic candidates for transplant.

The evaluation process

The transplant evaluation process is designed to (1) assess the patient's current physical condition, (2) determine all possible treatment options, (3) assess the suitability of the patient's condition for transplant, (4) share with the patient and family information regarding the transplant, including chances for survival and rehabilitation, and (5) allow them to make an informed decision regarding the surgery.[29]

Many patients with organ failure have been treated for years by their local physician or, in the case of renal failure, have been receiving long-term dialysis treatments. Because of a deteriorating course, a declining quality of life, or perhaps a feeling of helplessness on the part of the referring physician, the patient is referred to a transplant center. By the time patients become candidates for transplantation, many have been hospitalized many times, and their condition has deteriorated significantly.

Some primary physicians have difficulty openly discussing the idea of a transplant with their patients. Therefore, in some cases, the patient may not be told why he or she is being referred to the transplant center, other than for a second opinion or for the "latest treatments." It then comes as a shock to patients and families when the admissions clerk notes the admission diagnosis as heart or liver transplant evaluation. This can lead to intense anger, fear, and mistrust, intensifying an already stressful situation.

Even when patients are fully informed, the evaluation process is inherently stressful. Patients may be far from their homes and usual support systems. As one patient described it, "I went 500 miles from my home ... to a big university hospital, and underwent a great number of tests to see whether there was any hope."

The psychiatric evaluation is an integral component of the transplant evaluation. Many patients perceive this part of the evaluation as the time to convince the organ gatekeepers of their motivation, worthiness, and suitability for transplantation.[29] Patients may ask their family physicians, ministers, or local politicians to call the transplant team to convince the team of their worthiness. Because of their need to please, some patients downplay their fear or uncertainty about the surgery,[30] which can interfere with an accurate assessment. The psychiatrist may get a very different (and distorted) picture of the patient, who is attempting to look good, from that of the nurse who cares for the patient daily. Therefore it is important that nursing observations and assessments be shared with the transplant psychiatrist.

The box offers a suggested format for the clinical interview used by the transplant psychiatrist to begin the psychiatric evaluation. Understanding the interplay of psyche and soma, the psychiatrist evaluates how the physical illness may be affecting or even causing any emotional difficulties. Understanding the impact that the disease has on the patient's life is essential to understanding the patient's responses.

The patient evaluation includes a complete history, with emphasis on the medical, psychiatric, and substance abuse history; administration of the Mini Mental State examination[31]; discussion of attitude toward, motivation for, and expectations of transplantation; and a review of the patient's social support systems and resources.

Another purpose of the initial assessment is to identify psychologic factors that might impede or enhance patients' chances of survival.

PREOPERATIVE PSYCHIATRIC INTERVIEW

1. Chief complaint (in the patient's own words): "Why are you here?"
2. History of current illness: cause of organ failure, complications, current symptoms, current assessment of the patient's level of understanding of the illness, and previous compliance with treatment recommendations
3. Quality-of-life changes secondary to illnesses: "What can you not do now that you used to be able to?"
4. Past medical history: past surgeries, medical illnesses, assessment of coping mechanisms during earlier illnesses
5. Sexual history: past sexual experiences: "How has the illness affected your sexual activity?"
6. Alcohol and other drug use history: amount and frequency of alcohol or other drug use
7. Education and work history: highest grade or degree completed, jobs held
8. Support systems: family, friends, religious and financial resources
9. Current economic status: income, disability status, current employment
10. Social history: marriages, divorces, social supports, current living situation
11. Legal history: arrests, including DUIs
12. Family history: medical/psychiatric/alcohol or other drug problems in the family
13. Family of origin: ethnic background, patient's early developmental history, information about parents, siblings, current family relationships
14. Mental status examination (including Mini Mental State examination score)[31]

Patients who have extended family support, who are able to discuss the possibility of death openly, and who want to prolong life to do specific things seem to have fewer psychologic difficulties after the transplant. The motivation for transplant is carefully examined, especially in light of reports that patients who have specific plans for the future after transplant make a better psychosocial adjustment.[32] After surgery these patients seem better able to achieve their preoperative goals and integrate their new self-image. They are more compliant with treatment and adjust well to their changing role within the family. Conversely, patients who view surgery as a mutilating physical assault are at higher risk for psychiatric morbidity.[32]

During the preoperative psychiatric assessment (which may take several sessions), the ways in which patients and their families deal with the recommendation of transplant are examined. Patients and their families react in a variety of ways—from total denial to acceptance and relief that an alternative to death is available.[33] The coping mechanisms that patients use to deal with their chronic illness are also noted, because they are fairly reliable predictors of how patients will react to transplantation.[34-36] This initial meeting is also useful in determining a patient's competency to make decisions and his or her ability to give informed consent.

Because transplanted patients need to comply with a rigorous medical regimen, dietary restrictions, and exercise programs, all candidates are evaluated for the motivation to comply, as well as for a proven history of such behavior. Noncompliance is discussed in greater detail later in this chapter.

During the evaluation special attention is paid to the identification of any possible psychiatric contraindications to transplant. Specific psychiatric contraindications have been poorly defined in the literature. Empirical evidence is difficult to obtain, and the topic remains controversial. Although the specifics may differ from center to center, the list presented in the box above, right may be used as a guideline for identifying psychiatric contraindications to transplantation.

Although the evaluation process differs from institution to institution, it is generally true that after the psychiatric evaluation is completed, a confidential written evaluation is prepared and shared with appropriate members of the transplant team. The discussion typically focuses on the presence or absence of risk factors, the patient's potential for compliance, and the patient's ability to cope with the psychosocial stressors associated with transplantation. The transplant psychiatrist may make specific rec-

---

PSYCHIATRIC CONTRAINDICATIONS TO TRANSPLANTATION

Absolute contraindications
Psychosis
Active suicidal ideation
Active substance abuse/dependence
History of serious noncompliance

Relative contraindications
History of a psychotic episode
History of a suicide attempt
History of substance abuse/dependence with less than 6 months of abstinence
History of relative noncompliance
Axis II (personality disorder) diagnosis
IQ of less than 70
Poor social supports

---

ommendations concerning patient education, medications, psychotherapy and, occasionally, psychiatric hospitalization. Although a great number of patients with organ failure may need a transplant, not every patient is a suitable candidate, nor does every patient choose this option. Christopherson noted, "The final goal of the transplant evaluation should not be to persuade a 'good' candidate to choose surgery, but to provide the necessary information and freedom through which the patient and family can reach the decision that is best for them."[37]

PSYCHIATRIC DISORDERS FREQUENTLY ENCOUNTERED IN TRANSPLANT PATIENTS

The most common psychiatric disorders encountered are anxiety, depression, organic brain dysfunction, and psychosis. These reactions may represent a more serious psychiatric condition or may solely represent an adjustment disorder related to the patient's medical condition and the recommendation for transplant. In a prospective study of 247 consecutive candidates for liver transplant, 18.6% had delirium, 19.8% had an adjustment disorder, 4.5% had major depression, 9.0% had abused alcohol, and 2.0% were dependent on or had abused drugs.[38] Other researchers have reported that 95% of liver transplant patients experience preoperative psychologic distress and that 100% experience postoperative psychologic distress.[4]

Anxiety

Most patients faced with the need for a transplant exhibit some degree of anxiety. Frequently these patients are thought of simply as "hyper" or nervous types. Anxiety, however, may interfere with patient education, informed consent, comprehension of treatment explanations, and therefore the patient's compliance.[39]

The anxiety may be manifested by agitation, fear, a sense of losing control, or a fear of impending doom. Anxious patients may complain of insomnia and may show depressive symptoms. Anxiety may be accompanied by marked motor restlessness and autonomic hyperactivity that are unresponsive to treatment.[40] Although a diagnosis of extreme anxiety can generally be made on a clinical basis, objective testing, including measures such as the State-Trait Anxiety Inventory,[41] are useful in making a quantitative assessment of the patient's anxiety and following it over time.

For patients who have mild-to-moderate anxiety, relaxation techniques, imaging techniques, hypnotherapy, and biofeedback are sometimes helpful. Benzodiazepines may help to relieve extreme anxiety, but they are contraindicated in patients who also have delirium or cognitive impairment. Further, benzodiazepines are largely protein bound; that is, they depend on liver metabolism for degradation and excretion by the kidney. Metabolites can accumulate in patients who have renal or hepatic insufficiency, so they should be used with caution in patients with these conditions.[42,43] The box below summarizes frequently used pharmacologic agents for use with anxious patients.

Benzodiazepines also reduce the ventilatory response to hypoxia,[44] so they should be used

---

PHARMACOLOGIC AGENTS FOR TREATMENT OF PSYCHIATRIC SYMPTOMS

Antipsychotic drugs
Class of drugs
Neuroleptics
Major tranquilizers

Partial list of drugs available
Chlorpromazine (Thorazine)
Thioridazine (Mellaril)
Fluphenazine (Prolixin)
Trifluoperazine (Stelazine)
Perphenazine (Trilafon)
Thiothixene (Navane)
Loxapine (Loxitane)
Molindone (Moban)
Haloperidol (Haldol)

Indications for use
Schizophrenia, psychotic depression, organic brain syndromes (delirium), extreme agitation

Mechanism of action
Postsynaptic blockade of central dopaminergic activity

Continued.

Side effects

Anticholinergic, extrapyramidal, sedation

ANTICHOLINERGIC SYMPTOMS: Dry mouth, constipation, blurred vision, urinary hesitancy and retention, exacerbation of glaucoma

CENTRAL ANTICHOLINERGIC SYNDROME: Warm and dry skin, anxiety, restlessness, agitation, confusion, stupor and sometimes coma; dilated pupils, no bowel sounds

EXTRAPYRAMIDAL SYMPTOMS: Acute dystonic reaction — an involuntary, sustained contraction of skeletal muscle; occurs most commonly during the first 2 days of treatment

Parkinson-like syndrome — more common in older patients; usually occurs during the first weeks of treatment:

Tremor (irregular tremor)

Rigidity (cogwheel rigidity starts with shoulders)

Akinesia ("zombielike" slowness)

Akathesia (patients are fidgety)

Rabbit syndrome (involuntary chewing movements)

Tardive dyskinesia (slow ticlike movements)

Drug interations

Antacids may inhibit absorption of oral antipsychotics

Tricyclic antidepressants raise plasma levels

Antidepressant drugs
Class of drugs

Tricyclic antidepressants (TCA)

Monoamine oxidase inhibitors (MAOI)

Partial list of drugs available

Amitriptyline (Elavil)

Desipramine (Norpramin)

Doxepin (Sinequan)

Imipramine (Tofranil)

Nortriptyline (Aventyl)

Proptriptyline (Vivactil)

Indications for use

Depression, panic disorder

Mechanism of action

Increases central nervous system neurotransmitters

Side effects

Anticholinergic (dry mouth, blurred vision, constipation, urinary hesitancy)

Autonomic (tremor, sweating)

Cardiac (orthostatic hypotension, tachycardia, ECG changes, conduction disturbances)

Other: sedation, restlessness, insomnia, rashes, weight gain, confusion

Drug interactions

Plasma level increased by antipsychotic drugs, exogenous thyroid, and guanethidine

Plasma level decreased by barbiturates, alcohol, and smoking

Central nervous system depression occurs with antipsychotic drugs, sedatives, anticonvulsants, and alcohol

Impaired antihypertensive effect of methyldopa, guanethidine, and bethanidine

Marked hypertension can be caused by sympathomimetic drugs (e.g., isoproterenol, epinephrine, phenylephrine, amphetamines)

May dangerously increase the half-life of anticoagulants (e.g., dicumarol)

List of monoamine oxidase inhibitors

Phenelzine (Nardil)
Isocarboxazid (Marplan)
Tranylcypromine (Parnate)

Indications for use

Atypical depression, panic disorder, patients who do not respond to TCA

Mechanism of action

Block monoamine oxidase throughout the body

Side effects

Drowsiness or stimulation, insomnia, hypotension, hypertensive crisis in response to ingested tyramine

Drug interactions

Hypertensive crisis in response to amphetamines and sympathomimetic amines, catecholamines and sympathomimetic precursors
Severe hypertension in response to meperidine (Demerol)
Central nervous system depression potentiated by alcohol and major tranquilizers and sedative hypnotic drugs

Antianxiety drugs
Partial list of drugs available

Chlordiazepoxide (Librium)
Diazepam (Valium)
Oxazepam (Serax)
Chlorazepate (Tranxene)
Lorazepam (Ativan)
Flurazepam (Dalmane)
Alprazolam (Xanax)
Prazepam (Centrax)
Midazolam (Versed)
Triazolam (Halcion)

Indications for use

Short-term treatment of restlessness and anxiety
Alcohol withdrawal, seizure disorders, and muscle relaxant

Mechanism of action

Enhance inhibitory neurotransmitters; limbic system depressant

Side effects

Central nervous system depression
Tolerance and physical addiction
Disinhibition
Exacerbation of schizophrenia and depression

Drug interactions

Increased sedative effect when combined with alcohol
Disulfiram (Antabuse) raises plasma levels
Food and antacids decrease the rate of absorption

cautiously in patients who have cardiac or pulmonary disease. Benzodiazepines that have shorter half-lives, such as midazolam, triazolam, lorazepam, temazepam, and oxazepam, accumulate less with multiple doses and are more rapidly cleared after the medication is stopped. Drugs that have longer half-lives, such as diazepam, flurazepam, chlordiazepoxide, and clorazepate, can be given effectively on a once-a-day schedule but may cause excessive daytime sedation. In addition, they are less likely to cause severe withdrawal symptoms if they are abruptly discontinued.[45]

For patients who complain of difficulty sleeping, flurazepam, temazepam, and triazolam may be particularly helpful. Triazolam, because of its ultrashort half-life, is often used for this problem. However, it has been associated with amnestic episodes, dissociated and confusional states, and rebound insomnia. For the patient who is unable to take oral medication, lorazepam and midazolam can be given by intramuscular injection. Lorazepam given before painful procedures may be helpful, because it has amnestic properties.

An alternative medication option for extreme anxiety in transplant patients who cannot take benzodiazepines is a low dosage of the high-potency neuroleptics, such as haloperidol or fluphenazine. These should, however, be used with caution in liver failure patients, because they are metabolized by the liver.

Before these or other psychotropic medications are prescribed or administered, the possible drug interactions should be considered. Transplant patients are typically taking numerous medications, some of which may either prolong another drug's half-life or decrease the amount of the active medication by inducing microsomal enzyme induction.

Depression

Although the exact incidence and prevalence of depressive disorders in transplant patients have not been well established, they are very common both before and after transplant surgery. While mild depressive states usually resolve on their own, prolonged periods of depression that meet the criteria for a major depressive episode require psychiatric intervention.[15]

Most transplant patients show some evidence of depression, but it may be difficult to assess because many of the typical vegetative symptoms of depression (e.g., anorexia and weight loss, insomnia and fatigue) can also be explained by physical factors. A therapist skilled in differentiating between medical symptoms and symptoms of depression should evaluate changes in a patient's mood and mental status. The Beck Depression Inventory is a useful self-reporting instrument that can be used to follow depressive symptomatology.[46]

At certain times, depression is more likely to occur. When a patient dies, for instance, all those who know the deceased are affected. If the deceased was waiting for a transplant, other patients who are waiting may become depressed and withdrawn and fearful that they too will die before a suitable organ can be found. In the most severe cases, they may become so despondent that they give up and refuse a transplant. The transplanted patients may feel guilty for having "taken" an organ that could have saved the deceased's life. If the person who died had already received a transplant, the waiting patients may become depressed and wonder whether it is worth it. Other newly transplanted patients may become despondent because they are fearful of the same thing happening to them.

A defense machanism commonly used against depression is rationalization. Patients who rationalize find the differences between themselves and the patient who died, pointing out that he or she was sicker, older (or younger), or less compliant than they.

Suicide is always a risk in the chronically ill patient who is depressed. In a survey of 127 dialysis centers, the suicide rate was 100 times higher in dialysis patients than in the general population.[13] Many patients with organ failure feel they have no control over their lives, and some see suicide, albeit a very destructive option, as controlling one's destiny.

Some patients become depressed after they leave the intensive care unit. As they begin to assume more of their own care, they may realize that their responsibilities are greater than they originally believed. They may become discouraged at their slow progress, the number of medications they require or the number of procedures necessary. Although many factors may contribute to this postoperative depression, it is severe when the expectations about the transplant are unrealistic.[13]

Depression is also likely to occur when rejection is suspected or has been diagnosed. Patients fearing the loss of their newly transplanted organ may react with grief, anger, sadness, irritability, regression, or withdrawal. They may become angry at the staff and may stop participating in their care.

Depression in the transplant patient warrants prompt intervention. Patients who become depressed preoperatively are at an increased risk for surgical morbidity,[47] and it has been suggested that depression affects the patient's adjustment after discharge and also affects survival.[48] In general, before starting any antidepressant, the psychiatrist should consult with the transplant team concerning the patient's medical condition. Unfortunately, the use of tricyclic antidepressants, such as amitriptyline (Elavil), desipramine (Norpramin), doxepin (Sinequan), imipramine (Tofranil), or trazodone (Desyrel) is often contraindicated in liver and heart transplant candidates, because of decreased liver metabolism or the risk of congestive heart failure and dysrythmias.

Starting doses for patients with end-stage liver disease and renal failure are low. Dosages can be increased every 2 to 5 days to a therapeutic level only if the patient is tolerating the current dosage.[45] Because of the long half-lives of these drugs and their sedative properties, a once-a-day dose in the evening is generally recommended. Many patients with organ failure can tolerate an average daily dosage that is one third to one half the usual therapeutic dosage in healthy patients. Careful monitoring of these patients, however, is essential. Although tricyclic antidepressants are not dialyzable and are not metabolized by the kidney, the same starting dosages and maximum dosages are generally applicable for patients with end-stage renal disease.

Because severely ill patients are taking multiple drugs that may enhance or impede the metabolism of antidepressants and thus lead to either toxicity or subtherapeutic drug levels, plasma levels of tricyclic antidepressants should be monitored closely. Therapeutic blood levels may not be reached for 2 weeks, but levels should be drawn 12 hours after each change in dosage and again when a steady state has been reached.

For cardiac transplant candidates, tricyclic antidepressants can have serious side effects. They can cause an increase in the PR interval, QRS duration, and QT interval, and a flattening of the T wave. In patients who have preexisting bundle branch block, atrioventricular heart block may develop. Many pretransplant patients are on type I antidysrhythmic medications (quinidine, disopyramide, procainamide), which may have additive effects on conduction if used concurrently with tricyclic antidepressants.[49]

The cardiomyopathy patient with unstable disease should be hospitalized before starting tricyclic antidepressants, and generally these should be given only if the depression is life threatening. Tricyclic antidepressants may have a mild negative inotropic effect, which may destabilize marginally compensated patients. Before starting any antidepressant, the psychiatrist should verify that the patient does not have any residual conduction defects, congestive failure, dysrhythmias, or orthostatic hypotension. In general, tricyclic antidepressants are relatively safe in patients with stable cardiac function. After heart transplant, patients have healthy, denervated hearts, so vagal blockade is of no concern.

The first choice for antidepressant therapy in patients with cardiomyopathy is nortriptyline or doxepin, both of which cause less orthostatic hypotension, although impaired left ventricular function may potentiate tricyclic-induced orthostatic hypotension.[50,51] The other consideration in choosing an antidepressant is the potential for anticholinergic side effects, such as constipation, anticholinergic delirium, or urinary retention. The least anticholinergic of the antidepressants are desipramine and trazodone. They are preferred over amitriptyline, which is the most anitcholinergic.

Organic brain dysfunction

The transplant psychiatrist is often asked to see patients who have had a change in mental status. Up to one quarter of cardiac transplant patients are reported to have postoperative mental status changes.[28] Greenberg et al[20] found that 88% of 24 patients who were candidates for kidney transplantation or hemodialysis showed some signs of organic mental impairment. Because the cause of such changes is often difficult to assess in light of the patient's medical condition and numerous medications, delirium goes unrecognized in as many as 65% of patients.[52,53]

Delirium. Delirium is common, but failure to diagnose and treat it appropriately can have serious consequences. Mortality rates range from 23% to 33% within several months of the diagnosis of delirium.[53-55] A careful clinical interview with attention to the mental status examination, including the Mini Mental State Examination,[31] can help. Occasionally neuropsychologic testing may be used.

Often called an acute brain syndrome, delirium is a reversible madness, a toxic psychosis, or an acute confusional state.[56] It has also been described as a reversible global impairment of cognitive processes.[57] The onset is generally acute, and one's level of awareness fluctuates.[58] Delirium may present as a combination of the following signs and symptoms: incoherence, altered psychomotor activity, disorientation, perceptual disturbances, attention deficits, memory impairment, and sleep-wake alteration.[15]

Delirious patients may be delusional and have hallucinations, may be paranoid and hyperalert, or may be simply forgetful and slightly agitated. Unfortunately, they may mistakenly be thought to have ICU psychosis or may be labeled depressed, psychotic, or confused. In all cases of delirium, however, the EEG shows a generalized slowing.[59,60] The Mini Mental State examination,[31] Trailmaking Tests,[61,62] and serum albumin level assessment[63] may also prove helpful in making the diagnosis of delirium. Serum albumin level can be a particularly helpful indicator, because metabolism disorders leading to delirium can occur in patients whose nutritional state is poor.

Careful attention must be paid to the diagnosis, the cause, and the treatment of this condition. In transplant patients etiologic factors related to delirium might include a metabolic derangement (e.g., uremia or encephalopathy), a physiologic disturbance (e.g., cardiogenic shock), infection, rejection, drug reaction, or neurologic events.

Although delirium may occur in anyone (hence its nickname, everyman's psychosis[58]), certain factors are known to increase the risk: severe physical illness, history of substance abuse, history of myocardial infarction, and confusion.[64] Candidates for transplant are at risk for delirium. Hepatic encephalopathy is a common cause of organic brain syndrome. In 108 consecutive liver transplant candidates, 18 were found to have delirium.[63] According to another study, 6 of 33 heart transplant patients had at least one episode of delirium.[65] Finally, in a retrospective study of the neuropsychiatric sequelae in 83 heart transplant patients, seven (12%) developed metabolic encephalopathy and seven others developed acute psychosis.[23]

The management of delirium depends on its cause and manifestations. First and foremost, an attempt should be made to treat the underlying cause. Additionally, the patient should be oriented frequently by family and nursing staff. Familiar objects as well as orienting devices such as clocks and calendars may be helpful.

The pharmacologic treatment of delirium is highly individualized. If the patient is agitated, the quickest response is produced by intramuscular (IM) or oral (PO) haloperidol.[66,67] Haloperidol can also be given intravenously (IV) in an emergency setting. In contrast to PO and IM haloperidol, IV haloperidol has relatively few extrapyramidal side effects. Mild agitation usually responds to 0.5 to 2 mg of haloperidol, moderate agitation to 5 to 10 mg, and severe agitation to 10 mg or more.[45] If the agitation persists for more than 20 minutes after administration of the initial dose, another dose (double the initial dose) can be given. This medication is especially useful in heart transplant patients, because it has almost no pulmonary or cardiovascular side effects.[45,68] It should, however, be used with caution in liver failure patients, because it is metabolized by the liver.

Dementia. Dementia may be difficult to diagnose during a brief consultation because it is usually a diagnosis made over time. Its features include a loss of intellectual abilities sufficient to interfere with social or occupational functioning. Also typical are personality change, impaired abstract thinking and judgment, and other disturbances of higher cortical functioning.

Unlike delirium, dementia usually causes no alteration in attention.[15] Early in the disease there may be only mild personality changes, such as lack of initiative, irritability, and loss of interest. Family and friends may be the first to note these changes and bring them to the attention of the medical or nursing staff.

In evaluating transplant patients, it is best to test intellectual functioning, as part of a mental status examination, over time. Because of low cardiac output states, large doses of medications, or repeated episodes of hepatic encephalopathy or uremia, patients may experience a decline in intellectual performance. If deficits seem to be present, a full dementia workup, including the following, is indicated: a computed tomography (CT) scan, EEG, serum levels of folate and vitamin B_{12} and thyroid function tests, a neurologic consultation, and neuropsychologic testing.

Acute psychosis

Despite a history of effective coping and absence of psychiatric illness, the critically ill patient may develop an acute psychotic illness. This syndrome is thought to result from a combination of psychiatric pathologic factors including sleep deprivation, medication side effects, sensory deprivation, and alterations in the patient's metabolic and physical condition. Psychotic patients may have auditory and visual hallucinations, paranoid delusions, or confusion.

The literature contains numerous reports about psychotic symptoms in transplant patients.[38,69] Medications are frequently the cause. According to a recent review of 70 cardiac transplant patients, 10 manifested psychotic symptoms that were thought to be caused by steroids.[69] Steroid psychosis is observed in about 7% of transplant recipients but generally clears as the steroid dosage is reduced.[70] Others have suggested that a patient's difficulty in assimilating a stable internal body image may be responsible for a psychotic break after transplantation.[71]

Sometimes treatment must be instituted while the cause of the psychosis is still being sought. One of the first measures is to prevent patients from harming themselves or others. This can be done by providing a protective environment and controlling the patient's psychiatric symptoms with medications. These patients may be at risk for suicidal behavior because of their distorted reality and impaired judgment. Restraints (although not usually preferable) or one-to-one nursing care may be necessary to protect the patient and the staff. Communication with psychotic patients should be simple, direct, and repetitive.[72] Every attempt should be made to help these patients understand what is happening to them. Giving them a sense of control may decrease their anxiety or agitation.

Pharmacologic intervention is indicated if the patient becomes disruptive or out of control. The risks associated with undermedicating and inadequately supervising the patient are greater than the potential for overdosing the patient.[72] Haloperidol is the drug of choice in the treatment of acute psychosis. Tricyclic antidepressants are contraindicated in the treatment of steroid psychosis, because they tend to make this condition worse.[40]

THE PRETRANSPLANT PERIOD

After the decision is made to proceed with the transplant, the waiting period for a suitable donor may be long. As the availability of transplant technology and the number of eligible candidates have increased, waiting times have increased.[34,73,74] The wait may result in increased anxiety, depression, fear, anger, and competition among waiters. Patients may become frustrated at the delay and wonder whether they are really on "the list." One patient poignantly described the waiting period in the following way: "like being on a long-distance phone call and being placed on hold; the longer you wait, the more it costs you."

On good days, patients wonder whether they really need the transplant; on bad days, they wonder whether they will live until a suitable donor is found. The wait may be accompanied by a decline in health, further compromising the quality of life and leading to the fear that they will die waiting. Patients frequently have dreams about the transplant (often in disguised form), which can be very helpful in shedding light on the patients' fears and concerns.

By virtue of their unique role as transplant candidates, patients share many mutual concerns. Dependency on the family may increase, leading the patient to feelings of guilt from being a burden. Financial stress is a concern for most patients, because they are unable to work and families typically need to care for them at home. Patients often express feelings of helplessness and powerlessness. As the wait lingers, they may face intensified awareness of and fear of death.

A common topic for discussion among the waiters is their respective blood types, body sizes, and United Network for Organ Sharing (UNOS) computer classification. Competitiveness can therefore develop among patients.[34] When one patient undergoes transplant surgery, other patients may become preoccupied with details about the surgery and the organ donor, asking about the geographic origin and cause of death of the donor, details about the operation, and sometimes why that patient received a transplant before them. Patients may feel entitled to information about a newly transplanted patient.[34] Sharing the information, however, may not only violate patient confidentiality but may also prove upsetting and provoke expressions of anger or depression as the waiter continues to wonder "Why not me?"

If a nurse spends extra time with or bends hospital rules for a particular patient, other patients may fear that they are not as "special" or do not have as good "connections" with the transplant team,[34] and therefore will have to wait longer for a transplant. Favoritism, however subtle, will be picked up by these patients who are in a life-and-death struggle.

As the waiting period extends from days to weeks to months, patients often show signs of stress. They may want to see their physicians more frequently to get reassurance that they are not forgotten. The physicians, in turn, may want to avoid the patients, feeling they have nothing to offer since they cannot "give" the patient the organ that is needed for survival.[34]

A morbid type of humor—black, or gallows, humor—may be openly verbalized during the preoperative period.[34] Patients may joke about inclement weather, because it is then that fatal accidents are more likely.[75] Aware that many people drink and drive during holidays, waiting patients talk about sitting by their phones, wondering whether the projected number of fatalities will be correct and how many of them will be organ donors. One patient at our institution expressed embarrassment and guilt after blurting out that he was glad the legal speed limit had been raised to 65, because more people are likely to die in accidents. After waiting 7 months for a suitable liver, another patient was heard asking a new medical student her blood type, as casually as if he were asking her about the weather.

Black humor is heard not only from the waiters but from the families and the hospital staff. Seeing construction workers on high beams renovating the hospital, the wife of one of our transplant candidates remarked to a member of the transplant team: "They are in a high-risk job, you know; I wonder how often they fall. . . ." As they struggle to keep their patients alive, the nursing and medical staff are also affected by the long waiting periods.

The psychosocial impact of the waiting period varies, depending on individual patient differences. Patients who are able to remain at home and live a relatively normal life may adapt better to a lengthy wait. However, this same group feels distress at having "to put life on hold, never knowing when the beeper might go off." They are unable to leave town, take vacations, or make long-term commitments. They also worry that because they are not sick enough to be in the hospital, their UNOS classification is lower and hence they will be bypassed for transplant by someone who is more critically ill. They express concern that they have to get critically ill before someone will give them a transplant. Critically ill patients who must be hospitalized during the waiting phase express concerns about running out of time before a suitable donor is found, as well as fears about becoming too ill to continue as a viable transplant candidate.

Families may also show increased stress during the waiting period. They may feel the need to be strong for their critically ill relative, but at the same time feel inadequate to handle the increased financial stress and the physical and emotional needs of the patient and other family members. They have the difficult task of preparing for the possibility of the patient's death, and at the same time for the possibility of extended life with a transplant.

THE POSTTRANSPLANT PERIOD

Transplant patients ideally achieve better health and return to their preillness life-styles with improved quality of life. Research indicates that most patients who survive organ transplants return to happier, more productive, and much improved lives.[76] Many obstacles, however, must be overcome, including medical complications, psychosocial adjustment, and physical rehabilitation. As in the preoperative experience, patients go through several phases. Although the process is continuous, for purposes of study the postoperative period is divided into the ICU experience, transfer to the floor, early recovery at home, and finally, long-term recovery.

The ICU experience

For the first few days after transplant surgery, the patient may be groggy, wondering whether the transplant is really over. They are essentially immobile, surrounded by and tethered to beeping machines (Fig. 7-1). They may be frightened or confused, but unable to communicate effec-

I slept sounder than I remember to have done in my life . . . for when I awaked it was daylight. I attempted to rise, but was not able to stir; for as I happened to lie on my back, I found my arms and legs were strongly fastened on each side to the ground. . . . I likewise felt several slender ligaments across my body, from my armpits and my thighs. I could only look upwards . . . and the light offended my eyes. I heard a confused noise about me; but in the posture I lay I could see nothing.

Jonathon Swift
Gulliver's Travels

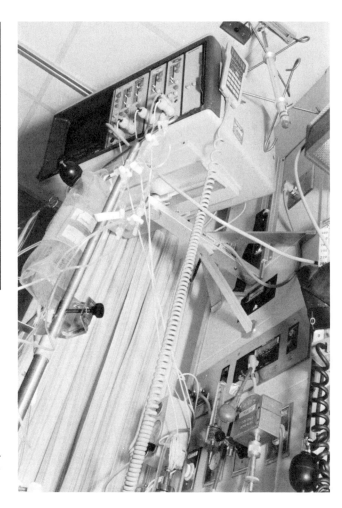

Fig. 7-1 View from patient's perspective in an intensive care unit. (From Beare PG and Myers J (1990). Principles and practice of adult health nursing. St Louis: The CV Mosby Co.)

tively because of the ventilator. Later on in their recovery, however, some patients have difficulty recalling time spent in the ICU. Others have vivid recall of even the smallest details of their care.

As patients become more aware, they are thankful for having received (and survived) the transplant procedure. Preoperative symptoms of angina, shortness of breath or extreme fatigue, and reliance on dialysis are gone. Family members are the first to note such external signs as a decrease in jaundice or a return to "normal color."

Occasionally narcotics, steroids, or other medications can contribute to an acute psychosis. This psychosis is often accompanied by a paranoid reaction made worse for many heart transplant patients because they cannot clearly see their family members or caregivers, who are covered by sterile hats, gloves, masks, and gowns.

During the first few days after surgery, patients may be disoriented and often become delirious. They may be frightened, anxious, agitated, euphoric, or withdrawn. Patients may talk about dreams, which may in fact be hallucinations or illusions that occur during their delirious states.

They often talk about the experience as being "reborn." This is a time when patients' fantasies about the donor are especially prominent. Many patients know the city where the organ came from and the age of the donor. Sometimes the family members of the transplanted patient find out through the local newspaper or television news station about a trauma victim and deduce the identity of the donor. If asked, they may express fantasies about the cause of death, the characteristics of the donor, and his or her family.

The immediate postoperative period has been described as the honeymoon period.[40] Patients are "in love" with their new organ. Many feel better than they have in years and want to write books, raise funds for the transplant team, and talk about their experience to anyone who will listen. The combination of medications and the normal euphoric state immediately after transplant can make a patient seem quite manic. Many patients at this time believe that they will be among the minority who have no complications, and that their organ will not reject. Grateful at the chance for a "second life," they may want to "fulfill a bargain made with God during the wait for a donor organ."[29]

Families may have difficulty accepting the fact that their loved one has an organ from a donor of the opposite sex or that the organ came from a person of an ethnically dissimilar background (see the discussion on p. 118). This anxiety may be handled with jokes about a wife's growing a beard or a father's taking up ballet. The spouse of one such transplant patient at our institution wondered nervously how her husband would be "changed," because he now had the heart of a 17-year-old woman.

One patient (a white male) was terrified that he had received an "unchristian heart"; another (a white male), having been told that the heart had come from a local inner-city hospital, was angry at the possibility that he had received a heart from a black man. Another patient, believing that he had a 19-year-old heart, expected to be able to quickly resume mountain climbing and marathon running, and was excited that he would no longer be impotent. A few days later, he became depressed after learning from an article in the local newspaper that he had received the heart of a young woman who had died in a tragic accident. For several days he lay in bed, not participating in his recovery, until he was able to share how guilty he felt for benefiting from the young girl's misfortune. Further, he now felt that his expectations about being a "jock" and being sexually potent were no longer possible because he had "a lady inside him."

Much attention is given to the donor organ, but it is also important to help patients resolve the loss of their organ. Although the organ to be explanted is no longer considered functional, it is keeping the patient alive. Realizing that one's beating heart or liver has been taken from one's body and replaced with that of a dead person can bring to the surface unconscious fears or anxieties that many patients, given the opportunity, are willing to express: "What did they do with my heart?" "Can I see it?" "Did they throw my liver away?"

Some patients deal with this loss by a reparative fantasy. One patient fantasized that his organ was at the National Institutes of Health, being studied by scientists, or being used to teach medical students and other physicians. It is important to explore these fantasies and to help the patient grieve for their loss so that they can accept the new organ.

Survivor guilt is commonly experienced by transplant recipients and is often evident in patients' dreams. Analyzing dreams is particularly useful, because patients do not repress their unacceptable thoughts in dreams. One patient who had spent months waiting for a suitable donor, and who frequently joked about killing a few people in the hospital parking lot, had a recurrent nightmare after his transplant that he was a Ninja warrior, killing everyone in sight, so that he might live and enjoy a sense of power. Another patient had violent nightmares about automobile accidents in which she was driving and her mother kept being killed. When asked about her associations with the dream, she replied, "I felt guilty. I wanted them to take my mother to the hospital. Instead, there was only one bed left, and I got it." This patient, who had been very ill at the time of surgery, felt that she did not deserve the transplant, since she had not waited as long as some of her peers who were not as sick as she.

Another patient, after her first liver transplant failed, dreamed that she could fly but that in her flight she would knock into other people and send them to their death. This patient felt guilty because she enjoyed the flying part of her dream. Dreams like these are not unexpected when we realize that these patients wait weeks, sometimes months, for someone to die so that they can survive.

Transfer to the floor

Some researchers have identified the psychologic difficulties during the period of hospitalization and immediately after discharge. Questionnaires sent to 11 transplant centers produced data from a total of 595 heart transplant recipients. All centers reported that during the initial hospitalization their patients experienced depression and mood alterations, an increase in family stress, problems with changing body image, and an increase in marital stress.[77]

When patients are transferred from the ICU, they may experience mild depression. This time of transition is sometimes described as an "emotional roller coaster."[5] Patients who have been extremely dependent are expected to begin assuming responsibility for their care. They may have become quite dependent on the nurses and equipment in the ICU and feel anxious and afraid about being transferred to the floor, where they will receive less monitoring and less intensive care. They may become disillusioned and angry and may experience periods of regression or rebellion, during which they want others to provide total care of them.

As patients adjust to life after transplant surgery, the process of incorporation takes place.[7] During incorporation, the patient accepts the new organ as part of his body. For some patients this creates psychologic difficulties and for most patients requires evolution through several stages, leading finally to acceptance. Patients from different cultural and ethnic backgrounds react differently. Generally, though, about two weeks after surgery patients begin to assimilate the new organ as their own. The organ can sometimes be viewed as having taken on human characteristics or a personality of its own. One patient whose biopsy showed signs of mild rejection said his liver was "being temperamental and refusing to cooperate" and that he was "going to have a talk with it." Another man who denied any feelings toward his new heart began sobbing during a heart biopsy when he saw on the catheterization screen that his new heart was sewn into his chest with staples. It was only then that he realized *his* heart was gone.

The first biopsy procedure is likely to cause the patient anxiety, because its outcome predicts to some degree the patient's immediate prognosis. Even a report of mild rejection may cause depression and feelings of hopelessness. Patients may blame themselves for not being "perfect enough" to avoid rejection.[29] Because the patient in early rejection may show no external signs of rejection and continue to feel well, he may refuse to accept the diagnosis. Because rejection is usually treated with high dosages of corticosteroids, this can place the patient more at risk for affective and cognitive disturbances.[40]

As the recovery process continues, efforts should be made to help patients reestablish family roles. There may be some resistance or reluctance, by spouses especially, to let the patient reestablish these roles that were altered as a result of chronic illness. Visits by a home health nurse during this period may help the family adjust. The home health nurse can also identify problems that require more formal family interventions.

Long-term adjustment and recovery

The recovery period extends far past the discharge from the hospital. Although patients are generally eager to leave the hospital, they may, when the discharge date approaches, begin to regress. Patients feel safe in the hospital, where immediate medical attention is obtained by pushing a buzzer. Patients may feel ambivalent as they prepare to leave the place where they were "saved" or "reborn." Consistent with the theme of rebirth, one patient described his impending discharge as "leaving the cocoon"; another described it as "leaving the womb." It is after their discharge that patients may begin to talk about a fear of life rather than a fear of death.[10]

Problems noted in the preoperative evaluation may continue into the postoperative period, the most common being anxiety and depression. Patients may begin to worry about mounting hospital bills and organ rejection, or they may begin to deal with an unresolved grief reaction to the loss of their diseased organ.[18] One patient who was doing well 3 months after his liver transplant was found dead from suicide. Although some of the reasons for his suicide remain a mystery, he had reportedly become upset over the hospital bill he had received that day.

Some patients who have become well entrenched in the sick role may have difficulty adjusting to a less dependent role. They may refuse to exercise or care for themselves and, more seriously, may refuse to take their medications. This kind of behavior may be a way to reassume the sick role and be taken care of again.

Because patients commonly view their transplant as a rebirth or a new life, it is not unusual for them to begin to talk about having been born on the day of their surgery and later to celebrate their transplant birthday. Some patients may actually begin to believe they are younger than their chronologic age. Some case studies from our institution illustrate this point. One patient reasoned that since the heart is the seat of life and he had received the heart of a 21-year-old, he was somewhere between 21 and 45 (his age). He began dressing and acting much younger and divorced his wife for a younger woman who could keep up with him. Another woman who had been married nearly 20 years, and ill for most of that time, became promiscuous after the transplant because, she stated, "I feel like a teenager now, and I am making up for lost time."

Body image changes may continue to be a problem for the patient after transplant surgery. Patients joke about the external signs of transplant, such as the midline zipper scar after a heart transplant and the Mercedes Benz scar after a liver transplant. Long-term use of immunosuppressants induces alterations in their physical appearance. Cyclosporine therapy induces abnormal hair growth (hirsutism), and a high-dose regimen of steroids can cause undesirable side effects such as moon facies, hirsutism, acne, and weight gain. Because our bodies give us a sense of self, these external changes are very important in terms of the way patients think about themselves. In what has been called the Frankenstein syndrome, they may perceive themselves as "damaged" or "pieced together."[78] Finally, reverse isolation, used to protect some transplant patients from infections, requires that the patients wear surgical masks while in public areas. The masked appearance may result in social stigmatization, and the fear from others that they are contagious.

Patients may have sexual dysfunction before transplant and wonder whether they can have sexual relations after surgery. One heart transplant patient who had been impotent before his surgery called the transplant psychiatrist 3 months after his transplant, wondering whether he could "put on his wedding ring." Discussion revealed the latent message: The patient had had an erection and wondered whether it was safe to have intercourse.

After the patient returns home, frequent outpatient follow-up visits to the treating physicians may prove reassuring. When frequent travel to the center is not possible, a system whereby the patient can call his physician, or nurse coordinator working with the transplant team, with questions or concerns may be helpful.

Although few long-term quality of life studies have been done on transplant patients, the self-reports of most heart transplant patients are encouraging. More than 90% of survivors of a heart transplant return to New York Heart Association class 1 cardiac status, and 82% to 92% of the heart transplant recipients at Stanford University who survive longer than 1 year have been classified as rehabilitated.[79,80] In a study of 75 heart transplant recipients, 89% rated their quality of life as good to excellent, and 82% were satisfied with that quality. There were positive changes in feelings about themselves, and patients were pleased with their independence and sense of accomplishment. Negative quality of life factors included financial strain and physical appearance.[81]

Varying degrees of depression, anxiety, anger, and behavioral regression are present after kidney and liver transplant. These problems affect the patient's self-report on overall quality of life. In a recent study comparing kidney and liver transplant recipients, 32% of kidney recipients and 100% of liver recipients were found to be experiencing psychiatric distress.[4] In kidney transplant patients the distress tended to abate when the patient's physical status improved. Unfortunately, liver transplant patients have longer hospital stays and longer dependent relationships with caregivers and, technically, this operation is more difficult. These factors often lead to more frequent complications, which may account for the reported differences in overall quality of life.

In a study assessing the quality of life in 859 patients with end-stage renal disease, 79% of kidney transplant recipients were able to function at nearly normal levels, compared with between 24% and 59% of those patients undergoing dialysis.[82] The functional ability of patients, including their physical activity, ability to administer self-care, life satisfaction, ability to work, and psychologic affect were studied. On three subjective measures (life satisfaction, well-being, and psychologic affect), transplant recipients had a higher quality of life than patients on dialysis.[82]

As the need for biopsies and clinic visits becomes less frequent and patients settle into their normal routines, they talk about the little things they are grateful for: their appreciation of a beautiful fall day, a picnic with a grandchild, or dinner with the spouse. There comes a day when identity shifts, and they are once again a mother, a husband, or a worker and no longer just "a transplant."

The special issue: noncompliance

"Noncompliance can be defined as any act or omission on the part of the patient that fails to conform to the advice and recommendations of his physicians."[83] Commonly cited as good predictors for future compliance are the ability to tolerate adverse conditions and the availability of emotional support from family and friends.[25] Conversely, noncompliers are said to have low tolerance for frustration and an inability to delay gratification.[84]

It is difficult to assess preoperatively whether a patient will be compliant postoperatively, because the pretransplant patient is often desperate to accept all treatment recommendations in exchange for a transplant. Certainly, a history of medication or dietary noncompliance and poor coping skills are indicators of potential problems. Unfortunately, few studies have examined noncompliance in transplant patients.

We know that excessive denial of one's illness can lead to noncompliance. Patients who tend to deny their illness do not accept the significance of treatment recommendations. For these patients an intervention may be necessary to break through the denial. A psychologic conflict may underlie other patients' noncompliance. Patients who feel unresolved anger or hostility over their illness may become noncompliant and act out in self-destructive ways. In its most severe form, a patient commits suicide either by being noncompliant with medicines and diet or by taking his life. It has been found that playing on the patient's fears in the hope of increasing compliance is ineffective and may actually hinder compliance.[85,86]

Patients who have little family support may form strong attachments to the staff, who meet many of their emotional needs. Discharging these very dependent patients abruptly or without consideration of their strong attachments may be seen unconsciously by the patient as abandonment or "being kicked out of the house." Noncompliance may be one way of gaining readmission to the hospital, where the patient can be taken care of by his or her medical family.

One teenaged patient from a highly dysfunctional family refused to take his medication despite the knowledge that this would result in rejection of his liver. His mother, an alcoholic, was unsupportive, and during a 7-month hospital stay in which he received three liver transplants, he was "adopted" by a caring and supportive nursing staff who became, in effect, mother surrogates. The institutional and staff transference reactions were pronounced. Although he did well while hospitalized, he refused to take his medication after discharge. His body ultimately rejected the liver, and he died.

Occasionally, noncompliance may signal a disruption in the patient-physician relationship. The patient may feel abandoned by the surgeon who transfers the patient's care to internal medicine physicians or other medical specialists after surgery. This perceived abandonment can have very serious, even life-threatening, consequences. Regular contact after discharge with the transplant clinical nurse specialist and surgeon improves knowledge and compliance in the following areas: medications, progression of physical activity, resumption of sexual activity, weight reduction, and reporting and treatment of pain.[87]

According to one study of compliance in transplant patients, educated patients in professional positions and those with manual skills were more able to comply with the demands of the posttransplant regimen than were others.[81] In one series of heart transplant patients, noncompliance contributed to graft failure in 21% and death in 26%.[13] According to this study, the risk for noncompliance increased for patients who had less family support, who were single or divorced, and who were less than 40 years of age.

Understanding some of the psychologic conflicts that contribute to noncompliance may decrease the incidence and morbidity of noncompliance. Prompt attention to noncompliance is certainly imperative. Noncompliance may be the red flag to the transplant team that patients are having psychiatric difficulty adjusting to and living with their new organ. It is the one sign readily seen by nonpsychiatric staff and, if observed, should alert the team to look for psychiatric difficulties.

REFERENCES

1. Ferguson RM (1988). The evolution of solid organ transplantation. In Gallagher TJ and Shoemaker WC (editors). *Critical care: state of the art*, vol 9, pp 1-21. Fullerton, Calif: Society of Critical Care Medicine.
2. Riether AM and Stoudemire A (1987). Surgery and trauma. In Stoudemire A and Fogel BS (editors). *Principles of medical psychiatry*, pp 423-450. New York: Grune & Stratton.
3. House RM and Thompson TL (1988). Psychiatric aspects of organ transplantation. *Journal of the American Medical Association, 260*, 535-539.
4. House RM, Dubovsky SL and Penn I (1983). Psychiatric aspects of hepatic transplantation. *Transplantation, 36*(2), 146-150.
5. Gulledge AD, Buszta C and Montague DK (1983). Psychosocial aspects of renal transplantation. *Urologic Clinics of North America, 10*, 327-335.
6. Lefebvre P and Crombez J (1977, August). *The one-day-at-a-time syndrome in post-transplant evolution.* Paper presented at World Congress of Psychiatry, Honolulu, Hawaii.
7. Mulsin HL (1971). On acquiring a kidney. *American Journal of Psychiatry, 127*, 1185-1188.
8. Freyberger H (1973). Six years experience as a psychosomaticist in a hemodialysis unit. In *Topics of psychosomatic research*. Basel: Karger.
9. Sutherland DER, Goetz FC and Najarian JS (1984). Pancreas transplants from related donors. *Transplantation, 38*, 625-633.

10. Kemph JP (1966). Renal failure, artificial kidney and kidney transplant. *American Journal of Psychiatry, 122,* 1270-1274.

11. Abram HS and Buchanan DC (1976-77). The gift of life: a review of the psychological aspects of kidney transplantation. *International Journal of Psychiatry in Medicine, 7*(2), 153-164.

12. Chapman CR and Cox GB (1977). Anxiety, pain and depression surrounding elective surgery: A multivariate comparison of abdominal surgery patients with kidney donors and recipients. *Journal of Psychosomatic Research, 21,* 7-15.

13. Dubovsky SI and Penn I (1980). Psychiatric considerations in renal transplant surgery. *Psychosomatics, 21,* 481-491.

14. Hong BA, Smith MD, Robson AM and Wetzel RD (1987). Depressive symptomatology and treatment in patients with end-stage renal disease. *Psychological Medicine, 17,* 185-190.

15. American Psychiatric Association (1987). *Diagnostic and statistical manual of mental disorders* (3rd ed, rev). Washington, DC: Author.

16. Lowry MR and Atcherson E (1979). Characteristics of patients with depressive disorder on entry into home hemodialysis. *Journal of Nervous and Mental Disease, 167,* 748-751.

17. Reichsman F and Levy NB (1972). Problems in adaptation to maintenance hemodialysis: a four-year study of 25 patients. *Archives of Internal Medicine, 130,* 859-865.

18. Penn I, Bunch D, Olenik D and Abouna G (1971). Psychiatric experience with patients receiving renal and hepatic transplants. *Seminars in Psychiatry, 3,* 133-144.

19. House A (1987). Psychosocial problems of patients on the renal unit and their relation to treatment outcome. *Journal of Psychosomatic Research, 31,* 441-452.

20. Greenberg RP, Davis G and Massey R (1973). The psychological evaluation of patients for a kidney transplant and hemodialysis program. *American Journal of Psychiatry, 130,* 274-277.

21. Simmons RG, Kamstra-Hennen L and Thompson CR (1981). Psychosocial adjustment five to nine years posttransplant. *Transplantation Proceedings, 13,* 40-43.

22. Castelnuovo-Tedesco P (1971). Cardiac surgeons look at transplantation—interviews with Drs. Cleveland, Cooley, DeBakey, Hallman, and Rochelle. *Seminars in Psychiatry, 3*(1), 5-16.

23. Hotson JR and Pedley TA (1976). The neurological complications of cardiac transplantation. *Brain, 99,* 673-694.

24. Glassman BM and Siegel A (1970). Personality correlates of survival in a long-term hemodialysis program. *Archives of General Psychiatry, 22,* 566-574.

25. Vaillant G (1977). *Adaptation to life* (pp 75-126). Boston: Little, Brown & Co.

26. Kübler-Ross E (1973). *On death and dying.* New York: Macmillan Publishing Co.

27. Eisendrath RM (1969). The role of grief and fear in the death of kidney transplant patients. *American Journal of Psychiatry, 126,* 129-135.

28. Rees WD and Lutkins SG (1967). Mortality of bereavement. *British Medical Journal, 4,* 13-16.

29. Christopherson LK (1987). Cardiac transplantation: a psychological perspective. *Circulation, 75*(1), 57-62.

30. Allender J, Shisslak C, Kaszniak A and Copeland J (1983). Stages of psychological adjustment with heart transplantation. *Heart Transplantation, 2,* 228-231.

31. Folstein MF, Folstein SE and McHugh PR (1975). Mini Mental State: a practical method for grading the cognitive state of patients for the clinician. *Journal of Psychiatric Research, 12,* 189-198.

32. Christopherson LK and Luunde DT (1971). Selection of cardiac transplant recipients and their subsequent psychological adjustment. *Seminars in Psychiatry, 3,* 36-45.

33. Tisza VB, Dorsett P and Morse J (1976). Psychological implications of renal transplantation. *Journal of the American Academy of Child Psychiatry, 15,* 709-720.

34. Levenson JL and Olbrisch ME (1987). Shortage of donor organs and long waits. *Psychosomatics, 28,* 399-403.

35. Thompson ME (1983). Selection of candidates of cardiac transplantation. *Heart Transplantation, 3,* 65-69.

36. Van Thiel DH, Schode RR, Starzl TE, Iwatsuki S, Shaw BW, Gavaler JS and Dugas M (1982). Liver transplantation in adults. *Hepatology, 2,* 637-640.

37. Christopherson LK (1979). Cardiac transplantation: need for patient counseling. *Nursing Mirror, 149,* 34-36.

38. Trzepacz PT, Brenner R, Van Thiel DH (1989). A psychiatric study of 247 liver transplantation candidates. *Psychosomatics, 30*(2), 147-153.

39. Freeman AM, Watts D and Karp R (1984). Evaluation of cardiac transplant candidates: preliminary observations. *Psychosomatics, 25,* 197-207.

40. Watts D, Freeman AM, McGriffin DG, Kirklin JK, McVay R and Karp RB (1984). Psychiatric aspects of cardiac transplantation. *Heart Transplantation, 3,* 243-247.

41. Spielberger DC (1983). *Manual for the State-Trait Anxiety Inventory.* Palo Alto, Calif: Consulting Psychologists Press.

42. Cutler NR and Narang PK (1984). Implications of dosing tricyclic antidepressants and benzodiazepines in geriatrics. *Psychiatric Clinics of North America, 7,* 845-861.

43. Basch SH (1980). Emotional dehiscence after successful renal transplantation. *Kidney International, 17,* 388-396.

44. Lakshminarayan S, Sahn SA, Hudson LD and Weil J (1976). Effects of diazepam on ventilatory responses. *Clinical Pharmacology and Therapeutics, 20,* 178-183.

45. Stoudemire A and Fogel BS (1987). Psychopharmacology. In Stoudemire A and Fogel BS (eds). *Principles of medical psychiatry* (pp 79-112). New York: Grune & Stratton.

46. Beck AT, Ward CH, Mendelson M, Mock JE and Erbaugh J (1961). An inventory for measuring depression. *Archives of General Psychiatry, 4,* 561-571.

47. Surman O (1978). The surgical patient. In Hackett TP and Cassem NH (eds). *Massachusetts General Hospital*

handbook of general hospital psychiatry (pp 65-92). St Louis: The CV Mosby Co.

48. Beidel DC (1987). Psychological factors in organ transplantation. Clinical Psychology Review, 7, 677-694.

49. Levenson JL (1985). Neuroleptic malignant syndrome. American Journal of Psychiatry, 142, 1137-1145.

50. Glassman AH, Johnson LL, Giardina EV, Walsh T, Roose SP, Cooper TB and Bigger JT (1983). The use of imipramine in depressed patients with congestive heart failure. Journal of the American Medical Association, 250, 1977-2001.

51. Roose SP, Glassman AH and Giardina EV (1986). Nortriptyline in depressed patients with left ventricular impairment. Journal of the American Medical Association, 256, 3253-3257.

52. Levine PM, Silberfarb PM and Lipowski ZJ (1978). Mental disorders in cancer patients: a study of 100 psychiatric referrals. Cancer, 42, 1385-1391.

53. Trzepacz PT, Teague GB and Lipowski ZJ (1985). Delirium and other organic mental disorders in a general hospital. General Hospital Psychiatry, 7, 101-106.

54. Rabins PV and Folstein MF (1982). Delirium and dementia: diagnostic criteria and fatality rates. British Journal of Psychiatry, 140, 149-153.

55. Weddington WW Jr (1982). The mortality of delirium: An underappreciated problem. Psychosomatics, 23, 1232-1235.

56. Stead EA (1966). Reversible madness. Medical Times, 94, 1403-1406.

57. Murray GB (1987). Confusion, delirium and dementia. In Hacket TC and Cassem NH (eds). Massachusetts General Hospital handbook of general psychiatry (2nd ed, pp 84-115). Littleton, Mass: PSG Publishing.

58. Lipowski ZJ (1987). Delirium (acute confusional states). Journal of the American Medical Association, 258, 1789-1792.

59. Engle GL and Romano J (1959). Delirium, a syndrome of cerebral insufficiency. Journal of Chronic Diseases, 9, 260-277.

60. Obrecht R, Okhomina FOA and Scott DF (1979). Value of EEG in acute confusional states. Journal of Neurology, Neurosurgery, and Psychiatry (London), 42, 75-77.

61. Reitan RM (1958). Validity of the Trailmaking test as an indicator of organic brain damage. Perceptual and Motor Skills, 8, 271-276.

62. Lezak MD (1983). Neuropsychological assessment (2nd ed). New York: Oxford University Press.

63. Trzepacz PT, Brenner RP, Coffman G and Van Thiel DH (1988). Delirium in liver transplantation candidates: discriminant analysis of multiple test variables. Biological Psychiatry, 24, 3-14.

64. Murray GB (1978). Confusion, delirium and dementia. In Hackett TC and Cassem NH (eds). Massachusetts General Hospital handbook of general psychiatry (1st ed, pp 93-116). St Louis: The CV Mosby Co.

65. Mai FM, McKenzie FN and Kostuk WJ (1986). Psychiatric aspects of heart transplantation: Preoperative evaluation and postoperative sequelae. British Medical Journal, 292, 311-313.

66. Dudley DL, Rowlett DE and Loebel PJ (1979). Emergency use of intravenous haloperidol. General Hospital Psychiatry, 1, 240-246.

67. Tesar GE and Stern TA (1986). Evaluation and treatment of agitation in the intensive care unit. Journal of Intensive Care Medicine, 1, 137-148.

68. Slaby AE and Cullen LO (1987). Dementia and delirium. In Stoudemire A and Fogel BS (eds). Principles of medical psychiatry (pp 135-169). New York: Grune & Stratton.

69. Freeman AM, Folks DG, Sokol RS and Fahs JJ (1988). Cardiac transplantation: clinical correlates of psychiatric outcome. Psychosomatics, 29, 47-54.

70. Helfrich GB, Chu-Aquino B, Pechan W and Moores C (1980). Are there too many complications from renal transplantation? In Schreiner GE (ed). Controversies in nephrology. Washington, DC: Georgetown University Hospital.

71. Castelnuovo-Tedesco P (1973). Organ transplant, body image, psychosis. Psychoanalytic Quarterly, 42, 349-363.

72. Groves JE and Manschreck TC (1987). Psychotic patients. In Hackett TP and Cassem NH (eds). Massachusetts General Hospital handbook of psychiatry (2nd ed, pp 209-226). Littleton, Mass: PSG Publishing.

73. Casscells W (1986). Heart transplantation: recent policy developments. New England Journal of Medicine, 315, 1365-1368.

74. Bustuttil RW (moderator). Discussants: Goldstein LI, Danovitch GM, Ament ME and Memsic LD (1986). Liver transplantation today. Annals of Internal Medicine, 104, 377-389.

75. Frierson RL and Lipmann SB (1987). Heart transplant candidates rejected on psychiatric indications. Psychosomatics, 28, 347-355.

76. Evans RB and Brodia JH (1985). Executive summary: National Heart Transplantation Study. Seattle: Battelle Human Affairs Research Center.

77. McAleer MJ, Copeland J, Fuller J and Copeland JG (1985). Psychological aspects of heart transplantation. Heart Transplantation, 4, 232-233.

78. Dubovsky SL, Metzner JL and Warner RB (1979). Problems with internalization of a transplanted liver. American Journal of Psychiatry, 136, 1090-1091.

79. Christopherson LK, Griepp RB and Stinson EB (1976). Rehabilitation after cardiac transplantation. Journal of the American Medical Association, 236, 2082.

80. Samuelsson RG, Hunt SA and Schroeder JS (1984). Functional and social rehabilitation of heart transplant recipients under age thirty. Scandinavian Journal of Thoracic and Cardiovascular Surgery, 18, 97.

81. Lough ME, Lindsey AM, Shinn JA and Stotts NA (1985). Life satisfaction following heart transplantation. Heart Transplantation, 4, 446.

82. Evans RW, Manninen DL, Garrison LP, Hart LG, Blagg CR, Gutman RA, Hull AR and Lowrie EG (1985). The quality of life of patients with end-stage renal disease. New England Journal of Medicine, 312, 553-559.

83. Cooper DKC, Lanza RP and Barnard CN (1984). Noncompliance in heart transplant recipients: the Cape Town experience. Heart Transplantation, 111, 248-253.

84. Stewart RS (1983). Psychiatric issues in renal dialysis and transplantation. *Hospital and Community Psychiatry, 34,* 623-628.

85. Eisenthal S, Emery R, Lazare A and Udin H (1979). 'Adherence' and the negotiated approach to patient-hood. *Archives of General Psychiatry, 36,* 393-398.

86. Matthews D and Hingson R (1977). Improving patient compliance. *Medical Clinics of North America, 61,* 879-889.

87. Marshall J, Penckofer S and Llewellyn J (1986). Structured postoperative teaching and knowledge and compliance of patients who had coronary artery bypass surgery. *Heart and Lung, 15*(1), 76-82.

8

Psychologic Stresses for Transplant Nurses

Anne Marie Riether

Much has been written about the indications for organ transplants, the surgical procedures, potential complications, and the recovery of the patient.[1-4] Little attention, however, has been paid to the psychologic effects that a transplantation program has on the nurses who care for these patients. When a hospital administration decides to begin a transplantation program, a great deal of excitement may be felt as the surgical team assembles and awaits their first patient. Unfortunately, nursing needs are often overlooked in these preparations, decisions, and subsequent planning. In this chapter the impact of a transplantation program on nurses is examined. Role conflicts, identity changes, and the common emotional reactions of nurses are discussed. Finally, some ways to help patients and nurses through the emotional rites of passage of transplant surgery are presented.

Patients who are being considered for transplant surgery are by definition in organ failure. Although they come from differing backgrounds and cultures and have different personalities and cognitive abilities, they have in common an intractable organ failure that cannot be treated by other, lesser surgical or medical means. Before the advent of transplant surgery, these patients ultimately faced death, and nursing's role was to assist the patient and family in this

process. However, some of these patients are now being given a better prognosis with transplant surgery. Today nurses have the difficult task of helping their patients adjust emotionally to an almost certain death if they do not undergo transplant surgery while helping them to prepare emotionally for their surgery and subsequent recovery after transplantation.[5]

Unfortunately, beginning transplantation programs may fail to address psychologic issues, possible conflicts, and identity changes that nurses may experience.[6] A nurse familiar with dialysis, atherosclerotic heart disease, or hepatitis may feel ill equipped to deal with a patient who is undergoing kidney, heart, or liver transplantation. These surgeries, unlike other types of operations, are radical and most times irreversible procedures. Nurses may question the ethics or morality of the surgery.[7] If they have seen multiple postoperative complications, life-style restrictions, and day-to-day side effects, they may question whether their efforts and those of the transplant team are worthwhile.

The nursing environment, as well as identity of the nurse, changes when a transplantation program is begun. An intensive care unit (ICU) that has housed a wide variety of acutely ill patients may suddenly become the "pretransplant unit," a type of critical care holding area for patients who are waiting for donor organs to become available.

☐ With special acknowledgment to Martha Zalewa Boudreau, RN, BSN, for her contributions to this chapter.

The selection of suitable transplant candidates is generally not determined by the nurses who care for these patients.[4,8] Regardless of their personal feelings about the suitability of a particular patient, nurses are charged with caring for the patient's medical, as well as emotional, needs.[5] During the wait for a suitable donor, patients may begin to deteriorate, and the nurse may feel conflict, reluctant to give up hope yet fearing that a donor will not be found in time. If an organ is found, nurses may feel guilt about the death of the donor, especially if the donor was a patient in the same institution or the same ICU.

If nurses are not given an opportunity to work through these emotion-laden issues, conflicts may arise that will affect the care of these patients. Although each patient's situation and personality are unique, the nursing staff caring for particular types of transplant patients share common experiences. A description of these patients and nursing interventions follows.

TYPES OF PATIENTS

Patients who are critically ill are often at the limit of their coping abilities. Emotionally as well as physically depleted, they cannot care for themselves and therefore look to their nurses and physicians for caring. Families are also in need of comfort and often cannot provide the much-needed support to patients during this stressful time. Some transplant patients exhibit maladaptive patterns of behavior that can open the door to a destructive relationship between nurse and patient.

The dependent patient

Nurses caring for dependent patients often feel like a parent caring for a small child. Dependent patients seem incapable of caring for even their most basic needs and want their nurse-parent to do it for them. They often become attached to a particular nurse, and if this "favorite nurse" is not caring for them, they may become withdrawn and despondent. Like small children who do not want to be left alone, these patients may call their nurses into their rooms, frequently for relatively minor requests. They may convince their nurses that no one else can care for them, leaving their nurses feeling guilty when they

leave at the end of their shift. Unconsciously, these patients expect their nurses to magically protect them from harm, just as children see their parents as omnipotent adults. They may blame their nurses for any complication that befalls them and become angry that their nurses are not using their influence with the transplant team to serve as advocate for them to get them an organ. Helping these patients to assume more of the responsibility of their care can often foster more mature behavior.

In the more severe stages, patients may "perform" only when their favorite nurse is present, not wanting to eat, talk, participate in physical therapy, or cooperate with their treatment at other times. Like adolescents acting out with a substitute teacher, they may throw temper tantrums when other nurses care for them. Showering their nurse with compliments, they expect total devotion and may become enraged if their favorite nurse is not there for them. As boundaries become blurred, separations can become difficult for the nurse as well as the patient. Nurses may begin visiting their patients during their off-time and thinking about their patients while at home. Falling into the trap of accepting the role of nurse-parent, they may feel guilty for taking a vacation and leaving this terminally ill "child," who might die before they return. Alternative, more healthy interactions encourage a shared team approach to the patients, allowing the patients to share in the responsibility for their own care.

Because of the intense dependence and neediness of these patients, nurses other than the primary nurse may have difficulty caring for them. They may also resent the patient's thinking that a particular nurse is the only one who can care for them. Once operating, these dynamics may be difficult to correct, because the primary nurse, as well as the patient, generally experiences a resistance to separating. Changing assignments is not always an easy solution. Nurses caught in this conflict may become overprotective and defensive about "their patient" and become critical of the care that their peers give. They may feel guilty about leaving their patient with a nurse who "doesn't understand the patient as I do." Classic signs of this problem are the nurse's feeling exhaustion before the shift starts, yet feeling unable to leave when the shift is over.

Patients also have difficulty with a change of assignment. Just as a small child becomes jealous when another child comes into the home, patients may become angry when "their" nurse is assigned to another patient. Patients who are already feeling vulnerable may feel abandoned and become quite despondent, requiring psychiatric intervention.

The best remedy for this situation is to identify these dynamics as early as possible. If nurses begin to feel that they are the "only ones" who can care for, or understand, particular patients, this should be addressed in a supportive environment such as a support group.

Unit policies concerning special privileges for patients, the giving and accepting of patient gifts, visitation, or visits by nurses during off-hours should be observed consistently by all staff. If these limits are not observed, splitting can occur; that is, patients label some nurses "mean" for not allowing them to break the rules and other nurses "nice" for being lenient.

The angry patient

Most nurses have had some experience with angry patients. They are easy to spot and seem to spend most of their time complaining. Nothing seems to please them. They are the patients who no nurse wants to take because they make the nurse feel useless and angry. They may have difficulty communicating the reason for their anger and may act out or become verbally abusive. These patients are often demanding, insensitive, and self-centered. It may seem that the more the nurse does for them, the more they expect. They may be critical of the nurse to the nurse's peers and to their family, making it frustrating to care for them and care about them. A small change in these patients' schedules may trigger an explosive rage, and once ignited, this anger often keeps others at a distance.

Angry patients may also become silent or refuse treatments and procedures. Because transplant patients may be fearful of angering the transplant team, the group of people who have the power to save their lives, they frequently turn their anger inward and do not comply with their treatment. Left untreated, anger can become self-destructive, even life threatening. These patients may fear abandonment if they openly express their anger at their primary nurse or members of the transplant team, and may simmer until a "float" nurse is assigned to care for them. Suddenly, the patient explodes with rage. Because the float nurse is not part of the transplant team, the patient considers it safe to ventilate anger. This sudden outburst may prove very therapeutic and cathartic for the angry patient but may be very upsetting to the nurse who is unaware of the underlying dynamics.

Although it is difficult to care for someone who shows these personality characteristics, a key to making the situation tolerable is to try not to take it personally. These patients may be using this style of coping to avoid getting close, or they may be angry at their medical situation. For some, nothing short of getting well will satisfy them. Linking their behavior to their feelings is particularly helpful. For example: "Mr. Jones, I see you are not eating and that you are complaining about the food. I am wondering if it is because you are upset about not being transplanted last weekend when a heart was available." This kind of interpretation links the patient's behavior to a situation and to emotions that the patient may have difficulty acknowledging directly. It opens the door to communication about the real issue rather than superficial talk about hospital food.

Another helpful intervention is the use of "I" messages. In this type of communication the nurse, using nonjudgmental statements that begin with "I," makes an observation about the patient's behavior and then expresses thoughts about that behavior, how it makes the nurse feel, and what she or he would like to happen. Using the example mentioned earlier, the nurse can very easily express concern to the patient by using I messages:

I see: Comment on the person's behavior

I think: Comment on what you think is going on

I feel: Comment on how the patient's behavior makes you feel

I want: Comment on what you would like the patient to change

Putting this together, you might say something like this:

"I see you are not eating and that you are complaining about the food. I think that you may be upset about not being transplanted last weekend when a heart was available. I feel sad and disappointed for you, but I would like you to at least try to eat some dinner."

Once in the habit of using I messages with patients, nurses find that they can be very empathetic communication tools. Consider the alternative, nonempathetic style of communication: "Stop complaining about the food. You know you need to eat something so you can get ready for your transplant."

When anger begins to interfere with nursing care, consultation with a psychiatrist or psychiatric clinical nurse specialist familiar with the issues of critically ill patients may be helpful. A patient's anger may be the only evidence of underlying depression or impending psychologic decompensation. Often these patients become more angry as their physical condition deteriorates. They may resort to unacceptable behaviors in an attempt to gain control of the situation, speaking critically of one or more nurses to manipulate the nursing assignment or "bribing" health care workers to obtain more fluids than their fluid restriction allows.

Caring for several of these patients simultaneously certainly intensifies the stress for nurses. Keeping these patients alive demands energy as well as skill. Caring for these angry patients can be exhausting, leading to feelings of unappreciation and abuse. After caring for these types of patients over a long period, nurses often complain of feeling disillusioned and burned out. The institution must plan effective ways to supplement routine coverage when several of these patients are unstable at the same time. Weekly support group meetings, discussed later in this chapter, are an effective way for nurses to ventilate their feelings about these patients. Leading these groups, the psychiatric clinical nurse specialist or the transplant psychiatrist can help the nursing staff understand the psychodynamic defenses of displacement that angry patients frequently use.

The controlling patient

Controlling patients like to run the show; they give those taking care of them "orders of the day" and like to give the impression that they are experts on everything. They may tell the nurses when they are available for procedures and "advise" them on the mixing of intravenous infusions and medications. They have a difficult time assuming the patient role and often come from a supervisory, military, or medical background. They may tell the transplant team when they want their transplant and have difficulty accepting the uncertainty of the waiting period. The more out of control these patients feel with regard to their destiny, the more they attempt to control their surroundings. They may order their family in for a conference or try to conduct business as usual from their hospital beds.

These patients can be either authoritative or patronizing to their nurses; the dynamics are the same. Comments such as "It must be frustrating for you not to know when or if you are going to be transplanted," or "I know it's difficult being a patient and having things done to you all the time" are useful. Allowing these patients some control over their day is also helpful. For example, allowing them to decide when they want to bathe, eat breakfast, and schedule appointments with physical and occupational therapy may be helpful. Exploring what their lives were like before they became ill can provide insight into their losses, including how their self-esteem is linked with being in control.

The apathetic patient

Unlike controlling patients, apathetic patients allow nurses to perform any intervention without question or protest. Their affects are usually flat or inappropriate. They may smile during painful procedures or show little response to pain. They often do not react to good or bad news about their condition and do not seem interested in actively participating in their care. They usually appear lethargic, without goals or plans for the future.

The nurses who care for these patients may begin to assume the feelings that seem to be absent. They may begin to hurt for their patients, worry for them, and cry for them. Nurses may talk for the patient and answer questions posed by the treating physician.

Sometimes nurses emotionally "fuse" with the patient. A clue that this process is occurring is the nurse's use of the plural rather than the singular: In giving a report, the nurse may say, "We are doing well today," or "We had another biopsy today." This emotional fusion is destructive both for the patient and the nurse. Psychiatric intervention may be needed to help separate the feelings of the nurse from those of the patient and to help the patient get in touch with his or her buried emotions.

As is true in any case of altered mental status, an organic cause for the patient's apathetic state should be sought in conjunction with contributory psychologic factors.[9,10] The patient may have an organic brain syndrome related to low cardiac output or may be encephalopathic. Cumulative doses of all medications should be recorded daily to ensure that the patient is not being overly sedated.

The denying patient

Patients who have not had serious limitations placed on their daily activities or changes in the quality of life as a result of their illness may have difficulty adjusting to the sick role. In contrast to the dependent, chronically ill patient, denying patients may refuse to accept the extent of their disease. People who have a sudden onset of organ failure may deny the extent of their disease, and this denial may interfere with their compliance. Although denial is a common defense mechanism and may be useful to decrease patients' anxiety about their condition,[10-12] total denial of their disease can be life threatening.[12] Denial can lead to noncompliance with treatment recommendations and refusal of the transplant option. The nurses caring for these patients may begin to feel angry, helpless, or hopeless. Having made repeated attempts to care for these patients, they may become irritated when patients reject their help because they are "not sick." Because denial is an unconscious defense mechanism to ward off anxiety or conflicts,[11] these patients may need psychiatric intervention to help them begin to accept their illness realistically and actively participate in treatment.

Confronting a patient's denial can be lifesaving; however, it can sometimes leave patients feeling helpless and desperate as the image that they held of themselves is dispelled. Patients should be watched closely for any suicidal ideation and appropriate measures taken if this occurs.

The manipulative patient

Often very intelligent and usually initially well liked by nursing staff, manipulative patients may try to impress the staff with their connections and seek special privileges from their nurses and other members of the transplant team. They may tell different versions of incidents, depending on what they have to gain from the situation, and they have a unique ability to get everyone involved in their drama, including top-level administrative officials. These patients may try to get nurses to grant special requests by flattery, promises of gifts, or special recognition by their friends in the administration. Often presenting themselves as victims, these manipulative persons have the uncanny ability to persuade people into willingness to rescue them from the system that has wronged them.

After caring for these patients for a while, the nurse may be left feeling conned or may begin to feel anxious or angry without knowing exactly why. Often it is not until much later that manipulation by the patient is recognized as the cause.

Sometimes it is not easy to avoid being manipulated; however, if patients consistently present themselves as victims when they seem to be capable and intelligent persons, nurses may wish to give their stories another look. It may be that these patients have been willing volunteers for all of their troubles so that they can get other people to take care of them and thus profit from their situation. Unfortunately, patients with this type of personality style are very difficult to treat because they are ego-syntonic, meaning that it causes little emotional distress or discomfort for them. It is the people who interact with these patients who become frustrated and angry at being used and manipulated.

The VIP patient

In some respects all transplant patients are VIP patients. They often get a great deal of publicity and are well known by many of the hospital personnel. They may receive special meals, private rooms, the attention of many consulting physicians, and are watched more closely than the average hospital patient. The patient's family treats him or her as a fragile member, often being quite overprotective.

Some transplant patients may take this status even further and may feel entitled to it. VIP patients may feel entitled because of their wealth, political power, or profession. As their requests are granted, they may get used to having what they want when they want it. They may get a larger room or sitters even when neither is warranted and does not seem in their best interest. They may use their influence to postpone procedures, extend visitation, and generally not follow unit rules. Nurses and physicians, afraid of confronting this behavior because of the patient's status and connections, may allow these patients to manage their own treatment. Unfortunately, the end result, ironically, is that often these entitled patients do not get the best care because of interference with their own treatment.

TEMPORAL RITES OF PASSAGE FOR THE NURSE

The nurse's role differs, depending on whether the patient is getting ready for transplant, has just undergone transplant surgery, or is preparing for discharge from the hospital. Nursing interventions are also individualized to the patient's medical and psychologic condition. The successful emotional resolution of each phase allows patients to go onto the next one. However, the hospital course of a transplant patient is often not straightforward. Readmission to the ICU or hospital can disrupt smooth transition through these phases.

A clinical nurse specialist, working with the transplant team, can help with the continuity of care by communicating the medical and psychologic needs of patients to all other appropriate nursing staff. Patient care conferences and rounds are effective ways of sharing this information among nursing staffs. Whenever possible, it is helpful for the nurses who will be on the receiving end of a patient transfer to visit the patient before the transfer. This practice can help get the patient's transition off to a good

start and keeps communication open between nursing staffs. The ultimate goal is a smooth transfer and continuity of patient care.

The pretransplant phase

Depending on the type of transplant, patients may or may not be admitted to the hospital for a transplant evaluation before the transplant surgery. If so, this allows the staff to assess the patient's and family's coping styles and emotional needs. Occasionally patients are admitted emergently for transplant, and there is no time for an extended social services, nursing, or psychiatric assessment (e.g., a patient with an acute myocardial infarction or acute hepatic failure). These patients are unstable, and much of the nurse's attention is rightfully directed toward stabilization of the patient.[13]

The patient may be obtunded or intubated, making communication difficult, if not impossible. In such cases, the nurse and other staff must rely on the family to obtain information about the patient. The transplant team must decide with the family whether the patient would want the transplant and whether he or she is a suitable candidate.

Patients who are critically ill in the pretransplant phase may be delirious or in shock from their failing organ, and their ability to understand and retain information is often impaired.[6] More nursing time is frequently needed to help these patients and their families through special procedures as well as routine events. They may be overwhelmed by the gravity of the situation, or they may deny their fears and thus minimize the seriousness of the situation.

Commonly, the nurse is the one who first leads family members through the maze of equipment in the ICU and who explains the patient's condition in realistic yet hopeful terms. The nurse is the liaison among the physician, the patient, and the family and may be the only one available to answer questions when a physician is unavailable. A treatment plan clearly understood between physicians and nurses can lessen misunderstandings and unrealistic expectations. Further, research has shown that the more effectively physicians and nurses communicate and work together, the greater the chance of patient survival. According to a study comparing the actual and predicted death rate of 5030 patients in 13 well-equipped ICUs, synergistic physician-nurse working relationships are more important than a hospital's latest high-tech medical equipment.[14]

Nurses have the sometimes difficult task of alternating among their roles as health care provider, educator, confidant, patient advocate, and coordinator for the other patient care services such as dietary, respiratory therapy, physical therapy, and occupational therapy.[6] The nurse may feel emotionally drained but hesitant to share these feelings with peers who are also caring for transplant patients.

Some patients idealize their nurse at this time. Difficulty arises, however, when patients become disillusioned or coping mechanisms fail or they become angry at the length of time they must wait for a donor organ. Suddenly the nurse may become the object of intense displaced anger. Nurses who do not receive support or have insight into the patient's behavior may blame themselves for the turn of events or become angry at this ungrateful patient.[15]

Some patients die waiting for a transplant. Both nurse and patient are aware of this possibility, but neither may wish to initiate discussion about it. Most critically ill patients, if given the opportunity, discuss their feelings about death. Surprisingly, many of them do not fear their death as much as their caregivers fear it. Patients may wish to make out a will and discuss funeral arrangements with family, or they may wish to speak with a member of the clergy.

Death may also be perceived by the transplant team as a failure. All the persons involved may avoid talking about the possibility of a patient's death lest they admit their powerlessness over the final outcome.

Finally, caring for these patients is likely to force nurses to confront their own mortality, because patients may be similar in age to the nurse or the nurse's family members. Listening empathetically yet objectively to patients' fears and fantasies about surgery is difficult, especially if the nurse has ambivalent feelings about transplantation.

The phase ends abruptly. When an organ is found, the patient leaves for the operating room in a matter of hours. As this phase ends, the patient is readied for surgery with last-minute laboratory tests and procedures. Although there may not be much time, it is important for the patient and nurse to spend a few minutes reflecting on their time together. The nurse has shared what has been a most difficult and uncertain time in the patient's life. Although they may see each other again in several hours, their relationship will never be the same again. After surgery the patient will have a new organ and, one hopes, a more certain future.

The middle phase

After surgery comes a period during which tremendous emotional changes occur (see Chapter 7). Some patients have a relatively brief stay in the ICU, whereas those who are less stable spend a much longer time in the ICU. These patients will show varying degrees of anxiety, depression, and fear. To ask a patient who is tearful or crying after surgery "How are you feeling?" is not empathetic. A more sensitive statement might contain "I" messages (see p. 146), or the nurse might share with the patient that many patients experience similar emotions related to the operation and medications.

Patients may be delirious from high dosages of steroids and act abusive toward the nursing staff. The nursing staff in turn may resent taking care of an ungrateful patient. As noted earlier, caring for difficult patients can be exhausting and lead nurses to feelings of anger, frustration, and a sense of inadequacy and burnout.

Families may feel that the surgeon has saved their loved one's life; therefore problems in the postoperative course may be blamed on the nurses. Further difficulties between nurses and families may arise when the nursing staff seek to impose visitation restrictions. The transplant clinical nurse specialist can facilitate a smooth transition by acting as a liaison between the family and the health care providers, thereby alleviating frustrations arising from insufficient or confusing communication. Many families have stayed in patients' rooms before transplant, and they may want to sleep on cots or in chairs outside the ICU door so that they can visit their newly transplanted relative around the clock. Depending on the size of the family and the number of transplanted patients in the unit, the ICU waiting area may begin to look like a shelter for the homeless.

Spouses may feel resentful and become openly hostile when asked to observe visiting hours or leave the room during procedures. With these, as with other situations, the nurse who is aware of the patient and family dynamics can defuse an emotionally charged situation. Nurses working closely with a transplant clinical nurse specialist and/or psychiatric liaison often become quite skilled in dealing with these situations. Underneath seemingly unreasonable requests by families are often very reasonable fears. These families have lived with the dread that their loved one could die at any time, and this fear does not go away in a few hours after surgery. One woman who had awakened in her husband's hospital room before surgery and found him in cardiac arrest understandably had difficulty leaving him after surgery.

As patients begin assuming more care for themselves and their conditions stabilize, they are transferred to a general medical or surgical floor. Termination, or closure, with the ICU nurse is very important, as is communication between nursing staffs about the patient's specific physical and emotional needs.

The final phase

When patients are discharged to a general medical or surgical floor, their ICU nurses may experience sadness about the separation, particularly if the patient had a lengthy ICU stay. Similarly, patients may miss their ICU nurses and may call or visit them after transfer.[15] Helping the patient to terminate with the unit does not suggest that the nurse no longer cares for the patient; rather, this acknowledges that the ICU nurse is no longer primarily responsible for the patient's nursing needs.

Patients accustomed to having all their needs met promptly and having one nurse while in the unit may have difficulty adjusting to being one of many floor patients. Gradually allowing patients more responsibility in their care, such as taking their own medicines, and promoting independence while in the ICU will help.

After the transplant, the patient may experience an emotional let-down. Walking or wheeling around the hospital with the patient will help restore confidence in the patient's ability to survive beyond the watchful eye of the nurse or the monitoring equipment. When the patient is medically ready, passes during which the patient visits home or goes out to lunch or supper can be very therapeutic in helping both the patient and the family to adjust to their new life.

Some patients are reluctant to walk any distance from their rooms. The patient's progress in this area as well as his or her increasing physical strength can be measured with a pedometer obtained from the physical therapy department. A graph plotting the number of steps walked per shift is a motivating and therapeutic way of measuring a patient's progress. For the difficult-to-motivate patient, a "goal" of so many steps per day can be included in the patient's daily care plan.

A number of "firsts" after transplant may be causes for anxiety or elation both for nurses and for the patient. There is the first biopsy, with its inherent risks. Realizing that this procedure is stressful and allowing patients time to express their feelings about it can help. There is the first regular diet (perhaps after years of restricted foods), and as mentioned, there is the first walk after surgery. This may be the first time in years that the patient has not been overcome by shortness of breath or pain.

Patients experience setbacks such as infections, metabolic disturbances, and rejection. Helping patients adjust to their progress (or lack of progress) can be difficult. A staff support group can be a useful forum in which to explore feelings related to these emotional and physical setbacks.

When patients die, the transplant team that is also grieving may be little support for the nurse, who may be the main support for the grieving family. Many patients' families spend long periods at the hospital and many come to view the nurses as their extended support system. Abruptly terminating this relationship when the patient dies may be another loss for the family. Family members may continue to write or call the primary nurse while grieving over the loss of their loved one. During this period of bereavement, they may feel the need to review with members of the transplant team or the primary nurse the hospital stay, the transplant, and the patient's final days. This may be painful for the nurse, who is dealing with her or his own loss and grief and who is also expected to be caring for the next transplant patient and family.[15]

Sometimes these feelings of grief and bereavement last 6 to 12 months after the death of the patient. Adequate resources to respond to emotional needs of the family and staff are necessary. Staff and family support groups led by a psychiatric clinical nurse specialist, transplant psychiatrist, social worker, or chaplain may be especially helpful.

Finally, nurses are primarily responsible for getting patients ready for discharge. Discharge planning and education involve both patient and family. Emotionally the patient is attempting to disengage from institutional living, which may be a difficult task. When the discharge date is set, the patient may begin to regress, making more and more demands on the nursing staff. Understanding the patients' psychologic conflict about leaving the hospital where they were "reborn" (see Chapter 7) is useful.

Patients may wish to express their gratitude to nurses with expensive gifts, or they may invite them to welcome-home parties. Although the decision is an individual one, it is generally better to thank the patient for his or her thoughtfulness and ask the patient to express their gratitude in words rather than in an expensive gift. Patients may find it easier to give a gift than to tell the nurse how much he or she has meant. In the long run, though, the latter is usually more meaningful. Accepting expensive gifts or invitations to dinner can blur nurse-patient boundaries and lead to difficulties for both.

SUPPORTING THE SUPPORTERS

The stress and anxiety felt by nurses who work with transplant patients place a tremendous strain on the nursing unit as a whole. Tension and conflict may become overwhelming themes. The nursing staff and other transplant team members experience the same rites of passage that each patient experiences (see Chapter 7). However, the nurse especially may have no defined psychosocial support system.

"Care for the caregiver" programs offer a solution. In some programs, a weekly meeting of the staff nurses with the transplant psychiatrist, clinical nurse specialist, or chaplain has been helpful. The facilitator of the group should be knowledgeable of the emotional needs of transplant patients and the nurses caring for them. The group's sessions, structured yet informal, allow the staff to express their feelings about specific patients and situations without fear of judgment or ridicule. Many nurses are surprised and relieved to find that others share the same intense feelings about a particular patient or situation. The role of the facilitator is to help the staff to clarify their feelings so that they can be put into perspective. Open discussion bridges communication gaps among staff members and between staff and patients. Providing a healthy outlet for frustration and discussing these emotional responses in a supportive environment can result in more therapeutic nursing care.

REFERENCES

1. Levett JM and Karp RB (1985). Heart transplantation. *Surgical Clinics of North America, 65,* 613-629.
2. Painvin GA, Frazier OH, Chandler LB, Cooley DA and Reece IJ (1985). Cardiac transplantation: indications, procurement, operation and management. *Heart and Lung, 14,* 484-494.
3. Grady KL (1985). Development of a cardiac transplantation program: role of the clinical nurse specialist. *Heart and Lung, 14,* 490-494.
4. Marsden C (1985). Ethical issues in a heart transplant program. *Heart and Lung, 14,* 495-499.
5. Lunde DT (1969, December). Psychiatric complications of heart transplants. *AORN Journal,* pp 86-91.
6. McCauley KM (1985). Preoperative instruction: nursing assessment and teaching guide. In McGoon D (ed). *Cardiac surgery: An interprofessional approach to patient care* (pp. 237-249). Philadelphia, Pa: A Davis.
7. Dimsdale JE and Hackett TP (1982). Effect of denial on cardiac health and psychological assessment. *American Journal of Psychiatry, 139,* 1477-1480.
8. Billing E, Lindell B, Sederhold M and Theorell T (1980). Denial, anxiety, and depression following myocardial infarction. *Psychosomatics, 21,* 639-645.
9. Nash ES (1984). Psychiatric aspects. In Cooper DK and Lanza RP (eds). *The present status of orthotopic and heterotopic heart transplantation* (pp 235-241). Lancaster, England: MTP Press.
10. Mai FM (1986). Graft and donor denial in heart transplant recipients. *American Journal of Psychiatry, 143,* 1159-1161.

11. Mai FM (1987). Liaison psychiatry in the heart transplant unit. *Psychosomatics, 28,* 44-46.
12. Kraft I (1971). Psychiatric complications of cardiac transplantation. *Seminars in Psychiatry, 3,* 58-69.
13. Cardin S and Clark S (1985). A nursing diagnosis approach to the patient awaiting cardiac transplantation. *Heart and Lung, 14,* 499-504.
14. MD-nurse cooperation tied to ICU survival. (1987, May 1). *AMA News,* p 32.
15. Riether AM and Boudreau MZ (1988, November). Heart transplant: impact on CCU nurses. *American Journal of Nursing,* pp 1521-1524.

PART THREE

The Practice

9

Tissue Transplantation

Janice Z. Cuzzell and George Rutherford

The term *transplantation* has become very much a part of our everyday language. When we use this term, we are most often referring to organ transplantation, such as is performed with kidneys, hearts, livers and other solid organs. There are, however, many types of tissue transplants performed every day, including bone, skin, ligament, fascia lata, dura mater, cartilage, artery, vein, and heart valve transplants. In fact, the greatest area of growth in transplantation lies in the transplant of human tissues. Approximately 500,000 tissue transplants are performed each year, including thousands of cadaveric skin grafts.[1]

Tissue can be transplanted by any of the three grafting procedures: autografting, allografting, or xenografting. *Autografts* involve the transplantation of tissue from one part of the body to another. Autografting is also referred to as autologous transplantation. When autologous tissue transplantation is possible, the problems of the immune response are avoided. Examples of autografting include bone, skin, and vein grafts and autologous bone marrow transplant. *Allografts* involve transplantation of tissue from one member of a species to another member of the same species. Replacing a section of a person's jaw with a piece of rib from another person is an example of allografting. *Xenografts* involve transplanting tissue from a member of one species to a member of another species. The use of bovine heart valves or bovine skin grafts as temporary biologic dressings is an example of xenografting.

The role of the nurse in tissue transplantation is crucial. Despite an increased awareness about organ and tissue transplantation among the public and health care professionals, as with solid organs, there continues to be a critical shortage of tissues for transplantation. Although the majority of tissue transplants are not lifesaving procedures, they do enhance the lives of recipients in many ways—by restoring lost body functions, body image, and self-esteem. The nurse is the vital link between the donor and donor family and the potential recipient.

Thus the nurse must be informed—about the need for tissue donation, the potential benefits to tissue transplant recipients, and the options for family members wishing to give the gift of donation. The intent of this chapter is to broaden the nurse's awareness in these areas so that he or she can make the critical difference.

The clinical applications of tissue transplantation are numerous. Therefore nursing implications for specific types of tissue transplantation and recipient care will not be addressed. The focus of this chapter is the current status of tissue transplantation, with a special emphasis on bone and skin transplantation.

HISTORY

Humanity has long had the desire to replace diseased or injured body parts with healthy tissues from animals and other humans. The early history of tissue transplantation is rich with accounts of such attempts, primarily involving bones and skin. The earliest account is more legendary than factual. Cosmas and Damian, the patron saints of medicine, were depicted replacing a human leg by fifteenth-century Italian artists.[2] It was not until the seventeenth century when Jobi Meekren used the cranium of a dog to repair a soldier's skull wound that tissue transplantation as a science had its beginnings.[2]

During the early nineteenth century several accounts of bone transplants were recorded.[3-5] Later Macewen performed the first successful bone allografts in children, and Ollier described the osteogenic properties of bone and refined the principles of bone grafting.[6] The twentieth century has been an active time of research and accomplishment in bone transplantation. In the early 1900s large bone allografting was attempted, but without success. Today patients are benefiting from massive bone grafts for limb-sparing skeletal tumor resection. Although techniques of allografting are highly refined, autografting is still the procedure of choice in many instances. The relative advantages and disadvantages of autografting and allografting are discussed below.

Skin transplantation has an equally rich history, beginning in 1809 with the pioneering efforts of the French physician Louis Reverdin. Reverdin eventually performed the first cutaneous allografts using grafts taken from his own arm.[7] But it was only after Thierock developed the technique for split-thickness skin grafting that skin transplantation moved beyond the very early experimental stages.[7] Gindner performed the first cadaver skin allografts in 1881.[7]

The technical advances of the 1800s were followed by biologic advances in the 1900s. While Loeb was able to determine that rejection was an inevitable phenomenon after skin grafting,[8] it was not until the 1940s that Medawar et al were able to elucidate the responsible mechanisms.[9] During the 1950s and 1960s various preservation and sterilization techniques were investigated, and the techniques of autografting and allografting were compared with respect to immune responses and graft survival.[10-14]

The United States navy is credited with establishing the first formal tissue bank in 1951.[15] The first preservation technique used, which proved to be impractical, was freezing.

The development of the technique of freeze-drying, a process involving the removal of water from tissue and then sealing the tissue under a vacuum, represented a major advance in tissue banking because it allowed for storage of some tissues at room temperature.

As the demand for transplantable tissue increased, the number of tissue banks also increased. In 1976 the American Association of Tissue Banks (AATB) formed with an initial membership of only 25 banks.[1] The current status of tissue transplantation is in part reflected by the fact that the AATB now has over 400 member banks. The AATB sets standards for the operation of and offers accreditation for all U.S. tissue banks.

Tissue banks are classified as casual, institutional, or regional.[16] *Casual* banks are small hospital-based facilities that serve tissue transplant surgeons at the respective hospital only. A 1987 survey revealed that there were 300 to 450 casual tissue banks in the United States. *Institutional* tissue banks are usually located in large medical centers with an academic affiliation. There are approximately 30 to 40 such banks in the United States, which, like casual banks, serve their own facility's tissue transplant needs. *Regional* tissue banks serve multiple hospitals within a given geographic region. They are usually affiliated with a medical center.

BONE TRANSPLANTATION

Virtually any bone with a potential clinical application can be recovered from a cadaver donor. The uses for cadaver bone are many. Bone grafts are necessary for surgical procedures for the correction or repair of congenital, traumatic, degenerative, and neoplastic skeletal disorders. Specific examples include spinal fusion, allographic knee joint replacement, and acetabular hip reconstruction, arthrodesis for scoliosis, correction of craniofacial and periodontal defects, and replacement of bone lost to neoplastic disease. Many individuals with rheumatoid arthritis could also potentially benefit from a bone transplant. Alternative procedures to bone transplantation include amputation or synthetic reconstruction. Although synthetic implants provide rapid return to function and activity, long-term function of implants is limited by physical wear and tear and often these are not the best treatment modalities for the younger active patient.

The biology of bone grafting

Incorporation of a bone graft into the recipient is an interactive process between the native recipient tissue and the graft. Recipient and graft tissues play important complementary roles in successful bone transplantation. Following graft implantation, the graft becomes encased in a hematoma that gradually transforms into a fibrovascular structure for the ingrowth of blood vessels that bring with them mesenchymal cells capable of differentiating into bone-resorbing and bone-forming populations.[6] This host response is called *osteoinduction.* The graft response of recruitment of osteogenic cells is called *osteoconduction. Osteogenesis,* or the growth of new bone, is facilitated by a protein (bone morphogenic protein) in allographic bone that causes remodeling of the graft bone, so that in time the graft bone becomes truly recipient bone. The graft functions as a scaffold onto which new biomechanically competent bone of host origin is formed.

Bone is composed of mineral, collagen, matrix, and cells. Mineral, collagen, and matrix components are nonantigenic or weakly antigenic. However, cellular components display major histocompatibility complex (MHC) antigens and have antibodies to class I and class II MHC antigens.[6] Fresh osteochondral allografts appear to be the most antigenic. Deep-freezing and freeze-drying processing of tissue appear to inhibit immune responses.

Bone allografting is preferred over autografting for several reasons. Autografting involves an additional surgical procedure for removal of the bone segment, thereby increasing patient morbidity and mortality. There is the potential for substantial blood loss, infection, and perioperative discomfort and damage to the autograft.

Bone grafts may be of bone segments, small or large, crushed bone, or entire bony structures. The iliac crest, ulna, and radius are sources of small bone segments, while the femur, tibia, and humerus are sources of large bone segments. The incus, malleus, and stapes are transplanted to improve or restore hearing, and the mandible is transplanted for repair of a jaw damaged by disease or trauma.

Small bone segment grafts

Small segments of the iliac crest are used, usually after trauma sustained in an automobile accident, for spinal fusion in the cervical or lumbar region, and in treatment of congenital defects such as scoliosis and spina bifida. These conditions involve a ruptured disk that leaves the victim with debilitating pain. Cloward pioneered the technique of spinal fusion, beginning in 1956.[17] In this procedure the disk between two vertebrae is removed and the resulting hole is filled with a bone graft. Over time, the two vertebrae fuse via the graft. Iliac crest bone is also used to repair craniofacial defects that have resulted in misshapen and malaligned jaws.[4]

Femoral head grafts are frequently used to support synthetic hip prostheses. Frequently the bone surrounding the acetabulum in a patient in need of a prosthetic hip replacement cannot adequately support the prosthesis. In this situation the prosthesis can break through the acetabulum, creating a condition far worse than the original one. Other methods to support the prosthesis, including cementing and wiring it in place, have not proved effective. Femoral head grafts are transplanted to build up the acetabulum and support the prosthesis, thereby increasing the chances of a successful surgery and restoring mobility and function. The overall success of segmental bone grafts is 90% to 95%.[18]

Large bone segment grafts

Autologous bone is, of necessity, in short supply. This is particularly true when large bone segments need to be replaced. In these cases large cadaver bone segments can be transplanted (Fig. 9-1). Large bone segments are transplanted to reconstruct major skeletal deficits resulting from trauma or limb-sparing skeletal tumor ablation.[6,14] The grafting of large bone segments requires that the donor and recipient bone sizes match. To ensure this match x-ray films of the donor bone segments are made to compare with eventual films of the recipient bone that is to be replaced. Massive osteochondral allografting presents a particular challenge

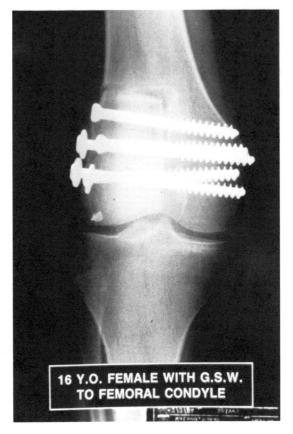

Fig. 9-1 Distal femoral hemicondyle used to repair the femur of a 16-year-old female; the femur had been shattered in an accidental shotgun blast. The patient regained full function of the knee. Without a bone graft, a knee fusion or a total knee replacement would have been necessary.

related to preservation of the graft (Fig. 9-2). Unlike bone, cartilage cannot regenerate and must be kept viable using the technique of cryopreservation. Despite this potential problem, the success rate of massive osteochondral grafting is approximately 90%.[19]

Crushed bone grafts

Crushed bone (pieces of bone about the size of small sugar cubes) is used most commonly to support prosthetic knee and hip replacements. It is also used to fill skeletal defects (Fig. 9-3). Sources of crushed bone include the iliac crest,

femoral head, and the cancellous bone found inside femoral and tibial shafts.

Bone can also be ground until it takes on the consistency of table salt. After is it ground, it is demineralized with hydrochloric acid. This process enhances the ability of the bone to incorporate and induce new bone formation.[13,20] The most common use for ground bone or "bone powder" is filling periodontal defects. The freeze-dried bone powder is reconstituted with sterile saline, and the pastelike substance that results is packed into the defect. Over time, new bone is formed.

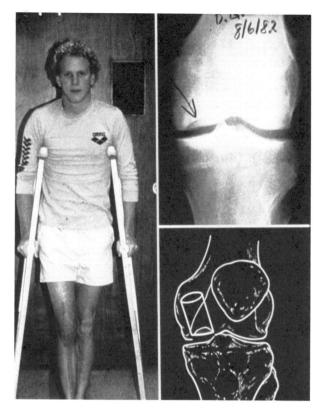

Fig. 9-2 Freshly recovered and cooled allograft used to treat osteochondritis dessicans. The infarcted area is excised and replaced with a plug consisting of cartilaginous tissue and cancellous bony matrix.

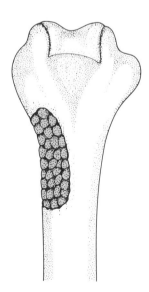

Fig. 9-3 Crushed bone graft. (Redrawn from Netter F. In Enneking WF and Conrad EU (1989). Common bone tumors. *Clinical Symposia, 41*(3), 1-32, New York: Ciba-Geigy.)

CARTILAGE, TENDON, FASCIA LATA, DURA MATER, AND HEART VALVE TRANSPLANTATION

Cartilage

Two types of cartilage are commonly transplanted: costal (attached to the ribs) and articular (found in the joints). Another source of cartilage is the nasal septum. Costal cartilage is used in plastic surgery to repair facial defects. Articular cartilage is used with large osteochondral bone grafts. The drawback with cartilage transplantation is the difficulty in preserving this tissue.

Tendon

We live in a sports-oriented society, and sports injuries, particularly to the tendons and ligaments, are common and increasing. A common injury is to the cruciate ligament of the knee. Tendon can be transplanted to repair this immobilizing injury. The patellar tendon is most commonly used because of its strength. The graft is threaded arthroscopically and attached to the tibia at one end and the femur at the other.

Fascia lata

Fascia lata is a thin membranous tissue covering the thigh muscles down to the knees. Fascia lata, because of its tremendous tensile strength, is also used for ligament repair. It is also used by plastic surgeons for repair of facial defects.

Dura mater

The dura mater is a thin, almost transparent tissue that is the protective lining between the brain and the skull. This soft tissue is very strong. The most common use of dura mater is for repair of the dura mater following head trauma, but it is also used for the repair of pelvic floor and abdominal wall defects.[21,22] It can be used to replace the bladder wall after removal of a tumor, to repair the pelvic floor and abdominal wall in gynecologic cancer patients, to support the vaginal apex in repair of vaginal prolapse, in periodontal repairs, and in reconstruction of the inner ear.[21]

Heart valves

Heart valve allografts have been used since 1962. Heart valves, like cartilage, must remain viable to function. They are removed from the donor heart within 12 hours after cardiac death and preserved within 24 hours by slowly freezing to $-135°$ C. When needed for implantation, they are slowly thawed to room temperature. Once thawed, they must either be used or discarded, because they cannot be refrozen.

DONATION

The criteria for bone donation can be found in Chapter 5. They are similar to those of solid organ donation, the major differences being the age range (from birth to 70 years) and the ability to do elective tissue recovery for up to 24 hours after cardiovascular death. After the bones are removed, the body is reconstructed with wooden dowels and plaster if necessary to its original conformity so that it is presentable at funeral services.

PRESERVATION TECHNIQUES

Tissues can be preserved for far longer periods than can solid organs. The three most common preservation techniques are freezing, freeze-drying, and cryopreservation.

Freezing

Most tissues can be preserved for many years by freezing to $-70°$ C. Freezer temperatures must be closely monitored to prevent thawing and refreezing (Fig. 9-4). Before transplantation frozen tissues are rapidly thawed. Once thawed they cannot be refrozen.[20]

Freeze-drying

Bone, tendons, fascia lata, and dura mater are preserved using freeze-drying, which involves the removal of water from tissue and sealing the tissue in a vacuum. This technique allows the tissue to be preserved and stored at room temperature for years.[23,24]

Cryopreservation

Tissues such as heart valves and skin must be frozen in a very controlled manner to preserve their viability. The technique used is cryopreservation. The tissue is immersed in a liquid protectant such as glycerol or DMSO and then slowly cooled at a constant rate, about $1°$ C per minute, to a final storage temperature of about

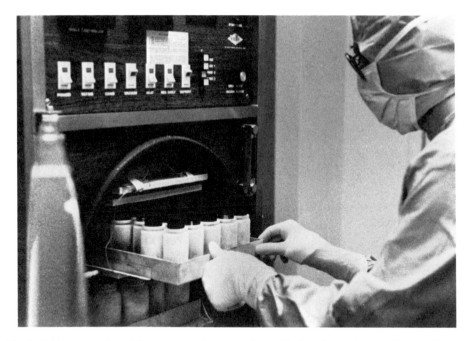

Fig. 9-4 Freeze-drying of iliac crest wedges, cancellous blocks, rib portions, and cortical struts.

−135° C. This temperature is achieved using liquid nitrogen.

Sterilization of bone grafts

One of the advantages of transplanted tissues over solid organs is that they are sterilized and cannot, with the exception of skin, transmit disease to recipients. Tissue bank personnel and tissue transplant surgeons are, however, at risk for disease transmission. There are three common methods of sterilizing tissues before preserving them: antibiotics, ethylene oxide (ETO), and gamma irradiation. Antibiotics are not true sterilants but do protect against bacterial contamination. Heart valves, skin, and articular cartilage are commonly treated with antibiotics. ETO kills bacteria and viruses but is a carcinogen and must be handled carefully.[25] ETO sterilization is contraindicated for tissues such as heart valves. Gamma irradiation is also effective against bacteria and viruses. This technique is somewhat impractical, because the tissue must be transported to and from a radiation facility and the radiation dose must be monitored carefully.

SKIN TRANSPLANTATION

Although seldom thought of as an organ, the skin is a functionally complex body system that serves as a selective barrier for heat, water, bacteria, and other variables important to the maintenance of a homeostatic environment. When skin trauma occurs, the body responds automatically by attempting to close the defect and thereby restore the integrity of this barrier. However, wound healing by the natural events of epithelization and wound contraction is a relatively slow process and one that is limited by the amount of tissue loss. As long as a wound remains open, heat and water readily escape from the internal environment, and potentially pathogenic microorganisms can enter. The degree to which skin loss contributes to physiologic alterations or overwhelming bacterial invasion is directly proportional to the size and depth of the wound and functional status of the immune system.

The need for skin transplantation

Skin grafting generally serves three major purposes; it is (1) sometimes a lifesaving intervention, (2) frequently used to restore structures cosmetically, and (3) necessary for restoration of function to injured body parts. Skin transplantation, like bone transplantation, employs the techniques of autografting, allografting, and xenografting. Autografting is limited in its capabilities when large areas of skin are lost, and xenografting is useful as a very temporary biologic dressing. Allografting, then, has obvious advantages. Skin allografts can be used as an immediate coverage of superficial burn wounds, to cover granulated areas between autografts, and as an immediate coverage after a major surgical excision. In the latter case allografts help to prevent infection, preserve deeper tissues, and provide timely closure of the wound.

Major burn injuries. By far, the most immediate need for skin replacement is seen in major burn injuries. The goal of treatment in burn trauma is timely closure of the wound, thereby controlling infection, decreasing pain, preserving remaining viable tissue, and maintaining joint function.[26,27] In deep partial-thickness and full-thickness burns, surgical debridement of nonviable tissue removes the potential source of infection. Debridement is followed by grafting of the patient's uninjured skin to the clean burn wound (autograft). If skin grafts are removed in thin enough sheets and the donor site is protected from injury and infection, healing will occur by secondary intention. Once healed, skin can be reharvested from the same site if needed.

Donor sites are limited in burn injuries involving large body surface areas. Consequently many successive autograft procedures are required to obtain wound closure. These procedures may take weeks to months, during which time alternative methods of wound coverage become necessary to minimize the complications associated with open wounds and "buy time" until donor sites heal.

Cadaveric skin allograft as a temporary skin substitute. Currently the biologic material of choice as a temporary skin substitute is human cadaver skin or *allograft.* Based on approximately 70,000 acute admissions to burn care facilities each year,[28] the annual national requirement for cadaver skin is estimated to be 3000 m².[29,30] In 1979 a national survey of skin banks found that only about 14% to 19% of human cadaver skin needed for burn treatment was being recovered.[31] Even if a significant increase has occurred in recovery rates over the past decade, efforts continue to fall short of the ever-increasing demand for allograft skin.

Although studies have addressed the importance of allograft viability at the time of transplantation,[32,33] the degree to which viability affects clinical outcome is yet to be determined. Nevertheless, every attempt is made to maintain the skin in a viable state until it is grafted to the recipient wound. Skin that is placed in refrigerated storage immediately after being removed and transplanted within 3 to 5 days appears to give the best clinical results. Long-term storage of viable skin can be accomplished by cryopreserving fresh tissue. Within 24 to 48 hours after harvest, the skin is packaged and placed in a freezing device that lowers the temperature at a controlled rate ($-1°$ C/min). The frozen skin is then stored at ultralow temperatures ($-80°$ C to $-196°$ C).

The viability of cryopreserved skin has been shown to be largely dependent on the specific methodology used to obtain and process the tissue.[33,34] This may account for reports that clinical results with cryopreserved tissue are less predictable than with fresh skin transplants. Although live familial donors have occasionally been used as a source of allograft skin,[35] the availability of cadaver donors makes postmortem tissue a more esthetically acceptable and cost-effective alternative.

To meet the demands for fresh and cryopreserved tissue, skin banks developed across the country in association with major burn centers. Standardization of skin banking techniques has greatly increased the availability of viable allograft as a skin substitute while minimizing the risk of disease transmission. As a result, the uses for allograft have expanded to include immediate coverage of areas of superficial skin loss and preservation of granulation tissue, tendon, and other viable tissues between surgical procedures. Allograft is also used as a "test" material before autografting and as a dressing for donor sites to promote healing and minimize scarring. Adherence of the transplanted skin to a wound indicates a relatively low bacterial count on the wound surface, increasing the likelihood of autograft vascularization or "take."[26,27,36]

Despite the fact that ABO and human leukocyte antigen (HLA) matched skin allografts have been shown to adhere longer to a wound surface,[37] tissue typing between donor and recipient is rarely performed. Matching of donor and recipient is usually limited to ABO compatibility. The demand for allograft as an intermediate intervention in the treatment of burn trauma has precluded the feasibility of keeping a large enough donor pool available for tissue typing. Therefore cadaver skin is one of the few transplanted organs in which rejection and its potential complications are expected. Its temporary usefulness serves to distinguish it from tissue and solid organ transplantation, where permanency is the goal.

CADAVERIC ALLOGRAFT SKIN PROCUREMENT
Donor screening

The quality of cadaver allograft and ability to function as an acceptable skin substitute depends on maintenance of cellular viability and structural integrity during recovery and processing. Skin remains viable for 3 to 4 hours after death without refrigeration and up to 18 hours with immediate refrigerated storage. After 16 to 18 hours tissue viability is variable, with only about 55% of metabolic activity remaining at 24 hours.[33] Therefore allograft skin should be recovered as soon as possible after death and no later than 24 hours.

Skin donor criteria are similar to those for other tissues. Contraindications to skin donation include disease states that can be transmitted to the recipient, including suspected or documented infections and malignancies. In addition, conditions that affect the integrity of the tissue are ruled out. These include inflammatory skin diseases, multiple skin lesions, unhealed wounds, and similar cutaneous impairments. Removal of skin is difficult in severely malnourished or obese donors, a factor that also needs to be considered during screening. Potential donors younger than 14 and older than 75 are usually evaluated on an individual basis, depending on body size (amount of retrievable tissue) and state of health.[29,30]

Obtaining consent for skin donation

The idea of donating one's skin as an organ carries with it certain psychologic implications. When approached for consent, family members frequently display either verbal or nonverbal aversion to the idea of skin removal. This probably results in part from association of intentional skin trauma with pain and disfigurement.

Questions asked by family members usually relate directly to concerns about disfigurement, specifically whether the body will be able to be viewed after donation. In such instances, it should be stressed that skin is removed in very thin sheets (only the outer layers), and from body areas normally covered with clothing. No skin is removed from the arms, face, neck, or upper chest unless prior approval is obtained. Funeral arrangements (including open-casket viewing of the body) are usually not disrupted.

Skin removal procedure

Cadaver skin allograft can be removed in any clean area where a sterile field can be established and maintained. The body is surgically prepared and draped, and thin (0.35 mm) strips of skin are taken with a dermatome (Fig. 9-5). Sterile saline may be injected subcutaneously to facilitate skin removal in areas of uneven contour, such as over bony prominences.

Skin specimens from multiple body sites are obtained. These specimens are later screened for bacterial and fungal contamination. A cadaver serum sample is usually obtained at this time for routine screening for infectious disease and ABO blood type (if desired).

Skin processing and storage

Recovered skin is placed in a sterile nutrient medium and transported to the skin bank on ice to discourage bacterial growth. At the skin bank, the tissue is prepared and packaged either for fresh storage or cryopreservation. Ultimate use of the recovered tissue depends on the results of serology and skin cultures. Tissue from donors found to be infectious is discarded.

Fresh storage requires packaging in sealed containers in nutrient media and temperature-monitored refrigerator storage at 4° C until used. May and DeClement have shown that the

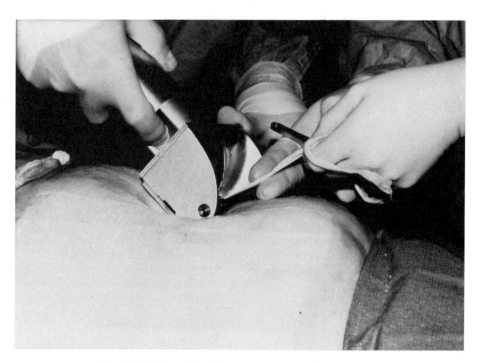

Fig. 9-5 Cadaver skin being removed with a dermatome.

viability of refrigerated fresh tissue decreases rapidly after 3 days of storage.[33] It is recommended by the Skin Council of the American Association of Tissue Banks that fresh allograft not used within 7 days be frozen or discarded.[29]

Controlled-rate freezing or cryopreservation of allograft theoretically protects cellular viability and allows extended storage using low temperature refrigeration ($-50°$ C to $-196°$ C). Expiration dates for skin frozen and stored at ultralow temperatures have yet to be determined. When allograft skin is needed, rapid thawing is indicated to further protect viability.[33,34] The thawed tissue is transported to the operating room in a balanced salt solution for grafting to the recipient.

CADAVERIC ALLOGRAFT SKIN TRANSPLANTATION
Skin transplantation procedure

Some skin banks elect to match the donor and recipient according to ABO blood type to ensure some degree of donor-recipient histo-compatibility. The donor skin is placed dermal side down on the debrided wound of the recipient and sutured or stapled in place (Fig. 9-6). Adherent allograft is usually changed every 5 to 7 days to prevent complete vascularization. If left in place longer, removal requires sharp debridement and is associated with excessive blood loss. Also, the longer the allograft is left in place, the greater the chance of rejection.

Clinical indicators of rejection

Once vascularization of the transplanted skin occurs, the onset of rejection is unpredictable. In patients with massive burns, an existing state of immunosuppression associated with the injury itself may delay rejection for weeks. Once established, the rejection phenomenon is often prolonged, lasting serveral days to weeks.

Local signs of tissue rejection may initially be confined to only a few grafted areas. Edema and cellular reaction produce granulation tissue that appears unhealthy and necrotic. The systemic

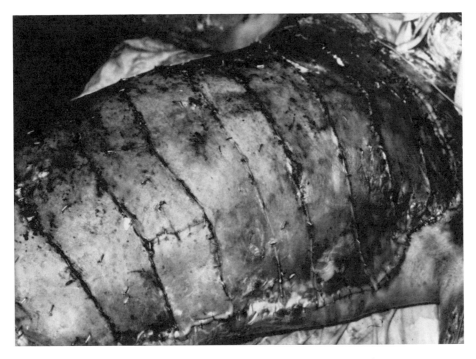

Fig. 9-6 Cadaver skin grafted onto a recipient's wound.

response is characterized by fever, malaise, and anorexia. Once rejection has begun, the wound is highly susceptible to invasive bacterial infection.

Treatment is supportive, because any further attempt to close the burn wound is unsuccessful until rejection is complete. In burns involving large surface areas, rapid clinical deterioration and death often occur as a result of invasive burn wound sepsis. On occasion the surgeon may elect to prolong the "take" of transplanted skin because of limited donor sites or other life-threatening complications. In these instances, immunosuppressant drugs are administered to prolong the onset of rejection.[35,38]

ALTERNATIVE SKIN SUBSTITUTES
Biologic dressings

Other biologic materials such as pigskin (xenograft) and amniotic membrane have been transplanted to serve as temporary skin substitutes. Antigenicity is not a problem because, unlike cadaver skin, they are nonviable and true

vascularization does not occur. Initially these materials appear more cost-effective than the procurement and processing of human tissue. However, clinical results have shown them to be less satisfactory in the treatment of extensive burns, with the potential for increased costs because of more frequent dressing changes and a longer hospitalization to obtain wound closure.[22,39]

Cultured skin

Under investigation is the growth of both autologous and allogeneic epidermal cells in vitro.[40-43] Small skin samples are obtained from either the prospective recipient (cultured autograft) or a human cadaver (cultured allograft). The samples are processed in a laboratory to separate the epidermal cells from the dermis. Single epidermal cells are then "seeded" onto media in petri dishes. In approximately 3 weeks the cells multiply and grow into a confluent epidermal sheet that can then be grafted to the wound bed.

Interestingly, cultured epidermal sheets grown from cadaver skin can be grafted onto a wound without the expected rejection that occurs when regular cadaver skin is transplanted. Cadaver epidermal cells grown in vitro lose human leukocyte antigen specificity and therefore are nonantigenic. Although the advantages of having a readily available and potentially permanent wound covering are obvious, to date the clinical results using cultured skin show the quality of healing to be less than optimal. Even after several months, the resulting epidermal cover is thin and poorly attached to the underlying tissue. In addition, the absence of a dermal layer promotes wound contraction and scarring.

Composite biologic grafts

With development of a composite biologic wound cover, recent studies have addressed the poor quality of healing observed with cultured skin.[44,45] Frozen cadaver allograft skin is transplanted to the recipient in the usual manner. After 4 to 5 days the epidermal layer of the vascularized cadaver skin is easily peeled away, leaving the dermal layer exposed and intact. The cadaver dermis is then grafted with either small (5 mm) pieces of autologous epidermis or cultured epidermal cells. Results to date show rapid outgrowth of the autologous grafts with complete healing and eventual skin repigmentation. The frozen dermis with the epidermal layer removed is thought to be so weakly antigenic that clinical signs of rejection are not observed. In addition, the composite graft appears to maintain its structural integrity, resulting in less scarring.

Composite synthetic grafts

Considerable attention has been given to the development of synthetic skin substitutes that are biologically inert and will permanently replace injured skin. Although not yet commercially available, the most promising of these materials is a biodegradable bilaminate membrane that serves as an "artificial skin."[46] When transplanted onto a clean wound, the "dermal" layer of this synthetic membrane readily vascularizes and acts as a framework for the deposition of collagen by fibroblasts. As new tissue is deposited in the wound space, the membrane gradually biodegrades. The result is scar tissue that biologically and physiologically resembles the dermis of normal tissue.

The outer layer of this material is composed of a transparent layer of silastic that can remain in place for several weeks while preventing the loss of water and heat. When donor sites are available, the silastic layer is peeled away and *very* thin (0.1 mm) autografts are placed on the new dermis. Although autografting is still required to attain wound closure, grafts can be taken in thin enough sheets to allow multiple recovery of the same site in a short span of time. For a massive burn injury, permanent wound coverage can theoretically be obtained quicker than with conventional interventions.

Although further study is needed, preliminary results of clinical studies are promising.[47] When artificial skin is used for wound coverage, the healed wounds are comparable to those treated with surgical excision and autografting. In addition, rejection does not occur with artificial skin. Investigation is progressing with the use of autologous epidermal cells to seed the "new" dermis and further decrease the amount of donor tissue needed for autografting.[48]

As a result of the high costs associated with procuring and processing human skin tissue, combined with the temporary nature of the tissue, the search for a permanent skin substitute has largely been confined to the specialty of burn care. Consequently the prognosis associated with extensive skin loss has continually improved with new technology. The future of skin transplantation holds even more exciting possibilities as the search for the ideal skin substitute continues. The implications such research holds for the rapid healing of all types of wounds are unlimited.

REFERENCES

1. Kim TF (1987). Tissue banking in midst of "revolution of expansion" as more uses are found for various transplants. *Journal of the American Medical Association, 258,* 302-304.
2. Beck EM (1968). *Source book of orthopedics* (p 243). New York: Hafner Publishing.

3. Burchardt H and Enneking WF (1987). Transplantation of bone. *Surgical Clinics of North America, 58,* 403-423.
4. Salyer KE and Taylor DP (1987). Bone grafting in cleft deformity: a craniofacial approach. *Australia-New Zealand Surgery, 57,* 67-75.
5. Head WC, Malinin TI and Berklacich F (1987). Freezer-dried proximal femur allografts in revision total hip arthroplasty: a preliminary report. *Clinical Orthopedics and Related Research, 215,* 109-120.
6. Friedlander GE (1988). Bone transplantation. In Cerilli GJ (ed). *Organ transplantation and replacement* (pp 617-624). Philadelphia: JB Lippincott Co.
7. Lutterman A and Curreri PW (1988). Skin transplantation. In Cerilli GJ (ed). *Organ transplantation and replacement* (pp 630-639). Philadelphia: JB Lippincott Co.
8. Flye MW (1989). History of transplantation. In Flye MW (ed). *Principles of organ transplantation* (pp 1-17). Philadelphia: WB Saunders Co.
9. Medawar P and Lehner T (1983). *Major histocompatibility system: the Gorer Symposium.* London: Blackwell Scientific Publications.
10. Abbot LC, Schottstaedt ER, Sanders JB and Bost FC (1947). The evaluation of cortical and cancellous bone as grafting material: clinical and experimental study. *Journal of Bone and Joint Surgery, 29,* 381-414.
11. Burwell RG (1969). The fate of bone grafts. In Aplet AG (ed). *Recent advances in orthopedics* (p 115). Baltimore: Williams & Wilkins Co.
12. Friedlander GE and Mankin HJ (1983). Bone banking: current methods and suggested guidelines. *Clinical Orthopedics and Related Research, 174,* 36-51.
13. Urist MR (1965). The bone induction principle. *Clinical Orthopedics and Related Research, 243,* 227-229.
14. Mankin HJ, Doppelt SH, Sullivan TR and Tomford WW (1982). Osteoarticular and intercancellary allograft transplantation in the management of malignant tumors of bone. *Cancer, 50,* 613-630.
15. Bright RD, Friedlander GE and Sell KW (1977). Tissue banking: the United States Navy Tissue Bank. *Military Medicine, 141,* 503-508.
16. Friedlander GE (1987). Bone banking in support of reconstructive surgery of the hip. *Clinical Orthopedic and Related Research, 225,* 17-21.
17. Cloward RB (1984). *Ruptured cervical intervertebral discs.* Randolph, Mass: Codman Publications.
18. Friedlander GE (1988). Bone transplantation. In Cerilli GJ (ed). *Organ transplantation and replacement* (pp 617-624). Philadelphia: JB Lippincott Co.
19. Tomford WW, Mankin HJ, Friedlander GE, Doppelt SH and Gebhardt MC (1987). Methods of banking bone and cartilage for allograft transplantation. *Orthopedic Clinics of North America, 18*(2), 241-246.
20. Jarrell MA, Malinin TJ, Averette HE, Girtanner RE, Harrison CR and Penalver MA (1987). Human dura mater allografts in repair of pelvic floor and abdominal wall defects. *Obstetrics and Gynecology, 70,* 280-285.
21. Rosomoff HL and Malinin TJ (1976). Freeze-dried allografts of dura mater—20 years' experience. *Transplantation Proceedings, 8,* 133-137.
22. Leary JH and Stanford EA (1976). *Freeze-drying today and tomorrow: international symposium on freeze-drying of biological products.* Washington, DC.
23. Perry VP (1976). Freeze-drying for the preservation of human tissues. *Transplantation Proceedings, 8*(2s), 189-193.
24. Hegstedt C, Aringer L and Gustavson A (1986). Epidemiologic support for ethylene oxide as a cancer-causing agent. *Journal of the American Medical Association, 255,* 1575-1578.
25. Pruitt BA and Curreri PW (1971). The use of homograft and heterograft skin. In Stone HH and Polk HC (eds). *Contemporary burn management* (pp 397-417). Boston: Little, Brown & Co.
26. Pruitt BA Jr and Levine NS (1984). Characteristics and uses of biologic dressings and skin substitutes. *Archives of Surgery, 119,* 312-322.
27. Frank HA, Berry C, Wachtel TL and Johnson W (1987). The impact of thermal injury. *Journal of Burn Care and Rehabilitation, 8*(4), 260-262.
28. American Association of Tissue Banks (1987). *Technical manual for tissue banking* (Sec 3: Skin Council).
29. DeClement FA and May RS (1983). Procurement, cryopreservation, and clinical application of skin. In Glassman AB and Umlas J (eds). *Cryopreservation of tissue and solid organs for transplantation.* Arlington, Va: American Association of Blood Banks.
30. May RS and DeClement FA (1981). Skin banking: Part 1. Procurement of transplantable cadaveric allograft for burn wound coverage. *Journal of Burn Care and Rehabilitation, 2,* 7-23.
31. Bondoc CC and Burke JF (1971). Clinical experience with viable frozen human skin and a frozen skin bank. *Annals of Surgery, 174*(3), 371-382.
32. May RS and DeClement FA (1981). Skin banking: Part 3. Cadaveric allograft skin viability. *Journal of Burn Care and Rehabilitation, 2*(3), 128-141.
33. May RS and DeClement FA (1980). Skin banking methodology: an evaluation of package format, cooling and warming rates, and storage efficiency. *Cryobiology, 17,* 33-45.
34. Burke JF, Quinby WC, Bodoc CC, Cosimi AB, Russell PS and Szyfelbiem SK (1975). Immunosuppression and temporary skin transplantation in treatment of massive third degree burns. *Annals of Surgery, 182,* 183-197.
35. Davidson BL and Hunt JL (1981). Human cadaver homograft in toxic epidermal necrolysis. *Journal of Burn Care and Rehabilitation, 2,* 94-96.
36. Higuchi D, Sei Y and Takivchi I (1981). Influence of histocompatibility antigens on skin homograft survival in an extensively burned patient. *Journal of Investigative Dermatology, 8,* 47.
37. Achauer BW, Hewitt CW and Black KS (1986). Long-term skin allograft survival after short-term cyclosporin treatment in patients with massive burns. *Lancet, 1,* 14-15.
38. Shuck JM, Pruitt BA Jr and Moncrief JA (1969). Homograft skin for wound coverage: a study in versatility. *Archives of Surgery, 98,* 472-479.

39. Gallico GG, O'Connor NE, Compton CC, Kehinde O and Green H (1984). Permanent coverage of large burn wounds with autologous cultured human epithelium. *New England Journal of Medicine, 311,* 448-451.
40. Hefton JM, Madden ME, Finkelstein JL and Shires GT (1983). Grafting of burn patients with allografts of cultured epidermal cells. *Lancet, 11,* 428-430.
41. Madden MR, Finklestein JL, Staiano-Coico L, Goodwin CW, Shires TG, Nolan EE and Hefton JM (1986). Grafting of cultured allogeneic epidermis on second- and third-degree burn wounds on 26 patients. *Journal of Trauma,* 26(11), 955-962.
42. O'Connor NE, Mulliken JB, Banks-Schlegel S, Kehinde O and Green H (1981). Grafting of burns with cultured epithelium prepared from autologous epidermal cells. *Lancet, 1,* 75-78.
43. Cuono C, Langdon R and McGuire J (1986). Use of cultured epidermal autografts and dermal allografts as skin replacement after burn injury. *Lancet, 1,* 1123-1124.
44. Heck EL, Bergstresser PR and Baxter CR (1985). Composite skin graft: frozen dermal allografts support the engraftment and expansion of autologous epidermis. *Journal of Trauma,* 25(2), 106-112.
45. Jaksic T and Burke JF (1987). The use of "artificial skin" for burns. *Annual Reviews in Medicine, 38,* 107-117.
46. Heimbach D, Luterman A, Burke J, Cram A, Herndon D, Hunt J, Jordan M, McManus W, Solem L, Warden G and Zawacki B (1988). Artificial dermis for major burns. *Annals of Surgery,* 208(3), 313-320.
47. Yannas IV, Burke JF, Orgill DP and Skrabut EM (1982). Wound tissue can use a polymeric template to synthesize a functional extension of skin. *Science, 215,* 174-176.

10

Cornea Transplantation

Delynn Heberlein and Gail Walsh

Although cornea transplantation is not considered a lifesaving procedure, it is certainly one that has great potential for enhancing life. The importance of this technology is underscored by the number of Americans, young and old, with impaired vision resulting from corneal damage. Defective corneas cause blindness in 30,000 Americans each year.[1] The advanced status of cornea transplantation and the fact that almost all patients who die meet the criteria for eye donation should have alleviated corneal blindness in the United States. However, even though more than 300,000 corneal transplants have been performed since 1961, the demand for transplantable corneas continues to outweigh the supply.[2]

HISTORICAL PERSPECTIVE

Corneal surgery has a long history (Fig. 10-1). In 1796 Erasmus Darwin pondered the idea of surgically removing damaged corneal tissues.[3] However, it was not until 1824 that keratoplasty (corneal replacement) was performed on chickens and pigs by Reisinger. The first human cornea transplants by von Hippel followed in 1886 but were plagued with infection and graft failure. Only after the development of microsurgical instruments and antibiotics was human corneal grafting successful. In 1905 Zirm performed the first successful human cornea transplant.[4]

Cornea transplantation in the United States was popularized in the 1920s and 1930s, primarily through the work of Elschnig.[5] By the

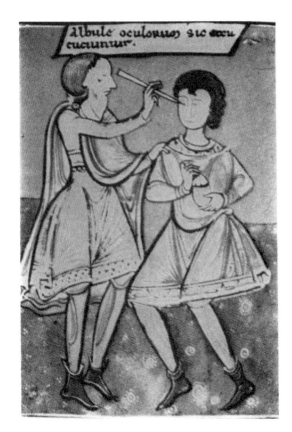

Fig. 10-1 Illustration from a medieval manuscript depicting ocular surgery for cataract. (From Casey TA and Mayer DJ (1984). Corneal grafting: principles and practice. Philadelphia: WB Saunders Co.)

1970s, the procedure was refined to the point that it was limited only by a lack of donor corneal tissue. Cornea transplants are now the most frequently performed transplant procedure. In 1987 nearly 36,000 were performed, and the success rate is 95%.[6]

CORNEAL ANATOMY AND PHYSIOLOGY

The eye is a relatively simple structure with a complex set of functions. Five sixths of the surface of the globe of the eye is covered by the white, fibrous, opaque sclera. The remaining area is covered by the cornea. The cornea is a transparent, avascular tissue that is continuous with the sclera and functions as a protective and refractive membrane through which light passes to the retina.

The pupil regulates the amount of light that enters the eye. Behind the pupil is a lens that focuses light on the retina. The retina then transforms light into nerve impulses that travel via the optic nerve from the eye to the brain. The brain interprets these impulses as images, thus producing sight. Clear corneas, therefore, are necessary for normal vision.

BLINDNESS

The causes of blindness are varied. Defective corneas are the leading cause of blindness, followed by macular degeneration, senile cataracts, optic nerve atrophy, and diabetic retinopathy.[3] Both glaucoma and cataracts can be successfully treated through early detection and the administration of medication, and surgery to remove the cloudy lens restores sight in 95% of cases.[6] Although investigation into methods of prevention and treatment is ongoing, effective treatments for macular degeneration, optic nerve atrophy, and diabetic retinopathy are currently unavailable.

Corneal blindness results when the normally transparent cornea becomes opaque from disease, injury, or a congenital defect. Disorders of the cornea result from alterations in production of the tear film, the conjunctiva, and the eyelids. Blinking is necessary to establish the tear film, which is necessary to keep the cornea oxygenated and hydrated. The tear film also acts as an immune defense by secreting protective immu-

noglobin. The eyelids maintain normal tear movement over the corneal surface, and the conjunctivae secrete mucin that bathes the cornea.

The leading indications for cornea transplantation are keratoconus (most common), keratitis, corneal dystrophy, trauma, and retransplantation.[3] All patients in need of a cornea transplant have in common an opacity of the cornea that prevents light from entering the eye. The goals of cornea transplantation are to improve vision, provide comfort to the patient with excessive lacrimation, photophobia, or pain, and improve physical appearance.

EYE DONATION

The potential eye donor is almost anyone who has suffered from either brain death or clinical death. When a family consents to the donation of a loved one's eyes, a technician from a local eye bank will recover the donated eye tissue. The technician first makes a gross examination of the eye with a slit lamp, looking for indications of ocular disease. The cornea is carefully examined for scars, trauma, or corneal disease.

Enucleation is a simple operation involving the transection of six ocular muscles and the optic nerve. Although the enucleation is not usually performed in an operating room (it may be done in the patient's hospital room), the procedure is a sterile one. The donor's skin around the enucleation sites is prepped with a bacteriocidal solution, and a sterile field is established and maintained throughout the procedure. The whole eye is then stored in a balanced salt solution. The corneal endothelium is examined by specular microscopy for cell density and regularity of size and shape. Finally, the cornea is rated on the basis of clarity, thickness, folds, and cell density. This information is then provided to the transplant surgeon.

Age as a criterion for cornea or eye donation is not as limiting as it is for solid organ donation. In general, there is no age limit that applies.[7] However, as with all tissue and organ donors, the younger donor is usually the healthier donor. Certain systemic diseases including serum hepatitis, syphilis, lymphoma, Crohn's disease, rabies, Jakob-Creutzfeldt disease, leukemia, AIDS, and other viral diseases prohibit the donation of tissue for transplantation. However, eyes can still be donated for research purposes that support the advancement of the technology of corneal transplantation.

Visual impairment is not a contraindication to eye donation. A donor who has worn glasses or contact lenses may have perfectly healthy corneas. A donor with ocular problems such as glaucoma, macular regeneration of the retina, or cataracts may donate eyes to research.

CARE OF THE POTENTIAL EYE DONOR

Optimal eye care of the potential eye donor is necessary to prevent infection, overexposure, and drying and irritation of corneal tissue. Eye care with cornea donation in mind should begin as soon as the potential donor is identified.

Tear production is decreased in the unconscious patient on a mechanical ventilator. Artificial tears or an ophthalmic lubricating ointment can be applied to prevent drying of the corneas. After clinical death, additional eye care that helps to preserve the integrity of the cornea includes irrigation of the eyes with a balanced salt solution. Between irrigations, the lids should be closed and lightly taped.

STORAGE OF EYE TISSUE

Before 1974 the primary method of storing corneal tissue for transplant was moist chamber whole-globe storage at 4° C. Maximum storage time using this method was 48 hours, although it was preferable to transplant the corneal tissue within 24 hours. A new technique known as *organ culture* allows corneal tissue to be stored at 37° C for up to 31 days.[8] This improved storage technique allows for the more optimal conditions associated with elective surgery.

EYE BANKING

Tales are told of eye banks that consisted of only a small refrigerator, a telephone, and a single volunteer. This is a far cry from the modern eye bank. The origin of eye storage can be traced to A. Magitot in 1911,[9] who first stored whole eyes in serum. The development of modern eye banking is credited to Vladimir D. Filatov of Russia in the early 1930s.[3] Filatov recognized

that corneas from cadavers could be successfully transplanted if removed within a few hours of death, stored at 4° to 6° C, and maintained under aseptic conditions.

The first eye bank in the United States, The Eye Bank for Sight Restoration, was organized in 1945 by Dr. R. Townley Paton.[4] Seven branch eye banks were established by 1956 with the common goal of providing donor eye tissue for transplantation and research purposes.

During the 1950s independent eye banks were formed, many with the support of Lions Club International. In 1955 the American Academy of Ophthalmology and Otolaryngology began discussing the formation of an association of eye banks.[3] The Eye Bank Association of America (EBAA) was established in 1961 and today has more than 90 member banks throughout 41 states, the District of Columbia, Puerto Rico, and Canada. Member eye banks look to the EBAA for standards for the recovery and distribution of eye tissue as well as for training and certification of eye bank technicians.

DISTRIBUTION OF DONATED EYE TISSUE

As prescribed by the Uniform Anatomical Gift Act of 1968, eye tissue may be donated for the purposes of transplantation, research or education. The first priority is to provide corneas for transplantation. If a donor cornea is not suitable for transplantation, the tissue will be used for research and/or educational purposes. If the cornea is used for transplantation, the remaining eye tissue is used for research or education. In these ways all donated eye tissue contributes to restoration of sight.

CORNEAL GRAFTING TECHNIQUES

There are several corneal grafting procedures. These include the techniques of penetrating keratoplasty and lamellar keratoplasty (nonpenetrating). Penetrating keratoplasty (Fig. 10-2) is the most common type of corneal transplant procedure performed.[10] In this procedure, after the center of the recipient's diseased cornea is removed, the full thickness of the diseased cornea is replaced with a clear donor cornea. A button of donor corneal tissue,

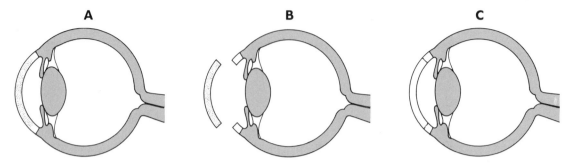

Fig. 10-2 Penetrating keratoplasty, in which (A) the entire clouded cornea is (B) removed and (C) replaced by a clear cornea.

slightly larger than the recipient opening, is sutured in place. Indications for full-thickness grafts include trauma, congenital corneal abnormalities, corneal degeneration and scarring, and metabolic diseases.

Lamellar keratoplasty (Fig. 10-3) is partial-thickness grafting. In this procedure, the anterior two thirds of the donor cornea is patched into the recipient cornea bed. This procedure does not involve entering the eye and is therefore associated with a decreased risk of infection and rejection. Lamellar patches can be used as a temporary measure until penetrating keratoplasty can be performed. Indications include restoration of normal corneal thickness, opacity of the anterior cornea, and disease of the cornea requiring deep excision. Patients with full-thickness disease or corneal endothelial dysfunction are not candidates for lamellar keratoplasty.

IMMUNOLOGIC ASPECTS OF CORNEA TRANSPLANTATION

The concept that the cornea, because it is avascular, is a "privileged" immunologic tissue, and therefore cannot be rejected by a foreign host, is outdated. All nucleated cells, including corneal endothelial cells, display histocompatibility surface antigens. The role that the absence of blood vessels in the cornea plays is in preventing the host from coming in contact with the foreign antigens carried on the transplanted tissue.

The efficacy of histocompatibility testing for corneal transplantation is controversial. Although sight is successfully restored in 90% of cases without HLA matching, retrospective and prospective investigations have revealed benefits in matching class I HLA antigen loci in patients at high risk for allograft rejection resulting from corneal vascularization that can

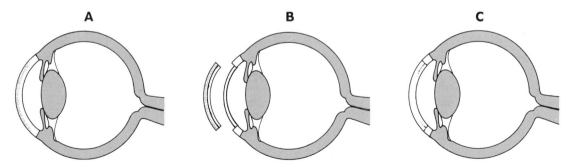

Fig. 10-3 Lamellar keratoplasty, in which (A) a partial clouded or diseased cornea is (B) removed in a layer and (C) replaced by healthy cornea.

occur as the injured cornea heals and before graft rejection.[11] In a 3-year prospective study, patients who shared two or more class I HLA antigens had an 18% rejection rate, while those who shared zero or one loci had a 39% incidence of rejection.[12] ABO compatibility has not been shown to increase success in corneal transplantation.[10]

IMPLICATIONS FOR NURSING PRACTICE

The nurse plays a vital role in eye donation. As in the case of potential organ donors, the nurse is in the best position to identify potential eye donors and facilitate this discussion with family members. The need for donor eye tissue continues to be the major limiting factor in corneal transplantation. As we become a nation of older Americans, there is a greater need for donor eye tissue. New procedures are being developed and others refined which require donor eye tissue. As a result, the demand may increase drastically in the future.

The contraindications to cornea donation are few and the potential yield is high. By offering the option of eye donation to bereaved families, it may someday be possible to cure conditions that render approximately 11 million Americans blind.

REFERENCES

1. Eye Bank Association of America (1986). *Fact sheet.* Washington, DC: The Association.
2. Swerdlow JL (1989). Matching needs, saving lives. Washington, DC: The Annenberg Washington Program.
3. Casey TA and Mayer DJ (1984). *Corneal grafting. Principles and practice.* Philadelphia: WB Saunders Co.
4. Rosenberg N and Snyderman R (1969). New parts for people. New York: WW Norton Co, Inc.
5. Trevor-Roper PD (1972). The history of corneal grafting. In Casey TA (ed). *Corneal grafting.* New York: Appleton-Century-Crofts (8).
6. Khodadoust A (1988). Corneal transplantation. In Cerilli GJ (ed). *Organ transplantation and replacement* (569-594). Philadelphia: JB Lippincott Co.
7. LifeLink of Georgia (1987). *Organ and tissue donation manual.* Atlanta, Ga.
8. Doughman DJ, Harris JE and Schmitt MK (1976). Penetrating keratoplasty using 37° organ cultured cornea. *Transactions of the American Academy of Ophthalmology and Otolaryngology, 81,* 778-793.
9. Polack F (1977). *Corneal transplantation.* New York: Grune and Stratton (237).
10. Smith RS (1989). Corneal transplantation. In Flye MW (ed). *Principles of organ transplantation.* Philadelphia: WB Saunders Co (625-529).
11. Bennett TO, Peyman GA, Tissot R and Cohen C (1975). Histocompatibility, penetrating keratoplasty. *Acta Ophthamologica, 53,* 403-407.
12. Gibbs DC, Batchelor JR and Casey TA (1973). The influence of HL-A compatibility on the fate of corneal grafts. In Porter R and Knight J (eds). *Corneal graft failure. A Ciba Foundation symposium.* Amsterdam: Elsevier (293-306).

11

Kidney Transplantation

Jennie P. Perryman and *Pamela U. Stillerman*

Diseases of the renal and urologic system affect more than 20 million Americans and claim more than 80,000 lives each year.[1] It is projected that by 1990 over 120,000 individuals will have end-stage renal disease (ESRD), requiring dialysis or transplantation to live. In 1988, 9123 kidney transplants were performed in 208 transplant centers.[2] Between January 1, 1980, and January 1, 1989, more than 63,000 people received kidney transplants in the United States (Fig. 11-1).

Kidney transplantation has come of age. No longer is it considered experimental. For the child, young adult, or patient with diabetes mellitus, transplantation is the treatment of choice. One-year patient survival rates of 95% to 97% exceed the 1-year survival rates of patients beginning dialysis.[3,4] Depending on transplant protocols, the 1-year graft survival of a living-related, nonidentical donor organ approximates 90%; for the cadaveric recipient, 65% to 85%.

According to the Task Force on Organ Transplantation (1985), recipients with successful transplants have achieved a superior quality of life when compared with the nontransplant ESRD patient population.[5] In the 1980s renal transplantation became the most cost-effective

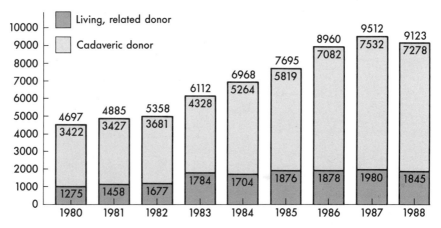

Fig. 11-1 Kidney transplantation in the United States, 1980-1988. (From Health Care Financing Administration, Washington, DC and United Network for Organ Sharing, Richmond, Va.)

therapy for treatment of ESRD. Eggers recently reported that maintaining persons on dialysis costs approximately three times as much as maintaining patients with functioning grafts.[6] This expenditure analysis included patients who are treated for graft failure, who may eventually return to dialysis.

THE PAST

The technology of renal transplantation today is rooted in a rich history spanning much of the twentieth century. At the turn of the century, 45 years before the advent of dialysis, there were sporadic attempts at kidney transplantation to sustain patients suffering from acute renal failure. A chronologic listing of the early signif-icant events in renal transplantation is found in the box below. In the eighth Human Kidney Transplant Registry, an analysis of the cumula-tive results through December 31, 1969, was summarized. A total of 3645 kidney transplant procedures were performed, with 40% per-formed during 1968 and 1969. The 1- and 2-year graft survival rates for living-related donor transplantation were 78% and 75%, respec-tively. Cadaveric transplants had a 52% 1-year and 41% 2-year graft survival rate. The good news was that two thirds of the patients were rated "completely normal" in their activities.[7] Progress was slowly but steadily being made.

The Courage to Fail: A Social View of Organ Transplants and Dialysis by Fox and Swazey

---

TIMETABLE OF EARLY ACHIEVEMENTS IN RENAL DIALYSIS AND TRANSPLANTATION

1900	Xenografting attempts by Lambert using kidney of a lamb, Rockefeller Institute, New York.
1906	Joboulay attempts xenografting goat and pig kidneys to arm vessels of human pa-tients.
1936	Voroney implants human kidney into patient's groin; patient succumbs in 48 hours.
1943	Kolff designs "rotating drum artificial kidney"; ten patients with acute renal failure survive.
1945	First clinical success: Lansteiner, Hufnagel, and Hume anastomose human cadaver kidney to radial artery and cephalic vein of toxemic woman in acute renal crisis; patient recovers.
1954	Merrill, Murray, and Hume perform transplant between monozygotic twins, Peter Bent Brigham Hospital, Boston. Recipient Richard Herrick lived 7 years. Hallmark of renal transplantation.
1959	Development of Quinton-Scribner AV external shunt; two patients begin long-term maintenance dialysis for ESRD.
1959	Murray in Boston and Hamburger in Paris almost simultaneously performed first successful nonidentical twin transplants. Both recipients had received prior total body irridiation.
Early 1960s	Identification of antigens by Terasaki and Najarian; use of microcytotoxicity for histocompatibility testing begins. Use of antilymphocytic serum by Woodruff in En-gland. Belzer develops perfusion technique.
1962	Burroughs Wellcome develops azathioprine, 6-mercaptopurine (Imuran). First suc-cessful nontwin transplant.
1963	Total of 194 kidney transplants reported; fewer than 10% of 103 nontwin trans-plants survived more than 3 months.
1964	Home dialysis started by Scribner and Curtis in Seattle, Merrill in Boston, and Shaldon in London.
1972	Passage of PL 92-603. ESRD patients are the first and only persons to be declared "victims of catastrophic illness" with federal funding available for medical treat-ment costs.

was published in 1974.[8] The title *The Courage to Fail* is quite descriptive of the transplant era of the late 1960s through the 1970s. According to Fox and Swazey, the 1970s was an era of continued high mortality and "devastating" unwanted side effects of chronic immunosuppression—cancer, gastrointestinal ulcerations, viral, bacterial, and fungal infections, hypersplenism, hyperparathyroidism, cataracts, bone disease, liver malfunction, hyperlipidemia, and vascular disease.

Immune modification techniques

Clinical research during the 1970s included attempts to effectively modify the immune response, so that the dosages of the immunosuppressive agents might be reduced. Manipulation of the immune response heralded an increase in the use of total body irradiation, splenectomy, and thoracic duct drainage. However, the untoward complications of these methods preclude their use as a standard for transplant management today. Total body irradiation was fraught with severe infections. Splenectomy, associated with a high morbidity and an increased incidence of thromboembolism, also had an appreciable mortality rate, especially in the diabetic population.[9,10] A recent review of Minnesota's experience with routine splenectomy before transplantation indicates that there is no significant difference in long-term graft survival between patients with and those without splenectomy.[11] With thoracic duct drainage, the lymphatic system was depleted of lymphocytes, thereby blunting responsiveness of the immune system. Timing of the transplant procedure to coincide with the recipient's depleted state is the major problem with this procedure, in addition to the potential for infection.

Transfusions. One immune modification technique, preconditioning patients with blood transfusions before transplantation, did have an impact on present protocols. The issue of blood transfusions for the potential transplant recipient has come full circle in the last 15 years. In the early 1970s transfusions were avoided in dialysis patients who were awaiting transplantation unless frank symptomology dictated otherwise. The physiologic basis underlying this practice was that the introduction of foreign antigens from blood transfusions would induce antibody stimulation. This increased level of circulating cytotoxic antibodies would potentially decrease the likelihood of a successful transplant. There was also the threat of viral transmission, especially hepatitis, with the transfusion.

In 1976 Opelz and Terasaki[12] published data suggesting that nontransfused patients had poorer graft survival than those who had been previously transfused. One-year graft survival in the transfused group was 80%, whereas the nontransfused patients had a 40% graft survival rate. Theories have been developed over the years to explain this phenomenon. One such theory is that pretransplant transfusions induce a state of immune modification in many recipients by down-regulation of the effector mechanisms, thereby reducing the potential for rejection and improving graft survival.[20]

Conversely, in potential recipients who have never been exposed to histocompatibility antigens through previous pregnancies, transfusions, or a prior transplant, the renal allograft will act as an immunogenic stimulus and as a target for the immunologic assault.[13] Consequently the development of cytotoxic antibodies against the graft will ensue, leading to graft loss within 3 months of transplant surgery.

Into the 1980s the transfusion effect on graft survival was repeatedly documented.[14-17] Programs using transfusion conditioning protocols with conventional immunosuppression regimens after transplantation reported improved graft survivals of 10% to 30% in comparison with patients who did not receive transfusions before transplantation. Furthermore, it appeared that the transfusion effect lasted through the first 3 to 6 months after transplantation, the critical period for graft loss caused by rejection.

But success and improved survival rates for some brought problems for other potential transplant candidates. Approximately 30% of the patients who received random donor transfusions became sensitized or developed antibodies specific to immunizing antigens in the transfusions.[13] Therefore three of every ten persons who were transfused decreased if not eliminated the chances of finding a donor kidney for which they did not have preexisting cytotoxic antibodies.

In the early 1980s, advancements were made in living-related transplantation with the introduction of deliberate donor-specific blood transfusions. Salvatierra[18] revealed that graft survival results comparable with those of HLA-identical donors could be achieved with parent donors and mismatched siblings when recipients were conditioned before transplantation with transfusions of donor blood. Once again, however, the original Salvatierra protocol had a sensitization rate of 35%. In time, stored blood proved to be less immunogenic than fresh blood and thus less likely to stimulate the production of antidonor antibodies.[19,20] Some programs administered azathioprine before transfusion to further decrease the incidence of antidonor antibodies.[21] As a result the sensitization rate decreased to as low as 8%, and graft survival in the living-related nonidentical HLA transplants at 1 year reached 90% to 93%.

THE PRESENT

Immune modification with blood transfusions significantly improved early graft survival rates when conventional immunosuppression with azathioprine and corticosteroids was the mainstay of transplant immunosuppression. However, the 1980s heralded a new era—the cyclosporine era. With cyclosporine immunosuppression, patient survival rates are 95%, and graft survivals, at least for the first 2 years, are 10% to 15% improved over conventional therapy results.[22] With cyclosporine protocols graft survival rates are improved without the risk of sensitizing a group of potential transplant recipients through the induction of blood products.[23] The question today then becomes "to pretransfuse or not to pretransfuse?"

Many programs have abandoned the preconditioning transfusion protocols for patients awaiting a cadaveric transplant. One exception, however, might be the patient who has never been exposed to foreign HLA histocompatibility antigens. Controlled prospective clinical studies are in process to determine whether the donor-specific transfusion effect, in combination with various cyclosporine immunosuppressive regimens in the living donor transplant population, remains significant.

The 1980s have seen improvements in graft and patient survival resulting from clinical observations and research in the selection and preparation of potential patients. There have also been advances in organ recovery and preservation, diagnosis and treatment of rejection, use of immunosuppressive drugs, and management of complications. It has been an exciting time when data from large registries are being analyzed, clinical observations are being documented, and hypotheses tested in multicenter collaborative studies. It is a time of debate, scientific trial, and analysis. The cyclosporine era is fast becoming the era of transplant progress.

Patient selection

There is no one profile that would describe the individual who is a potential candidate for renal transplantation. The only consistent variable is that all candidates must have ESRD or are rapidly approaching ESRD. The most frequent causes of ESRD requiring transplantation are hypertension, glomerulonephritis, diabetic nephropathy, hereditary or congenital disorders, or systemic lupus erythematosis. However, this list is not inclusive. Also, a patient's response to ESRD is individualized and variable, depending in part on his or her physiologic and psychologic adaptation to illness. A patient may be totally functional, employed, receiving continuous ambulatory peritoneal dialysis or home hemodialysis, and experiencing only occasional periods of low energy. Or the disease may have caused such symptomatology that the patient is severely depressed and exhibits "failure to thrive syndrome" while undergoing dialysis. A third example is the individual who has never received dialysis treatments but becomes a candidate for transplantation as the primary therapy while he or she is essentially free of the chronic side effects of the disease. Depending on the length of time that the patient has had ESRD, multiple symptoms may appear. The complexion may be sallow as a result of urochrome deposits in the skin; the patient may complain of lethargy, lack of energy, and an inability to walk even short distances or climb stairs without exhaustion. This is usually attributed to the effects of anemia caused by the lack of erythropoietin production. Baseline hematocrit levels may hover in the 23% to 25% range. Many patients are hypertensive.

Some may verbalize disgust with medication regimens, dialysis schedules, and dietary restrictions, or dependency issues relating to family and friends, staff, or the dialysis machine itself may be described. Especially if they are unemployed, patients may express anxiety about financial issues. Women and many men of child-bearing years may speak of a desire to have children and note frustrations with decreased libido, impotence, and even marital discord.

When patients are asked, "Why do you want a transplant?" any of the above issues might surface as the candidates describe a desire for more normalcy in their lives. Studies have been reported comparing transplant recipients' and dialysis patients' quality of life, using such factors as rehabilitation, life satisfaction, psychologic affect, and sexual activity.[24-28] Results have consistently shown that persons with a successful transplant have significantly higher scores on the factors studied. Furthermore, Evans[26] noted that the quality of life of transplant recipients compared well with that of the general population.[26]

In 1968, Merrill listed several factors to include as criteria for selection of patients for renal allotransplantation.[29] Among the factors listed were a failure to respond to conservative management, presence of a normal urinary outflow tract, absence of major extrarenal complications (malignancy, systemic disease, cerebral or coronary artery disease), and age considerations. Absence of active infection, severe malnutrition, and pancytopenia were also absolute considerations. Some programs expanded these criteria to include psychiatric and socioeconomic parameters.

In the late 1980s, the previous stringent criteria were relaxed. No longer must a patient have been unsuccessfully dialyzed to be considered for transplant surgery. Transplantation is now presented as an option at the time that the ESRD diagnosis is made. In several U.S. programs transplantation is considered the primary therapy for patients with diabetic nephropathy. Yet years ago, neither dialysis nor transplantation would have been options for this patient population.

In the past the upper age limit for kidney transplantation was 50. Today several centers will include the 60-year-old as a candidate, contingent on an otherwise stable state of health. At least one prospective study is in progress to compare the effects of transplantation and dialysis therapies on the older patient, examining potential risks, morbidity, and quality of life. For children transplantation is universally accepted as the primary mode of treatment for ESRD. However, some centers do have a weight minimum of 9.5 to 10.0 kg, because the small recipient size may limit the availability of donor organs.

On June 30, 1988, the American Society of Transplant Physicians adapted a Statement on Criteria for Selection of ESRD Patients for Renal Transplantation. The philosophy on which the statement evolved was that "all ESRD patients should be considered as candidates for transplantation unless there is a specific contraindication."[30] Examples of specific contraindications are outlined in Table 11-1.

Guidelines for patients with AIDS and hepatitis are in evolutionary stages. The patient who is HIV positive yet asymptomatic poses an unresolved issue for transplant centers. The basis for individual program policies regarding this issue is now founded on recently published guidelines from UNOS. UNOS policy states[31]:

Testing for HIV-Ab should be a condition of candidacy for whole organ transplantation, except in cases where such testing would violate applicable state or federal laws and regulations. A potential candidate for organ transplantation who tests HIV-Ab seropositive but is in an asymptomatic carrier state should not necessarily be excluded from candidacy for whole organ transplantation. However, a potential candidate for organ transplantation who tests HIV seropositive and has AIDS or AIDS-related complex should be excluded from candidacy for whole organ transplantation.

Table 11-1 Contraindications to selection of ESRD patients for renal transplantation

Absolute contraindications	Variances
Active infections	
Active HIV (ARDS, ARC)	
Active TB	Once infection is controlled, resume evaluation
Active systemic infection	
IV drug abuse	Free of substance abuse for 1 year
	Extensive psychosocial evaluation
Advanced cardiopulmonary disease	
American Heart Association class III and	May require cardiac catheterization, angio-
IV disease	plasty, or coronary artery bypass surgery
	before becoming a candidate
High risk candidates for any surgical procedure	
Advanced chronic obstructive pulmonary disease	
that places patient at risk for intubation	
Smoker in presence of lung disease	
Malignancy (except skin cancers)	
Patients at high risk for recurrence of malig-	Tumor free for a minimum of 2 years
nancies	
Active vasculitis/glomerulonephritis	
Active systemic lupus erythematosis	Candidates after manifestations quiescent
Wegener's granolomatosis	Goodpasture's—when anti-GBM antibodies
Goodpasture's syndrome	disappear
Psychosocial	
Reported repeated inability to comply with pre-	
scribed medical regimen	
Mental incompetence	
Marked obesity	
High risk for surgery	Candidate after acceptable weight loss
Positive current T cell lymphocytotoxic cross-match	Not a candidate for that particular donor

Since 1986 three patients who were HIV antibody seropositive have received kidney transplants.[32] Only one has survived for more than 6 months. In light of this poor prognosis, Rubin recommends that "all potential recipients of organ transplantation should be screened for antibody to HIV. All positive patients should be verified by Western blot analysis."[32] Furthermore dialysis rather than transplantation appears to be the best treatment for ESRD in patients who are seropositive for HIV antibody.[32]

There is some question about the advisability of transplanting patients who are hepatitis B surface antigen (HBsAg) positive. Rubin reports that the leading cause of death in patients with functioning renal allografts is liver dis-

ease.[32] The risk of death from liver-related complications in this patient population is approximately 5% per year. After a usually favorable initial postoperative course, there is a definite decline in patients who are chronically HBsAg positive beginning 1 to 2 years after transplantation. The use of azathioprine and other hepatotoxic drugs may be implicated.

Evaluation

Evaluation of a candidate for transplantation includes an extensive medical evaluation, a psychosocial assessment, and histocompatibility studies.

Medical evaluation and interventions. The medical evaluation includes a complete history and physical examination, with a detailed history for renal disease and concomitant complications. Patients with ESRD are prone to hypertensive disease, atherosclerosis, and hyperlipidemia. The hyperlipidemia can be further compounded with corticosteroid immunosuppression after transplant surgery. The leading cause of morbidity and mortality in patients with ESRD is cardiovascular in origin. Analysis of the Health Care Financing Administration (HCFA) data of the 1980s revealed that 20% of the patients on dialysis had ESRD secondary to hypertension. An additional 25% had diabetes mellitus with a potential for cardiovascular involvement. Helderman further noted that "cardiac disease in general and hypertensive cardiovascular disease in particular are exceedingly common among potential renal transplant recipients."[33]

For this reason it is recommended that an extensive cardiac evaluation be done on all patients older than 45 years of age, patients with a history of cardiac symptoms, and all patients with diabetes mellitus. A thallium stress test is indicated in the high-risk group. Further evaluation may include echocardiography and cardiac catheterization. Such interventions as percutaneous coronary angioplasty (PTCA) or coronary artery bypass surgery may be indicated based on the evaluation before acceptance of the patient for transplantation. Studies have shown that with proper evaluation and treatment of cardiovascular disease before transplant surgery, 2-year diabetic patient survival rates after transplantation are now comparable to nondiabetic survival rates.[34-36] The evaluation should also include studies to determine the patency of the iliac vasculature because of the tendency toward atherosclerosis and peripheral vascular disease in patients with diabetes mellitus.

Hypertension is usually controlled by medication and sodium and fluid restrictions in the ESRD patient. However, hypertension refractory to medical management may be a consideration for a pretransplant nephrectomy. Polycystic kidney disease with large swollen kidneys and infected cysts, severe pain, or hematuria; recurrent urinary tract infections or recurrent pyelonephritis; and ureteric reflux with history of infection are also indications for further evaluation and consideration of nephrectomy. As a rule, native bilateral nephrectomies are avoided whenever possible because of the increased morbidity among anephric patients. Without any source of erythropoietin, anemia is a constant problem for the anephric individual. Rather than electively creating an anephric patient, some centers will consider extensive antihypertensive drug therapy for the first year after transplant, before reevaluating the need for surgical intervention.[37] Whenever possible, attempts will be made to isolate a single kidney to be nephrectomized rather than bilateral procedures.

Another complication of ESRD is hyperparathyroidism caused by poor control of calcium and phosphate metabolism over the years. In renal failure the excretion of phosphate via the urinary system is diminished, causing phosphate retention. Serum phosphate and calcium are inversely proportional, so in the presence of an elevated serum phosphate level, the ionized plasma calcium level decreases to compensate. The parathyroid gland consequently secretes parathormone-stimulating osteoclasts to resorb calcium and phosphate from the bones to the plasma. Secondary hyperparathyroidism often develops, causing further bone demineralization. Aluminum hydroxides or phosphate binders are administered to control the calcium and phosphate imbalance of renal failure. Evaluation of the degree of parathyroid involvement is necessary before transplantation. In the event of elevated parathyroid hormone levels not responding to medical management, a subtotal parathyroidectomy may be indicated to prevent hypercalcemia after transplantation.[10]

Although a "normal" urinary tract is not a prerequisite for transplant, evaluation of bladder function and ureter patency is highly recommended. Cystoscopy, cystometrics, and voiding cystograms may be indicated, depending on the history obtained. Surgical intervention may be required for bladder reconstruction, correction of bladder strictures, or other bladder augmentation procedures. A diabetic recipient with a neurogenic bladder is taught a clean self-catheterization procedure.

Candidates with a history of peptic ulcer disease and diverticuli may require further gastrointestinal evaluation because of the potential for life-threatening complications after transplant with corticosteroid immunosuppression. Aggressive medical management with histamine antagonists is the first line of treatment today. Pyloroplasty and vagotomy are no longer performed electively for roentgenographic evidence of active disease or scarring.[10]

Other organ systems are evaluated on an individual basis, depending on what the history reveals. Smokers with diabetes mellitus or with chronic obstructive pulmonary disease are encouraged to stop smoking. All candidates are queried about previous bouts of infection and communicable disease. Active infections are treated before transplant.

Routine oral and dental evaluations are done on all patients to assess for periodontal disease, dental caries, or abscesses that could become sources of infection with the initiation of immunosuppression. Any corrective work necessary is performed before transplant.

Psychosocial assessment. Although there are no standard criteria for the psychosocial evaluation, this assessment is as important as the medical and physical assessments when evaluating a candidate for transplant. Of concern to the transplant team are the potential psychiatric side effects of the steroids and the chronicity of the medical management over time. Does this patient's history indicate an ability to cope with the added stress of transplant and long-term management? Are the typical coping behaviors that the patient expresses adaptive or maladaptive? If maladaptive, has there been a positive response to medical or psychiatric interventions? Does this candidate have a support system? What are the family dynamics? What are the expectations of the patient and significant others regarding transplantation? Are these expectations realistic? (For further discussion, see Chapters 7 and 8.)

Finally, patient and family education is initiated during the evaluation phase. Topics include a discussion of the transplant process and typical course; purpose, use, and side effects of immunosuppressive drugs; survival rates; and follow-up requirements. It may be in one of these discussions that transportation needs are identified for the first time. It is at this time that discussion about the donation process is broached. The expected outcome of the transplant evaluation is that motivated, informed, and stable individuals are selected for transplantation.

Histocompatibility studies. Transplantation success, measured by maximum length of graft and patient survival, depends on the recipient's immunologic acceptance of a "nonself" or foreign graft (see Chapter 3). One means of facilitating this is for the kidney donor and recipient to be histocompatible, thereby minimizing genetic disparity. The two major antigen systems for transplantation in man are the ABO system and the human leukocyte antigen (HLA) system.

In transplantation, as with blood transfusions, the major blood group, ABO, must be compatible between the donor and potential recipient. It appears, however, that the role of some minor blood groups such as Rh factor are insignificant. The rule of compatibility for ABO is that AB is the universal recipient and O the universal donor. However, because more than 50% of the individuals awaiting a kidney on the UNOS list are of the O blood group, UNOS policy for allocation and distribution states that O kidneys must be placed in O recipients, except in the case of six antigen-matched individuals who have a blood group other than O.[38]

HLA compatibility testing. During the evaluation, blood tests are done to determine the candidate's genetic typing. This typing is often referred to as tissue typing or HLA typing. (For further discussion of transplantation immunology and HLA, refer to Chapter 3.)

A mixed lymphocyte culture (MLC) is also performed with recipient and living-related donor sera in a culture to confirm HLA identity and to determine genetic disparity, specifically to the D-DR locus. Lymphocytes exposed to nonidentical HLA antigens respond by increased stimulation, DNA synthesis, and blastic formation. If blastogenesis occurs during the 5- to 7-day incubation period, incompatibility of the donor and recipient is determined. However, if there is a lack of blastogenesis, the test is suggestive of HLA-D locus matching and compatibility. At present, because of the incubation period, this test is performed as an evaluation for living donor transplantation only.

Immediately before any renal transplant and as part of the initial testing for a living donor transplant, a white blood cell cross-match is performed. Donor lymphocytes are exposed to recipient sera. This test detects the presence of preformed circulating cytotoxic antibodies to donor antigens. A positive cross-match precludes transplant with that particular donor. Transplant in the presence of a positive cross-match would result in hyperacute rejection of the graft.

Cross-match testing procedures continue to be refined. Cross-match testing differentiating T cells from B cells is available in some laboratories. The above scenario describes a positive T cell cross-match. Studies are in progress to determine the ramifications of a positive B cell cross-match in the presence of a negative T cell cross-match using either donor lymph nodes or peripheral blood specimens.[39]

The issue of matching. Another major question that has been debated in the cyclosporine era involves the issue of HLA matching. Over the last 20 years, the use of HLA matching for living-related donors is well established. As early as 1969 Terasaki has been a proponent of matching, reporting 6-month graft survivals of 95% in HLA identical siblings compared with 68% in mismatched living-related grafts.[40] It has been further established that matching of living-related individuals by HLA-A and -B antigens alone is not predictive of graft survival. Likewise, HLA-A and -B matching in unrelated donation appears to be of little benefit.[39] Instead, predictive matching depends on the number of shared chromosomes, or *haplotypes.*

Haplotype matching in a 1969 study showed not only short-term but also long-term effects on graft survival. Graft survival at the end of 1 year was 90% for HLA-identical siblings (two haplotypes), 70% for parental kidneys (one haplotype), and 45% for cadaveric donors (zero haplotype).[41] Over a long period data are calculated in units of half-life, which has been shown to be an effective measure of the graft loss rate. Long-term survival of these same grafts was a half-life of 7.5 years for cadaveric kidneys, 11 years for the parental grafts, and 34 years for the HLA-identical grafts.[41] Excellent results between nonidentical family members using the MLC to confirm typing and reactivity to a new locus, the HLA-DR, were documented by the late 1970s. Results were comparable to that of HLA-identical transplantation.

Matching for cadaveric kidney transplantation has been received with much less enthusiasm. One must acknowledge that even in a population of unrelated persons, individuals may share portions of two HLA haplotypes, thereby potentially increasing graft survival by matching at least some of the antigens. However it was not until the early to mid-1980s that concensus was reached in the transplant community that HLA matching was associated with increased graft survival in cadaveric transplantation. Part of the hesitancy may be attributed to the knowledge that there is only a 10% improvement in 1-year graft survival in U.S. transplant centers when comparing the best- and worst-matched grafts.[42] However, Terasaki has repeatedly documented improved long-term survival with HLA matching. In 1989 data were presented showing that the half-life of well-matched cadaveric kidneys has increased from 8 to possibly 11 years for kidneys transplanted with cyclosporine protocols since 1985.[43] For the HLA-identical sibling donors the half-life is 25 years; for the parental, it is 13 years.

Retrospective studies using MLCs with cadaveric transplantation found that those with lower degrees of stimulation did indeed have a superior graft outcome.[44] More feasible, less time-consuming tests for D locus matching have recently been developed. Many groups are reporting that matching with the HLA-B locus, which is located close to the HLA-D locus, is more important than matching with the HLA-A locus.[45] General consensus is that matching to the HLA-C antigen is of no value in transplantation. It appears that in the present arena, close attention will be given to the matching of HLA-B and DR loci, looking at one and two DR matches.

The United Network for Organ Sharing (UNOS) recently initiated a study to compare phenotypically identical cadaveric graft–recipient pairs and six antigen cadaveric graft–recipient pairs to various degrees of mismatched pairs of graft-recipients. Early graft function, frequency of rejection episodes, and graft and patient survival data will be correlated to type of match and various possible antigen groupings in an attempt to clarify and possibly validate the importance of HLA matching and cadaveric renal transplantation. Preliminary analysis of initial data show that there is no significant difference in 3-month survival or early function of identically matched kidneys when compared with lesser matched ones.[46] However, the analysis is of a sample of only 500 identical matches, compared with 5000 mismatches. Data will continue to be collected over the next several years before any conclusions are reached.

The kidney donor

The living-related donor. Unlike most other solid organ transplant recipients, the kidney transplant recipient has two sources for potential organs — the usual cadaver donor pool and a living donor pool. Since the first successful transplant of the Herrick twins in the 1950s, volumes have been written regarding superior survival rates of living-related donor (LRD) kidneys in comparison with cadaveric (CAD) ones.

In 1986 the national 1-year graft survival rate for living-related kidney transplants was 88%; for cadaveric kidney transplants, 71%. Patient survival was 96% for LRDs and 91% for CADs.[47] These survival rates were not stratified for immune modification techniques, HLA matching, or immunosuppression protocols. However, there was a 17% improved graft survival rate of living-related in comparison with the cadaveric grafts.

Of the 9123 kidneys transplanted in 1988, 1845 were from living-related donors.[2] The practice of transplanting living-related donor kidneys, although an accepted practice, has generated controversy over the years. In 1963 Thomas Starzl read the following statement in a presentation at the Western Surgical Association meeting[48]:

The use of volunteer living donors to provide kidneys for homotransplantation has many medical, legal, and social implications. The infliction of major operative trauma upon healthy and well-motivated donors cannot be dismissed lightly since the chance of ultimate viability of the homograft in its new environment is highly speculative. In the long run, justification for continued use of volunteer donors depends upon the demonstration that the donor operation carries a negligible risk and that the benefit to the recipient patient is substantial and predictable.

Twenty-three years later at Presbyterian-University Hospital, Pittsburgh, under the direction of Starzl, only one of the 193 kidneys transplanted were from living-related donors.[49]

Nationwide, the proportion of living donor transplants has declined from more than 30% of all transplants in 1982 to about 20% since 1986. This may result in part from the doubling in number of cadaveric donor kidneys in that same time period — 3681 in 1982 to 7532 in 1987.[50]

In a survey of 159 transplant centers in 1986, Spital and Spital[51] noted that of the 83 respondents, all reported performing living donor transplants. Concerns that Starzl addressed in 1963 appear to have been satisfactorily answered. Keown states that the use of living donors is justified on three grounds[52]:

1. The increase in graft survival exceeding that obtained by cadavers of 10% to 15% at 1 year and increasing with continued follow-up
2. The chronic inability of cadaveric donation to fulfill the demand
3. The ability to arrange the transplant expeditiously and at the optimum moment

In December 1988 there were 13,947 renal patients on the UNOS waiting list, even though there were 9123 kidney transplants performed during that year. The supply of kidneys historically has not met the demand. In 1986 the usual wait for a kidney transplant was 6 to 12 months, with an 18-month wait for at least 20% of the patients.[53] With the large volume of patients on the UNOS computer waiting list today, one might speculate that the wait may be even longer.

Unilateral nephrectomy for the purpose of donation in a healthy adult incurs a mortality risk of less than 0.1%.[54] The long-term health and life expectancy of the living donor is not adversely altered by donation. Life expectancy is comparable to the general population when stratified by age, sex, and similar presurgical health status. There have been concerns that continued hyperfiltration of the remaining kidney may jeopardize long-term renal function as documented in experimental animal studies. A recent 10-year follow-up study of 52 donors showed that renal function is comparable to predonation levels. In several men there was a slight degree of hypertension and proteinuria. This was not statistically significant when the subjects were matched by age and sex to control subjects.[55]

As with any surgery, there are inevitable risks. In a series of 238 consecutive donors, Penn et al[56] observed the following postoperative complications: atelectasis, 14%; pneumothorax, 11%; urinary tract infections, 10%; small pleural effusions, 5%; and transient hypertension, 4%. Similar complications with varying rates have been reported by others.[56] According to Penn et al, 3 weeks after nephrectomy, creatinine clearance levels were 70.5% of the preoperative norm.[57] Follow-up studies of donors 10 to 20 years after nephrectomy show that the mean serum creatinine levels do not increase significantly over time from postnephrectomy values.[58] Similarly, in a study of individuals who had unilateral nephrectomies in childhood, the creatinine clearance levels averaged >4.3% of normal after a mean follow-up of 23 years.[58]

Most donors state that what is gained far outweighs the potential risks. Studies have shown that donors experience an improved self-image and have reported a closer relationship with the recipient.[59]

To further affirm that potential risks to the donors are negligible, the selection criteria for living donors are stringent. Of potential candidates desiring to donate, 30% to 50% are ruled out during the selection process.[17,37] Donors are usually between the ages of 18 and 60 and without any known health problems. On rare occasions the donor candidate may be younger, as in the situation of an identical twin. Absolute contraindications include objective findings of renal disease, atherosclerosis, or other systemic diseases. Relative contraindications are mild or moderate problems with other organ systems.[10] The potential donor must be ABO compatible and have a negative preliminary serum crossmatch.

A thorough medical evaluation is done, including a history and physical examination and a battery of routine tests (see the box below). Depending on the donor candidate, additional tests may be done such as pulmonary function tests, cardiac stress tests, and renal tomography. Because of the potential risks associated with an arteriogram, the renal arteriogram is performed last, after all noninvasive tests have been completed and reviewed. The arteriogram is done to evaluate the anatomy of the urinary system and to rule out any unsuspected disease or anomalies.

A second but equally important phase of the evaluation is the psychologic assessment. It is imperative that the motivation of the donor is sincerely altruistic and that there are no known attempts of coercion, either emotional or monetary. Additionally, there is usually an evaluation of the candidate's emotional maturity and stability. Expectations of the transplant are addressed to determine whether they are realistic.

TESTS FOR LIVING DONOR EVALUATION

ABO typing
HLA typing
Mixed lymphocyte cultures
BUN, creatinine, electrolytes, serum glucose
Liver function tests
CBC, clotting studies
Hepatitis and HIV screen
24-hour urine collection for creatinine clearance
   and total protein
Urinalysis and urine cultures
ECG, chest x-ray examination
Renal ultrasound and renal arteriogram

Other discussions include a review of the transplant process, potential risks involved, and financial aspects related to donation. The cost of the evaluation, transplant nephrectomy hospitalization, and immediate medical follow-up are usually reimbursed by the recipient's insurance. However, lost income while hospitalized and through convalescence is not. Also, there may be additional expenses if child care arrangements are necessary. All of these hidden lifestyle expenses with which the donor might be confronted are discussed openly before donation to avoid undue financial hardships during the hospitalization and convalescent phases.

The living-unrelated donor. The controversy about living donors has been further complicated in the last few years with the use of unrelated donors. Improved graft survival rates with cyclosporine immunosuppression are reported even with poorly matched kidneys. Because the supply of donor kidneys still does not meet the demand, the emotionally related or genetically unrelated living donor has become a limited but potential source of kidneys available for transplantation.

The number of living-unrelated donors is small. At present there is no mechanism to track this donor population. Categories of donors on transplant registries are either living-related or cadaveric. Therefore, depending on the transplant center's practice, the living-unrelated donor transplants are reported in either category. Usually, the living-unrelated donors are spouses, in-laws, step-relations, or friends. With pretransfusions, some centers report 1-year graft survival rates of 80%, comparable to haploidentical living-related donor transplants.[60] The advantage over cadaveric transplants is decreased time waiting for a suitable donor organ.

Support continues to grow regarding the use of genetically unrelated donors. Spital and Spital[53] conducted a survey to determine attitudes about the living donation issue. The survey was nonrandomized, local to Rochester, New York, and consisted of 732 physicians and 470 adults who were not physicians. More than 90% of those surveyed would donate to a family member, 86% would donate to a spouse, and 60% to close friends. Furthermore, 75% noted that donation to strangers should be allowed. These findings were consistent with a randomized Gallup poll of 1022 adults in the United States that was conducted in conjunction with the nonrandomized Rochester survey.[53]

There is concern by some professionals that there is an increased potential for the selling of one's kidney with the living-unrelated donor. Therefore monetary coercion by either the potential donor or recipient must be ruled out. Although the buying and selling of organs is practiced in Eastern countries such as Turkey and India, it is presently illegal in the United States.[5] (See Chapter 1 for further discussion.)

The cadaveric donor. By far the largest potential donor pool for transplantation is from beating-heart cadaver donors. Approximately 80% of renal allografts are from such donors. In 1988, 7278 kidney transplants were performed with cadaver kidneys.[2]

Before a fatal incident that caused brain death, this donor was a healthy individual. In addition to the general criteria for organ donors, the kidney donor's age range is 3 months to 65 years. The potential donor's history must show no renal disease or chronic hypertension, urine output must be greater than 1 ml/kg/hr (adult) and the serum creatinine must be within normal limits or returning to normal.

• • •

Regardless of the type of donor, cadaveric, living-related, or genetically unrelated, a final white cell cross-match is done immediately before surgery to determine the presence of preformed cytotoxic antibodies in the recipient sera that would react against the donor's antigens and consequently the graft.

Transplant surgery

Living donor nephrectomy. The standard approach for the living donor nephrectomy is through the flank. An alternate method used by some surgeons is an intraperitoneal approach, but with the increased potential for complications and risks, this method is the exception.

After the patient is adequately anesthetized, the donor is placed in the lateral position with the left or right flank anterior. An incision is made along the twelfth rib. Some surgeons

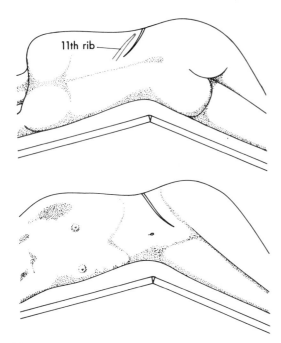

11th rib

Fig. 11-2 The donor nephrectomy incision. Anteriorly, the incision for the living donor nephrectomy is extended downward to permit extended exposure of the ureter. The twelfth rib may be resected, or the incision may be between the eleventh and twelfth ribs. (Redrawn from Lawson R (1983). Live-donor nephrectomy. In Glenn JF (ed). *Urologic surgery,* 3rd ed. Philadelphia: JB Lippincott Co.)

remove the twelfth rib for ease of access; others operate between the eleventh and twelfth ribs (Fig. 11-2). The kidney is thus exposed, with the vessels and ureter isolated.

Mannitol or other volume expanders are administered to facilitate adequate urine output. Care is taken to avoid unnecessary manipulation of the kidney and arterial vessels to prevent vascular spasm. Spasm can result in poor cooling, inadequate preservation, and ischemic damage to the kidney. Damage to vessels could result in thrombosis or stenosis of the affected vessel. After the nephrectomy the sole blood supply to the ureter arises from the renal artery. Damage to this vessel can cause necrosis of the distal ureter, urinary leakage, infection, and loss of the transplanted graft.[42]

Heparin, 2500 units, is administered via the renal vessels. Then, after adequate diuresis, the renal vessels are clamped. After the ureter, renal vein, and renal artery are dissected, the kidney is removed and perfused immediately with iced Euro-Collins solution. The purpose of the perfusion is to remove formed blood elements and decrease the core temperature of the graft. The kidney is then placed in a sterile container of solution and taken to the recipient's operating room for transplant.

After suturing the stumps of the donor's artery and vein the donor incision is closed. The patient recovers in the postanesthesia care unit and then returns to his or her room. The surgery does not usually require transfer of the patient to the intensive care unit postoperatively.

Nursing care of the donor involves usual postoperative management: prevention of infection, pain management, and aggressive pulmonary prophylaxis. Adequate hydration is essential, as is monitoring of renal function. Emotional support for this patient is imperative, because feelings of loss are not uncommon. Also, at this time, the focus tends to be redirected to the progress of the transplant recipient. To compound this further, the donor's convalescence is typically more stressful than the recipient's in that the recipient's surgery does not even involve incision into the peritoneum. Conversely, in the donor, major muscle groups have been incised and the thorax itself is involved. Recovery is therefore slower and much more painful. Fortunately, the pain experienced by most has been better controlled with the advent of *patient-controlled analgesia* (PCA) pumps and the use of epidural/intrathecal anesthesia in some recipients. For the donor, the hospital stay is generally 5 days with convalescence of up to 6 weeks.

Cadaveric donor kidney recovery. It is imperative that the cadaveric organ donor be managed to ensure adequate perfusion of the kidneys both before and during recovery of all the transplantable organs. Failure to provide oxygenation and hydration will result in serious damage to the kidneys with acute tubular necrosis (ATN) and delayed function or nonfunction after transplantation. Usually heparin

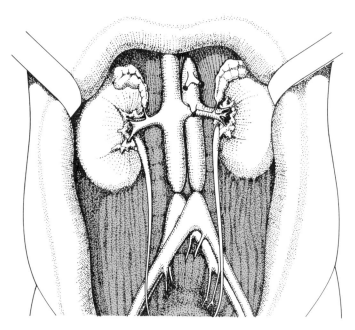

Fig. 11-3 Exposure of the structures removed in an en bloc cadaver renal recovery. (Redrawn from Whelchel JD (1987). Renal transplantation. In Grabar GB (ed). *Anesthesia for renal transplantation,* vol. 14. Norwell, Mass.: Cluwer Academic Publishers).

is administered to prevent clotting of the renal microvasculature. Diuretics may be administered to increase urine flow. In addition, phentolamine mesylate (Regitine) or phenoxybenzamine hydrochloride (Dibenzyline) is often administered to diminish renal vasospasm.

The most frequent method of renal graft recovery is the en bloc technique through a large abdominal incision (Fig. 11-3). This technique permits rapid removal of the organs, thereby reducing the possibility of warm ischemic damage with resultant irreversible anoxic damage, renal vascular spasm, and dissection injuries.[42] The aorta and vena cava are ligated at the level of the inferior mesenteric artery and cephalad to the renal vessels. The kidneys and ureters are dissected with the ureters ligated as close to the bladder as possible. Careful surgical technique is required to avoid excessive manipulation of the kidneys or damage to the vessels and ureters.[42] The dissected unit with portions of the

aorta and vena cava containing the renal vessels, kidneys, and ureters is then removed to a separate sterile table.

Preservation of the grafts begins immediately. The kidneys are flushed with a hyperosmolar, hyperkalemic, and hypothermic preservation solution (i.e., Euro-Collins or Viaspan) via an aortic cannula. Portions of the aorta and vena cava are then divided with each section containing the vessel attachments, corresponding kidneys, and ureters. Following the flush and dissection, the kidneys are preserved by one of two methods. The simplest and least expensive is the hypothermic method: The organs are aseptically packed in additional iced solution and packaged in sterile iced containers. In this hypothermic state, metabolism is slowed and ischemic damage is minimized. Kidneys have been stored for up to 48 hours using this technique. Ideally, however, to diminish the potential for ATN secondary to ischemia, many centers attempt to transplant kidneys within 24 hours of donor recovery. The second method of preservation involves pulsatile perfusion of a cooled solution via a pump through the renal vasculature. The solution consists of albumin and other nutrients. Not only is metabolism slowed with this method, but also nutrients and oxygen are delivered while metabolic wastes are removed. Kidneys are viable for over 60 hours in humans and 72 hours in animals using this method.[42]

Unlike other types of solid organ transplants, these longer preservation times for kidneys provide time for tissue typing. After typing, the kidney is matched to the thousands of potential recipients on the UNOS waiting list. The present UNOS policy for kidney allocation and distribution requires that any kidney that is either phenotypically identical or matches all six antigens must be offered to that matched recipient on the list.[62] If the distance between donor and potential recipient is great, the long preservation time permits transport of the graft to the receiving center. If there is no six antigen or phenotypically identical match nationally, the kidney is placed locally or regionally with the patient having the most accumulated points on the local listing.

Recipient surgery. With the hallmark transplant of 1954, the standard placement of the transplanted kidney has been extraperitoneal, in the right or left iliac fossa (Fig. 11-4). This position is advantageous in view of the close proximity to major vessels and the bladder. It also facilitates ease of assessment of the graft by

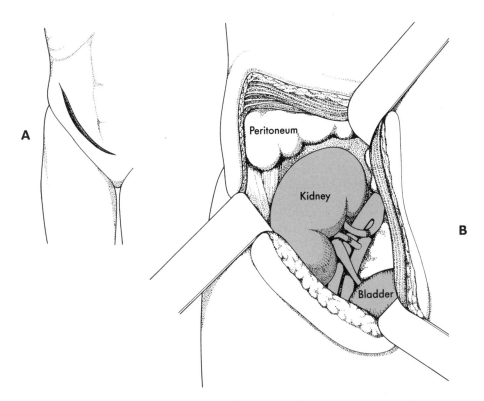

Fig. 11-4 Placement of the renal graft into iliac fossa. **A,** The incision is depicted for the right side of the abdomen, representing graft implantation in the right iliac fossa. **B,** The iliac vessels are exposed.

palpation, auscultation, and biopsy. Should removal or exploration of the graft be necessary, it is readily accessible.

The recipient's right iliac fossa is usually the site of choice, because exposure of the iliac vessels is generally easier. Although the left iliac space can be used, its use is avoided in patients over 40 years of age because of the increased potential for diverticulitis.[10] Differential diagnosis between graft tenderness resulting from acute rejection and tenderness of the underlying inflamed colon may be difficult to discern. When a patient has failed transplant grafts in both iliac spaces and the third transplant is performed, a transperitoneal approach facilitates more direct ease of access to undissected portions of the iliac vessels.[10] This intraperitoneal site is also used when transplanting kidneys into small children.

After the patient is anesthesized, either with general or regional anesthesia, an indwelling urinary catheter is inserted into the urinary bladder and irrigated with a sterile antibiotic solution. The abdomen and pubic area are then prepped and a curved incision is made in the right or left lower quadrant between the pubis and iliac crest.

The abdominal musculature and fascia are then divided. The intact peritoneum is freed from the retroperitoneal attachments and retracted medially.[10] The iliac vessels are exposed and the renal vein is sutured end-to-side to the external iliac vein. Typically the renal artery is anastomosed end-to-end to the internal iliac artery (Fig. 11-5). If the kidney is from a cadaver donor, the aortic cuff including the renal artery can be sutured end-to-side to the external iliac artery (Fig. 11-6). With a graft from a living donor, the hypogastric artery may be the vessel of choice for anastomosis.[37] This preference is

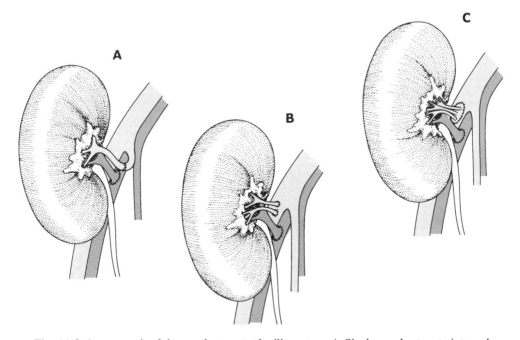

Fig. 11-5 Anastomosis of the renal artery to the iliac artery. **A,** Single renal artery to internal iliac artery and renal vein to external iliac vein. **B,** Multiple renal arteries to external iliac artery. **C,** Carrel patch containing multiple renal arteries to external iliac artery. (Redrawn from Whelchel JD (1987). Renal transplantation. In: Grabar GB [ed]. *Anesthesia for renal transplantation,* vol. 14. Norwell Mass.: Cluwer Academic Publishers.)

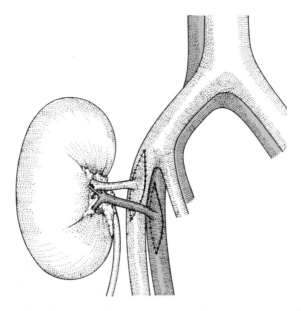

Fig. 11-6 Anastomosis of the cadaveric donor renal vessels to the recipient iliac vessels using carrel patches of donor aorta and vena cava. (Redrawn from Salvatierra O (1987). Renal transplantation. In Glenn JF (ed). *Urologic surgery,* 3rd ed. Philadelphia: JB Lippincott Co.)

because of ease of surgery and because this vessel is of similar size to the renal artery, thereby decreasing the incidence of stenosis. It has been reported, however, that in second transplants there is an increased incidence of sexual impotence in males when the contralateral hypogastric artery is used.[63]

During the surgery, care is taken to prevent kinking or angulation of the donor vessels, which could lead to compromise of renal blood flow. Revasculation of the kidney usually takes approximately 30 minutes. After the anastomosis is complete, the kidney usually "pinks up" rapidly. In a matter of minutes urine begins to trickle out of the ureter. Occasionally urine production may be delayed because of ATN, a condition usually associated with prolonged cold ischemia of the graft.

After vascularization is complete the surgeon begins the graft's ureteral anastomosis with one of three techniques. The most common is a ureteroneocystostomy (Fig. 11-7). An incision is

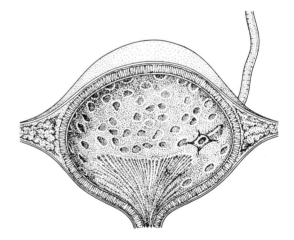

Fig. 11-7 Ureteroneocystostomy reconstruction of the urinary tract. The donor ureter is passed through a posterior bladder wall tunnel and anastomosed to the bladder mucosa. (Redrawn from Whelchel JD (1987). Renal transplantation. In Grabar GB (ed). *Anesthesia for renal transplantation,* vol. 14. Norwell, Mass.: Cluwer Academic Publishers.)

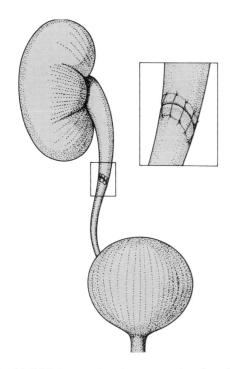

Fig. 11-8 Ureteroureterostomy reconstruction of the urinary tract. The proximal donor ureter is anastomosed directly to the recipient ureter.

made into the dome of the bladder. The ureter is then tunnelled through the posterior bladder wall, through the mucosal layer of the bladder, where it is then sutured end-to-side into the mucosal opening. The tunnel acts as a one-way valve preventing reflux of urine up the ureter with each bladder contraction. The potential for bacterial contamination of the kidney is therefore reduced.

Occasionally, when there have been multiple bladder surgeries or there are known bladder contaminants, a ureteroureterostomy is performed. In this procedure the transplanted ureter is attached to the ipsilateral native ureter[37] (Fig. 11-8). Recently anastomosis of the ureter directly to the dome of the bladder without a formal tunnel—the anterior ureterovesical anastomosis—has been shown to be an acceptable alternative.

Meticulous surgical technique is essential for this immunocompromised patient population. Patients usually receive preoperative immunosuppression therapy and may receive an additional infusion of corticosteroids during surgery. During the operative procedure it is critical that blood volumes remain expanded to facilitate rapid resumption of renal function after reperfusion. It is recommended that systolic blood pressures remain slightly elevated over preoperative levels unless contraindicated.[37]

Depending on the surgeon, a drain may or may not be placed near the kidney hilum. After closure, a light sterile pressure dressing is applied. Intraoperative mortality is low—reported to be less than 0.1% in most programs. Depending on the program's protocol, the recipient is then transferred directly to an intensive care unit or to the transplant floor for close monitoring.

Postoperative nursing care

The postoperative nursing care of the renal transplant recipient is essentially the same as the care prescribed for any patient who has undergone major surgery with general or spinal anesthesia. Care in the immediate postoperative period is predicated on the nurse's ability to assess, diagnose, and intervene promptly.

The renal transplant recipient has been suffering from renal failure, defined as "that stage of renal function in which the kidney is no longer able to maintain the integrity of the internal environment of the organism."[64] Thus systematic assessment of all body systems is paramount in the postoperative period. Because of the kidney's role in the normal maintenance of internal homeostasis, the following complications may be anticipated: (1) potential for fluid imbalance and (2) potential for electrolyte imbalance. Related to the surgical procedure, the following complications may be anticipated in the immediate postoperative period: (1) potential for vascular or urologic complications, such as hemorrhage or urologic leaks, respectively, (2) potential for pain, (3) potential for pulmonary compromise, and (4) potential for altered urinary and bowel elimination. In addition, immunosuppressive therapy predisposes the patient to the potential for infection. This is particularly evident in the critical care setting with use of invasive technology. Finally, but most formidably, the patient has the potential for rejection as a result of immunologic responses.

Each of these potential complications will be addressed with particular emphasis on assessment parameters and nursing interventions. Getting beyond these potential complications in the immediate postoperative period is only the beginning for the patient learning to live with a new kidney and incorporating it into his or her self-image. Knowledge deficit is a universally addressed nursing diagnosis for renal transplant recipients. Knowledge deficit related specifically to self-care activities such as home monitoring, administration of medications, and follow-up medical care is addressed. Assessment in this area actually begins in the pretransplant evaluation period and extends into the immediate postoperative period. One method of uniformly instructing recipients will be presented. General guidelines regarding follow-up will conclude this section.

Potential for fluid imbalance. The patient's fluid balance is determined by the level of renal function after transplantation. One of the following conditions may exist: (1) There may be immediate function characterized by the immediate formation of urine and massive diuresis; rapid restoration of function is also evidenced by declining BUN and serum creatinine levels. (2) The condition of ATN may exist, characterized by prolonged oliguria or even anuria for 5 to 60 days. As noted earlier, ATN may develop because of cold ischemia times greater than 24 hours. There is no treatment for ATN; only time may allow regeneration of tubular cells. To maintain homeostasis until recovery from ATN occurs, dialytic therapy may be temporarily reinstituted. The incidence of ATN occurs in less than 3% of patients undergoing living donor transplantation and in approximately 10% to 30% of patients after cadaveric renal transplantation.[42] (3) There may be no significant renal function, necessitating the patient's return to dialysis.

In each of these conditions, the patient's volume status must be carefully assessed. Common noninvasive assessment parameters include daily weights and strict intake and output records. Daily weights should be measured at the same time using the same scale. If the patient is undergoing peritoneal dialysis, he or she should be weighed during the drain cycle. If the patient gains more weight than preset parameters, the physician is notified. For the first 24 to 72 hours, the patient's urine output is drained via a closed urinary drainage system. The urine output is measured at frequent intervals for the first 24 hours. Some programs measure the urine output as often as every 30 minutes for the first 24 hours. If the urine output diminishes to less than prescribed parameters, the physician is notified. The most common cause of decreased urine output in the immediate postoperative period is occlusion of the urinary catheter secondary to clot retention. The nurse should have supplies readily available for aseptic irrigation of the urinary catheter. If irrigation attempts are unsuccessful, the urinary catheter should be replaced aseptically. Generally, the patient is replenished with intravenous (IV) fluids based on urine output. When urine volumes are extremely high, the IV fluids may be titrated to a prescribed central venous pressure (CVP), if a CVP line is placed.

Further volume assessment parameters include inspection of neck veins for distention, inspection of skin turgor and mucous membranes for dehydration, and inspection of extremities and the sacral area for edema. Auscultation of the chest is performed to determine the presence of any adventitious breath sounds such as crackles, indicating the presence of volume excess. Likewise, heart sounds are auscultated for the presence of an S3, indicative of intravascular excess.

Blood pressure and CVP readings, if a line is available, are correlated with clinical findings. The rate of IV fluids is generally titrated to replace urine output and maintain a CVP between 4 mm Hg and 12 mm Hg. For patients who have undergone spinal or epidural anesthesia, the CVP readings are leveled, calibrated, and measured with the head of the bed flat or at 30 degrees, respectively. Albumin may be ordered for a persistently low CVP. To ensure adequate perfusion of the newly grafted kidney, the systolic blood pressure should be maintained at greater than 110 mm Hg.

For the patient exhibiting signs of volume excess with decreasing urine output, IV diuretics such as furosemide may be used. If diuretics are unsuccessful, the rate of IV fluids is reduced to a "keep vein open" rate. If the infusion rate is not reduced promptly, the patient may develop respiratory difficulty associated with pulmonary edema, necessitating emergent dialysis. Emergent dialysis, particularly hemodialysis, is undesirable in the immediate postoperative period because of the potential for hemorrhage secondary to heparinization. The signs and symptoms of pulmonary edema include dyspnea, cough, tachypnea, crackles, and hypoxemia. Thus the nurse's role in volume status assessment is vital to maintaining adequate perfusion to the allograft as well as in preventing intravascular volume excess and pulmonary edema.

Potential for electrolyte imbalance. Like fluid balance, the patient's electrolyte balance is influenced by the level of renal function after transplantation. Because the kidney normally plays a role in the regulation of all electrolytes, there is the potential for numerous electrolyte disturbances. Commonly encountered are the electrolyte imbalances of potassium and glucose. Hyperglycemia caused by the effects of corticosteroids on glucose metabolism and the use of large volumes of dextrose-containing IV fluids intraoperatively may compound problems with fluid and electrolyte balance. Electrolyte imbalances in the renal transplant patient may be potentially life threatening and require the nurse to possess astute assessment skills for recognition of problems and to promptly administer appropriate interventions.

Imbalances of potassium may range from hyperkalemia (greater than 5.5 mEq/L) to hypokalemia (less than 3.5 mEq/L). In the setting of ATN, with the superimposition of acute rejection, hyperkalemia may present. Potassium accumulates as the renal tubules are temporarily damaged and are thereby unable to excrete excess potassium ions. Other contributory factors to hyperkalemia include excessive potassium administration and the use of stored blood for transfusion perioperatively and intra-

operatively. Also, there is increased cellular destruction with release of potassium ions secondary to the surgical procedure. Likewise, use of cyclosporine may exacerbate hyperkalemia. Metabolic disorders associated with acidosis and hyperglycemia may cause shifting of the ions, leading to hyperkalemia.

In contrast to hyperkalemia, hypokalemia may develop when potassium loss exceeds intake. This is particularly evident in the setting of massive diuresis in the early postoperative period. In addition, hypokalemia may be exacerbated by diuretic therapy. Abnormal gastrointestinal losses may also contribute to hypokalemia. It is important to correct hypokalemia promptly, because a persistently low potassium level may prolong a postoperative paralytic ileus should it occur. For patients receiving digitalis, the effects of digitalis are enhanced, increasing the potential for digitalis toxicity. In addition, cardiac dysrhythmias abound in the setting of hypokalemia.

The physical assessment findings in all electrolyte imbalances are fairly generalized, featuring abnormal neuromuscular function such as irritability, hyporeflexia and hyperreflexia, seizure activity, weakness, and cardiac dysrhythmias. A cephalocaudal physical assessment may elicit any of the following findings: (1) mental status assessment may elicit apathy and confusion, (2) cardiac assessment may demonstrate conduction abnormalities with a propensity for dysrhythmias, (3) gastrointestinal assessment may demonstrate problems with motility leading to cramping, diarrhea, or ileus, (4) genitourinary assessment may reveal polyuria or oliguria, and (5) neuromuscular assessment findings may range from irritability to flaccid paralysis and numbness of extremities.[65]

Nursing interventions center around prevention of hyperkalemia. Physical assessment and diagnostic monitoring with serum studies and electrocardiogram (ECG) monitoring are paramount. Laboratory values are monitored every 8 hours initially, or as needed for evaluation of therapy. Continuous ECG monitoring is recommended. The ECG changes are progressive in hyperkalemia. T waves appear tall and peaked. QRS complexes will then widen, associated with bradycardia and hypotension. Finally, the

P wave disappears, progressing to an idioventricular pattern to asystole and cardiac arrest.

There are two interventions that permanently correct hyperkalemia but require sufficient time to employ. These measures should be implemented when serum potassium is elevated but less than 6.5 mEq/L. Hemodialysis or peritoneal dialysis will permanently remove excess potassium. Also, sodium polystyrene sulfonate (Kayexalate) administered with sorbitol will reverse hyperkalemia by exchanging on a ratio of one-to-one sodium ions for potassium ions in the bowel cell wall. Sorbitol serves as an osmotic diarrheal agent that contributes to potassium loss via the bowel. Kayexalate with sorbitol may also be given as a retention enema for those patients who have not progressed to oral feedings. For maximal effects, the patient should retain the enema for at least 30 minutes. It is imperative that the patient expel all of the Kayexalate/sorbitol mixture to prevent obstruction and perforation of the bowel. A cleansing enema administered before and after the Kayexalate enema is employed to ensure complete expulsion.

An emergency situation develops when the serum potassium exceeds 6.5 mEq/L or when there are ECG changes indicative of severe hyperkalemia. Intravenous glucose, insulin, and bicarbonate may be employed emergently and temporarily to drive the potassium into the intracellular spaces. It is imperative to follow this measure with a permanent intervention such as Kayexalate/sorbitol administration or dialysis. Intravenous calcium chloride or calcium gluconate may be used to enhance cardiac contractility but are contraindicated in patients receiving digitalis. If hyperkalemia remains a problem for the patient, a reduced potassium diet is ordered. Evaluation of interventions for treating hyperkalemia is accomplished by monitoring the ECG and serum potassium levels.

In contrast to the hyperkalemic patient, the hypokalemic patient generally exhibits more symptomatology and clinical findings. Typically the patient complains of generalized muscular weakness and malaise. Lower extremity muscular cramps are characteristic of hypokalemia. In the immediate postoperative period, the patient may develop abdominal distention, nausea and vomiting, and decreased peristalsis exemplified by faint or absent bowel sounds.

The ECG changes, in general, demonstrate increased myocardial excitability or irritability. Dysrhythmias abound in hypokalemia, featuring premature atrial and ventricular beats, paroxysmal atrial tachycardia, atrioventricular blocks, and ventricular tachycardia. The increased irritability enhances the digitalis effect, predisposing the patient to digitalis toxicity. The ECG will demonstrate depression of the ST segment, a flattened or inverted T wave, or the presence of a U wave.

Interventions for treating and preventing hypokalemia include monitoring serum potassium levels, observing for potential ECG changes, and administering oral or parenteral potassium supplements as indicated. Measurement of intake and output can facilitate estimation of potassium lost via the gastrointestinal tract (in cases of gastric suction drainage, vomiting, or diarrhea). Potassium supplements should be diluted to facilitate absorption and to prevent gastrointestinal irritation. Intravenous potassium chloride supplements should always be slowly infused under continuous ECG monitoring.

Hyperglycemia is not uncommon in the immediate postoperative period. In patients with preexisting diabetes mellitus, hyperglycemia will be more difficult to control because of the effects of corticosteroids. ESRD secondary to diabetes mellitus is the third most common indication for renal transplantation and accounts for approximately 10% of the renal transplant patient population.[42] One active center reports the incidence as high as 30%. Another transplant center reports a 50% incidence.[66] Because of this incidence and the potential for steroid-induced hyperglycemia, it is important that the nurse monitor the blood glucose frequently and be familiar with the clinical signs of hyperglycemia.

In steroid-induced diabetes mellitus (SIDM), corticosteroid therapy aggravates a preexisting familial tendency for diabetes. Corticosteroid therapy leads to decreased utilization of insulin by the peripheral tissues; consequently excessive and prolonged hyperglycemia ensues, providing a sustained stimulus for insulin secretion.

The transplant recipient will become "insulin resistant" as persistent insulin secretion reduces the number of insulin receptor sites. A reduction in insulin production eventually occurs but will never completely cease. Consequently patients with SIDM are not prone to ketosis.[67] Also, because of the catabolic action of corticosteroids on amino acids, there is sustained negative nitrogen balance. Glycogenolysis occurs in the liver because the body cells lack adequate amounts of glucose for energy usage. The hyperglycemia, or insulin resistance, in patients with SIDM deprives cells of glucose, leading to glycogenolysis. Glycogenolysis perpetuates this by further elevating serum glucose levels.[68]

Studies have shown the incidence of SIDM to range from 5% to 46%.[69] This variation is thought to be related to the prevalence of risk factors in patients. Kahan et al[70] noted a 13% incidence of SIDM in 402 renal transplant patients. Seven percent of those developed SIDM during the first 2 months after transplantation. SIDM promptly disappears with the discontinuation of steroid therapy and, in some cases, when the dosage is reduced to maintenance levels. Unfortunately, in most cases, renal transplantation requires the use of corticosteroids throughout the life of the graft; thus the disappearance of SIDM is unlikely.

Assessment parameters for SIDM include the monitoring of serum glucose at intervals and correlation with clinical signs and symptoms of hyperglycemia. For nondiabetic pretransplant patients, the fingerstick method using a portable bedside monitor is performed before meals and at bedtime. Pretransplant diabetic patients are generally followed by an endocrinology team of specialists who control glucose with continuous IV insulin infusion. The method of insulin administration is changed from IV infusion to subcutaneous administration as the patient progresses to oral feedings. Serum glucose is then monitored before each meal and at bedtime.

The fasting serum glucose for patients with SIDM is moderately elevated, greater than 140 mg/dl. Random serum glucose levels are usually greater than 180 mg/dl. Typical signs and symptoms of hyperglycemia include polydipsia, polyuria, polyphagia, blurred vision, and lethargy. Polyuria caused by osmotic diuresis can contribute to dehydration, which can be deleterious to the newly grafted kidney. Volume assessment parameters such as inspection of skin turgor and mucous membranes, measurement of CVP, blood pressure, and urine output cannot be overemphasized in detecting signs of dehydration in the setting of hyperglycemia.

Insulin therapy is usually initiated when serum glucose levels are greater than 180 mg/dl for more than two weeks.[71] Short-acting regular insulin is used as the initial therapy. The patient's need for insulin will remain variable in the immediate postoperative period because of the daily tapering of steroid dosages. Therefore the nurse's assessment, monitoring of serum glucose levels, and evaluation of interventions must be ongoing.

Potential for complications related to the surgical procedure. When a patient undergoes renal transplant surgery, there is the potential for technical problems, such as vascular complications, urologic complications, and complications associated with the wound. Fortunately, vascular complications are uncommon. Occlusion of the renal artery or vein occurs in less than 1% of patients.[42] When it does occur, early surgical intervention may salvage the graft. The medical diagnosis is made with use of the radionuclide scan or arteriogram of the renal vessels demonstrating no perfusion to the graft. This situation necessitates prompt surgical exploration with transplant nephrectomy if the thrombosis cannot be corrected.

Vascular leaks may occur in the early postoperative period and are life threatening. Vascular leakage may be the result of problems at the site of anastomosis, complicated by delayed wound healing secondary to corticosteroid therapy. The nurse must be alert to physical assessment cues that might indicate postoperative bleeding. Emergency transplant nephrectomy may be required to save the patient's life in the event of hemorrhage. Rupture of the transplanted graft rarely occurs, but may occur as a result of swelling of the graft caused by acute rejection. Surgical removal of a ruptured graft is necessary in almost all cases.

The signs and symptoms of a vascular leak or

graft rupture are the same as those associated with postoperative hemorrhage: change in mental status, cool clammy skin, pallor, decreasing urine output, tachycardia, hypotension, abdominal swelling or tenderness, and bleeding along suture lines. The nurse recognizes these cues through periodic physical assessment or further assessment whenever the patient exhibits any of these signs and symptoms.

Urologic complications after renal transplantation may be serious and require prompt recognition and early intervention. There are several types of urologic complications.[42] First, ureteral obstruction caused by periureteral adhesions or improper placement of the ureter through the bladder tunnel may occur. Second, ureteral leakage secondary to ureteral necrosis may develop as a result of interruption of the blood supply to the ureter during implantation. Third, a vesical or ureteral fistula may form. Each of these conditions occurs as a result of poor tissue healing or poor vascularization. To medically diagnose a ureteral leak, a radionuclide renal scan, intravenous pyelogram study, or cystogram is performed that confirms the extravasation of urine.

To recognize the signs and symptoms of urologic complications such as obstruction or leaks, the nurse must periodically assess the urine output, the incisional suture line, and the patient's complaint of any new abdominal tenderness or swelling. In the event of obstruction or leak, the patient's urine output will decrease. There may be urine leakage into the wound or abdomen causing pain, or through the incision.

The patient undergoing renal transplant surgery may have wound complications. Development of a perinephric hematoma, urinoma, abscess, and/or lymphocele can be detrimental to the graft's function by creating external pressure on the kidney and/or on its ureter. Each of these conditions can become a medium for infection in view of the recipient's immunocompromised state.

Wound infections are classified as deep or superficial and occur in 1% to 2% of patients.[42] Deep wound infections usually require prompt surgical drainage. When the deep wound infection occurs in the presence of prolonged ATN or impaired renal function of unknown cause,

transplant nephrectomy is the treatment of choice.[42] Superficial wound infections occur in 1% of patients and cause little risk in terms of graft and patient survival.[42]

A medical diagnosis of a lymphocele, urinoma, hematoma, or abscess is made through ultrasonography. A lymphocele is a collection of lymphatic fluid in the perirenal space, causing compression or angulation of the ureter. It usually occurs 3 to 6 months after transplantation. The patient may develop an asymptomatic lymphocele or may have ill-defined abdominal discomfort or ipsilateral lower extremity edema. Mild to moderate impairment of renal function may develop, with increased BUN and serum creatinine levels. Surgical intervention is accomplished with internal drainage into the peritoneal cavity.

The nurse must be alert for signs of complications related to the wound. The wound is inspected for signs of infection and poor wound healing. The abdomen is inspected and palpated for swelling and tenderness. The extremities are inspected and palpated for the presence of edema, particularly ipsilateral edema.

The prevention of wound infections begins preoperatively with an antimicrobial shower, scrub, and shave of the patient. Perioperative prophylactic antibiotics are administered in many centers and, of course, strict asepsis is maintained during surgery. Postoperatively, aseptic technique is employed in caring for the incision. If a surgical drain has been left in place to facilitate drainage, aseptic technique is used when the drain is handled.

Potential for pain related to the surgical procedure. As with any patient who has undergone a major surgical procedure, the renal transplant patient will experience pain. Fortunately, the pain experienced by most has been better controlled with the advent of PCA pumps and the use of epidural/intrathecal anesthesia in some recipients. These patients may receive morphine sulfate (Duramorph) intrathecally, with its effect lasting for approximately 24 hours.

Regardless of the method of analgesia, the nurse is responsible for assessing the patient's level of pain, intervening when relief is needed, and evaluating the patient's response to pain management interventions. Both verbal and nonverbal cues indicative of pain are investigated. The nurse assesses all verbal complaints by ascertaining the exact location, nature, duration, and intensity of the pain and any aggravating and alleviating symptoms related to the pain. The nonverbal cues that are indicative of pain include restlessness, tachycardia, hypertension, splinting, and guarding of the incision with decreased respiratory efforts.

Depending on the type of analgesia prescribed, the nurse intervenes by administering analgesics and providing comfort measures. Pain management measures are evaluated by observing the patient's response. If the measures are successful, the patient's verbal and nonverbal cues will abate and the patient will obtain an acceptable level of pain relief.

Potential for pulmonary compromise. As the patient experiences postoperative pain, she or he develops the potential for pulmonary compromise. Pulmonary compromise may be related to splinting and guarding of the incision, thereby preventing the patient from coughing and taking deep breaths. The type of anesthesia the patient received and administration of analgesics may precipitate respiratory depression, which can also lead to pulmonary compromise.

To ensure adequate oxygenation to the tissues and to prevent pulmonary compromise, the nurse periodically assesses the patient's respiratory function by inspecting the patient's color for cyanosis, pallor, or ruddiness and chest movement for rate and depth of respirations. Immediate postoperative assessment is performed every 30 minutes for the initial 8 hours, then hourly for 24 hours, and then at 2-hour intervals. Breath sounds are auscultated every 4 hours for the presence of decreased breath sounds and adventitious sounds. Arterial blood gases are obtained as needed to assess oxygenation and ventilation. Chest x-ray films are ordered periodically to detect evidence of atelectasis and pulmonary infiltrates.

Numerous nursing interventions may be employed to prevent pulmonary compromise. Prevention of respiratory depression in the patient who has received epidural/intrathecal anesthesia may be prevented by titrating IV naloxone

according to protocol. Oxygen may be delivered via nasal cannula or face mask, depending on the patient's arterial oxygen level. The patient is encouraged to cough, turn, and take deep breaths at least every 2 hours. Analgesics are judiciously administered not only to control pain but also to enhance the patient's efforts in deep breathing and coughing. Splinting the incision with a pillow while the patient coughs alleviates some of the patient's discomfort, allowing for a more vigorous cough. The physician is notified for any change in the color or consistency of expectorated sputum. Usually, an incentive spirometry device is ordered to be used hourly while the patient is awake. In addition, early mobilization and ambulation on the first postoperative day greatly enhances respiratory efforts.

Potential for altered urinary and bowel elimination. The renal transplant surgical procedure may predispose the patient to the potential complications of altered urinary and bowel elimination. Depending on the type of ureteral anastomosis, an indwelling urinary catheter may be maintained for 1 to 5 days postoperatively. Because of the implantation of the ureter into the bladder, the patient may pass large blood clots that can cause catheter occlusion. If the urinary catheter occludes, the patient's bladder may become distended, causing pain and stress on the ureterocystostomy site. As the nurse assesses the urine output, she or he should readily diagnose this problem and intervene promptly by aseptic irrigation of the catheter. If this is unsuccessful, a new urinary catheter is aseptically inserted.

Additional problems the patient may experience postoperatively include spasms and frequency of urination when the catheter is removed. Bladder spasms may be alleviated with the use of agents such as B & O suppositories and oxybutynin chloride (Ditropan). Frequency of urination improves with time as the bladder accommodates larger volumes of urine.

The patient's gastrointestinal motility may be delayed because of the side effects of anesthesia. The patient may develop a paralytic ileus, necessitating nasogastric suction to relieve distention, and nausea and vomiting. The nurse performs an abdominal assessment every 8 hours, inspecting the abdomen for the presence of distention, auscultating for the presence or absence of bowel sounds, percussing for areas of tympany or hyperresonance, and palpating for areas of tenderness. Oral liquids are not instituted until the patient has normoactive bowel sounds and is passing flatus. Once the patient is tolerating liquids well, the diet is progressed.

All stools are tested for occult blood because of the potential side effect of gastrointestinal ulceration related to high-dose corticosteroid therapy and the stress of surgery. The physician is notified of the presence of occult blood in the stool so that appropriate actions may be taken. Generally the patient is started on antacids and/or an H_2 receptor antagonist such as ranitidine. If antacids are used, the nurse must be alert to the patient's predisposition to develop constipation and/or hypophosphatemia. In the presence of gastrointestinal bleeding, immediate endoscopy is indicated, because prompt surgical intervention may be necessary.[42]

Potential for infection. Manipulation of the immune system with antirejection medications exposes the patient to the potential for infection. Despite the dramatic decline in the incidence of fatal infections associated with the early years of transplantation, infections continue to be an important cause of morbidity and mortality in the renal transplant population.[72] Conflicting data have been presented comparing cyclosporine with azathioprine in regard to the incidence and severity of infectious complications. Two multicenter studies found no differences in the incidence and severity of infectious complications when comparing cyclosporine-treated patients to azathioprine-treated patients.[73,74] In contrast, several studies report a decrease in the incidence and severity of infectious complications associated with cyclosporine versus azathioprine.[75,76] This has been explained by the relationship of the incidence and severity of infections to treatment for rejection episodes.[76] Since azathioprine-treated patients experienced more episodes of rejection requiring treatment, they correspondingly experienced an increased incidence and severity of infections.

There appear to be two major factors that predispose the renal transplant patient to infection.[77] First, the preexisting condition of uremia, with its multiple effects, predisposes the patient to infection. Any underlying systemic illness, such as diabetes mellitus, lupus, or malnutrition, further compounds the effects of uremia. Second, in transplantation, the body's defenses are altered or bypassed. The patient's first line of defense, the skin, mucous membranes, and body secretions, may be bypassed with the use of invasive monitoring devices, endotracheal intubation, and urinary catheterization. This violation of the first line of defense, coupled with alteration of the second line of defense, the immune system, predisposes the patient to infection.

The immune system prevents infection by involving both cell-mediated (T lymphocytes) and humoral (B lymphocytes) immunity. To prevent posttransplant graft rejection, this immune response is altered pharmacologically by corticosteroids, azathioprine, and cyclosporine. The net effect of these drugs is to decrease the numbers of circulating T and B cells and impair or disrupt T and B cell function. Consequently, one can understand why the use of immunosuppressive agents has been termed a "double-edged sword" in which the benefit-to-risk ratio is precariously balanced. Throughout the years it has been recognized that the greater the amount and duration of immunosuppression, the greater the propensity for infection.[78] The current philosophy is to risk losing the kidney and return the patient to dialysis rather than continue massive immunosuppression, which may expose the patient to potentially life-threatening infections. The life of the patient is valued over the life of the graft. Only in renal transplantation is there an alternative modality such as dialysis on which to rely.

Conventional and opportunistic infections are seen postoperatively. Rubin et al[78] identified a timetable in which the various infections occur. In this timetable they have included bacterial, viral, fungal, and protozoal sources for infection in the renal transplant patient (Fig. 11-9). Knowledge of these various infections and their expected timetable of occurrence is a valuable guide for nurses. Physical assessment skills plus this knowledge will aid the nurse in

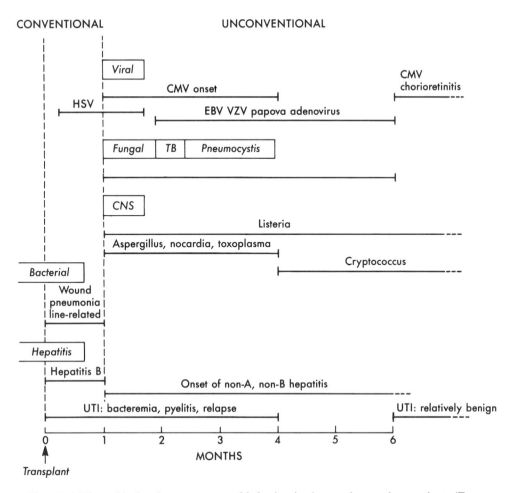

Fig. 11-9 Timetable for the occurrence of infection in the renal transplant patient. (From Rubin RH (1988). Infection in the renal and liver transplant patient. In Rubin RH and Young LS (eds). *Clinical approach to infection in the compromised host* (2nd ed, pp 557-621). New York: Plenum Medical Book Co.)

early recognition of infections and their prevention. (For a detailed account of the infections commonly seen in the posttransplant period, refer to Chapter 3.)

Assessment of the renal transplant patient for signs and symptoms of infection should be ongoing, systematic, and well documented.[77] The first step is evaluation of vital signs. Fever may or may not be present because of masking of the signs and symptoms of infection by corticosteroids. The nurse must be alerted to subtle changes in the patient's condition. Routine inspection of the skin and oropharynx is performed. Routine inspection of the mouth may demonstrate the vesicular lesions associated with herpes or the white, patchy, plaque-like lesions associated with candidosis. In that an organism may spread, causing infection throughout the gastrointestinal tract, any change in the patient's eating habits should be investigated. The patient should be routinely questioned about the presence of lesions in the mouth and on genitalia, dysphagia, anorexia, nausea, vomiting, abdominal cramps, diarrhea, melena, changes in stool, or rectal bleeding. If any of the symptoms are expressed, an infectious process in the gastrointestinal tract may be suspected.

In assessing the patient's respiratory function, the presence of pleuritic chest pain, cough, dyspnea, adventitious sounds such as rales, rhonchi, or wheezes, change in sputum characteristics, or fever requires further evaluation. A chest x-ray evaluation and arterial blood gas testing are done initially. Because of the numerous opportunistic organisms that can cause respiratory infection, careful investigation of the patient with any symptoms of respiratory embarrassment is paramount. Although the incidence of pneumonia has declined to less than 10% in many renal transplant centers, pulmonary infections remain a serious complication in the renal transplant population.[72]

When a central nervous system (CNS) infection is present, the changes may range from subtle to blatant. Any overt appearance of a neurologic sign or symptom requires immediate investigation. Symptoms that warrant evaluation include headache, personality changes, forgetfulness, irritability, agitation, disorientation, coarse tremors, nystagmus, motor impairment, focal changes, and obtundation.

General nursing interventions are guided by the knowledge of the patient's susceptibility to infection. The universal precaution of thoroughly washing hands before contact with a patient and in between patients cannot be overemphasized. The use of gloves for performing procedures or for the handling of body fluids decreases the risk of cross-contamination. Nurses with known infections should not care for immunocompromised patients, and visitors are carefully screened. As these measures are employed, their purposes should be explained to the patient.

Potential for rejection. Finally, but most formidably, the renal transplant patient may experience the potential complication of rejection. Despite histocompatibility testing, modulation of the immune system with pretransplant blood transfusions, and administration of cyclospor-

ine, most patients will experience at least one episode of rejection in the posttransplant period. Rejection is the body's normal response to foreign antigens on the allograft. Immunosuppressive agents are used in an attempt to keep these responses at bay, to prevent allograft rejection. The process of rejection is extremely complex and not fully understood. For a detailed explanation of the rejection process, see Chapter 3.

Renal transplant rejection is classified into four main clinical types defined by the length of time from transplant to the occurrence of rejection. The first type is hyperacute rejection, which occurs either immediately after restoration of blood supply or within 24 hours after transplantation. Hyperacute rejection results from preformed circulating cytotoxic antibodies and is unresponsive to treatment.[44] Irreversible rejection ensues, requiring transplant nephrectomy. This humoral immunologic mediated process causes immediate tissue destruction due to the antigen-antibody response and activation of the complement and coagulation cascade system. Thrombosis and necrosis of the kidney are the final results. Fortunately, current cross-matching techniques have prohibited this type of rejection from occurring with any frequency.[37]

A second type of rejection, accelerated rejection, may occur 2 to 5 days after transplantation between the immediate hyperacute rejection and the classic cell-mediated acute event. In accelerated rejection, biopsy may reveal both cellular and humoral components. The cellular infiltration may not be as intense as with pure cellular rejection, and vascular damage, often with necrotizing vasculitis, is seen. This type of rejection is extremely difficult to treat and may contribute to early graft loss.[79]

Acute rejection usually occurs 5 to 90 days after transplantation. This is the most common type of rejection and, fortunately, the most responsive to treatment. Immunologically, the process is primarily cellular, but humoral changes may be seen, or a combination of both.[42] Clinical findings may be subtle or blatant. The classic signs and symptoms are fever greater than 37.7° C, elevated BUN and serum creatinine levels, proteinuria, decreased urine output, weight gain, edema, hypertension, and a swollen, tender graft site.

The diagnosis of acute rejection is made more difficult when the patient is receiving cyclosporine. The nephrotoxic side effects of cyclosporine confuse the clinical picture. Reliance on trough cyclosporine blood levels is limited, because the patient may become toxic with levels considered to be in the subtherapeutic range. The diagnosis of cyclosporine nephrotoxicity is made by observing the trend in cyclosporine blood levels, serum creatinine levels, and the patient's clinical picture.

The renal transplant biopsy remains the hallmark in the diagnosis of acute rejection. Histologic findings indicative of a primary cellular response are heavy interstitial infiltrates of mononuclear cells and immunoblasts without a significant vascular endothelial lesion. Evidence of vascular inflammation with endothelial damage and minimal or no interstitial infiltration is characteristic of a primary humoral response. Fine-needle aspiration biopsy is being performed in many centers instead of core percutaneous biopsies. Attempts are being made to correlate fine-needle aspiration biopsy findings with core biopsy readings to ensure reliability. The core percutaneous renal transplant biopsy is not considered a benign procedure. The following complications may develop: microscopic and macroscopic hematuria, perirenal hematoma formation, clot retention, and hemorrhage. The complication of ATN after transplantation may further obscure the diagnosis of rejection. The renal transplant biopsy is employed to diagnose the superimposition of acute rejection on ATN.

Other diagnostic studies to confirm acute rejection include the radionuclide scan, which will demonstrate perfusion to the kidney and excretion into the bladder, and Doppler ultrasound of the renal blood vessels. Damping of the diastolic flow is indicative of rejection. Ultrasonography may also be employed to rule out obstruction from fluid collections that might be impinging on the graft or collecting system.

With the diagnosis of acute rejection confirmed, the patient may be treated with antirejection medications. Regimens most commonly used consist of either high-dose IV corticosteroid pulses or the monoclonal antibody OKT-3. Multicenter studies have documented a 75% reversal rate with high-dose steroids and a 94% reversal rate with OKT-3.[80]

The fourth type of renal transplant rejection is chronic rejection, developing insidiously over months to years after transplantation. Histologically there is chronic vascular inflammation with narrowing of the vessel lumen. The graft becomes deprived of blood supply, leading to replacement of the renal parenchyma with fibroblasts. This chronic process is unresponsive to any immunosuppressive treatment. The management of the patient with chronic rejection is primarily conservative, attempting to extend the life of the kidney while delaying the inevitable return to dialysis or retransplantation.

When the patient's renal function deteriorates to the point that dialysis is necessary, the patient's immunosuppressive therapy is discontinued. Cyclosporine and azathioprine may be abruptly discontinued, but the corticosteroids must be gradually tapered over time to prevent adrenal crisis. In emergent situations in which it is necessary to abruptly discontinue corticosteroids, a cortisol stimulation test may be performed to determine the level of functioning of the patient's adrenal gland.

Although a transplant nephrectomy may not be necessary for chronic rejection, it is frequently indicated for irreversible acute rejection. In these cases, as immunosuppressants are reduced, the patient may develop fever, acute pain, and inflammation of the graft, necessitating its surgical removal.

There are several nursing responsibilities to the renal transplant patient regarding the potential for rejection. First, the nurse should have the knowledge to assess for and recognize the signs and symptoms of rejection. The nurse should report any of the following findings to the physician: elevation of BUN and serum creatinine levels, proteinuria, new onset graft tenderness, temperature greater than 37.7° C, decreased urine output, edema, weight gain greater than 1 kg in a 24-hour period, and elevated diastolic blood pressure greater than

100 mm Hg. Other responsibilities include the administration of immunosuppressants to treat acute rejection episodes. Patient education about signs and symptoms of rejection and its prevention with maintenance immunosuppressants is an ongoing process initiated in the critical care unit and continued in the regular transplant nursing care unit. Emotional support for the patient and family needs particular emphasis when the patient is experiencing a rejection episode.

Potential for complications related to the administration of antirejection medications. When a patient is diagnosed with acute rejection, the nurse is responsible for implementing the treatment plan. The treatments for acute rejection require specialized nursing care for safe administration of pharmacologic agents. Each treatment is considered a "double-edged sword" capable not only of reversing the rejection, but also capable of eliciting toxic side effects and predisposing the patient to life-threatening infections. High dosages of IV corticosteroids, polyclonal antibodies, and monoclonal antibodies are the three methods of treating acute rejection. Each of these methods is described in detail in Chapter 4.

Knowledge deficit related to renal transplantation. Patient education is one of the most important aspects to include in the transplant patient's plan of care. Patient education is ongoing—initiated in the evaluation/pretransplant phase and continued throughout hospitalization and the outpatient follow-up phase. The success of the renal transplant is predicated on the ability of the patient to understand the medications, their purpose, proper administration, and side effects.

Most transplant centers employ a planned systematic educational program that teaches the patient and significant others self-care activities for posttransplant care. Careful attention must be paid to the renal transplant patient with specialized learning needs. Recipients who are blind, physically impaired, or unable to read or write need tailored educational programs. As the nurse implements the teaching plan, certain factors that may impede the patient's readiness to learn are considered. First, the mood swings, restlessness, insomnia, and possible personality changes associated with corticosteroids may limit the attention span and ability to concentrate. Second, dealing with the uncertainty of a successful renal transplant may hinder the patient's ability to concentrate. Third, the patient experiencing a prolonged uremic state, whether secondary to ATN or rejection, may have learning difficulties.

The process of teaching the renal transplant patient may be divided into three phases. The first phase comprises assessing the patient's learning needs and the mutual setting of short-term goals to achieve self-care. During this phase, the nurse assesses the patient's readiness to learn, observes for barriers to learning, and determines the best method of teaching the patient. Examples of short-term goals set during the first phase are noted in the box below.

The second phase is the active teaching phase, in which the above short-term goals are met and long-term goals are set. Most centers have developed a log in which the patient records daily vital signs, weight, and pertinent laboratory data. Digital blood pressure cuffs and digital thermometers are available for

---

SHORT-TERM TEACHING GOALS

The patient will:
1. Correctly identify the purpose, dosage, schedule, and side effects of each medication
2. Accurately record intake and output
3. Correctly measure and administer his or her own cyclosporine dosage
4. Record weight, temperature, blood pressure, and pertinent laboratory data (creatinine, BUN, WBC, potassium, and hematocrit values) in a daily log
5. Demonstrate the correct methods of taking his or her temperature and blood pressure
6. Identify which laboratory values should be monitored after transplant and describe the purpose of each
7. Be able to list the signs and symptoms of rejection
8. Be able to describe other signs and symptoms that warrant notifying the physician
9. Be able to identify work and activity restrictions

LONG-TERM TEACHING GOALS

The patient will:
1. Independently continue record-keeping at home and bring these records to follow-up appointments
2. Notify the physician of signs and symptoms of rejection while at home
3. Correctly taper the corticosteroid dose as directed
4. Independently administer his or her own medications

---

patients requiring them. One way to ensure continuity of teaching efforts is to provide the patient with a list of teaching goals and patient's accomplishments. The patient's progress can be followed daily by checking off the goals that have been met. This form can be posted at the bedside and serves as a ready reference for all nurses and other members of the transplant team caring for the patient. Examples of long-term goals that might be set during this phase are listed in the box above.

The third phase allows the patient to demonstrate understanding of various self-care activities. "Self-Administration of Medications" is a program used by several renal transplant programs, designed to validate the patient's understanding of medications before discharge. It is the joint responsibility of the nurse and the patient to determine when this program should be initiated. The pharmacy is notified to begin this program when a physician's order states "begin self-medication program." In one center, the patient is responsible for obtaining the medications from the pharmacy and returning the multidose vials when they are ready for refill. It is also the patient's responsibility to notify the nurse when it is time for the medications so the correct dosage and schedule can be validated. During this phase the patient is expected to independently record laboratory data, weight, and vital signs. This phase allows the patient to perform self-care activities in a controlled environment. The patient's confidence is boosted, diminishing some of the

insecurities associated with going home, where there is no constant vigilance.

During this phase the patient may attend a transplant support group that focuses on the "transition to home" with a multidisciplinary approach. A social worker, nutritionist, psychiatrist, transplant clinical nurse specialist, the patient, and any significant others may compose this group. One approach is for the group to begin as directed by patients' questions, then become more focused on specific, universally applicable topics. Topics covered may include medical follow-up, sexuality issues, life-style changes, dietary issues, reimbursement, and acquisition of medications. Information about activities and the risks of rejection and infection is reinforced. In addition, this is a time to explore the potential changes in role and family dynamics after renal transplantation.

Issues dealing with sexuality are discussed in the group setting. This may be a sensitive issue for many, but most patients benefit from the open, candid discussion. The patient's libido often returns after renal transplantation, as may fertility. Most men will be able to father children shortly after transplant. Women of childbearing age are encouraged to postpone pregnancy for at least 2 years after transplant to ensure stable renal function. The contraceptive methods of condoms, diaphragm, and foam are encouraged. Oral contraceptives and intrauterine devices are undesirable because of the risks of phlebitis and infection, respectively. The risk of sexually transmitted diseases is also openly discussed. Patients may engage in sexual intercourse at any point after transplant but need reassurance that the activity will not harm the kidney. Patients and their partners are encouraged to have a sense of humor as they reinitiate sexual intercourse trying to find comfortable positions.

Life-style changes in general are discussed in the group setting. Because of the initially high dosage of immunosuppressives, patients are encouraged to avoid large crowds in closed spaces for the first few weeks. They are instructed to avoid all persons with known infections, visiting construction sites, and tending to any fowl because of the risks of bacterial and fungal infections. Also, reinforcement regarding the typical posttransplant diet, with low sodium and low-concentrated sweets, is given at this time.

The social worker usually addresses questions about Medicare reimbursement policies and the acquisition of medications after hospitalization. Currently Medicare will pay for 80% of Medicare-approved charges for prednisone, azathioprine, and cyclosporine for 1 year after discharge following transplant. This benefit is subject to Medicare coinsurance and deductible provisions.

Issues of changes in role and family members' or the significant other's expectations are explored in the group setting. Changing from the "sick role" to the "well role" may cause a disturbance in family dynamics. Open communication between family members is encouraged. Having to adjust to the uncertainties of a successful transplant is addressed. "Don't be a slave to your kidney" is a permeating theme, encouraging the patient to enjoy each day with the new kidney without focusing on the uncertainties.

The patient's medical follow-up may either continue at the transplant institution or the patient may be referred back to her or his local physician. Regardless of the arrangements, the patient is seen quite frequently for the first 3 months after transplantation, when chances of rejection are greatest and when the immunosuppression dosage is the highest. During follow-up visits, the patient's laboratory data, vital signs, physical well-being, and compliance to and understanding of prescribed medications are assessed. It is important also during follow-up visits to emphasize health maintenance issues, such as dental and gynecologic health. Antibiotic prophylaxis for any dental procedure is ordered. Female patients are encouraged to have biannual pelvic examinations with a Pap smear. Patients experiencing visual acuity changes are encouraged to wait 6 months after transplant surgery to have lens prescriptions changed because of the effects of corticosteroids on the cornea. Patients are reminded also to wear sun block creams while exposed to the sun for extended periods to decrease the risk of skin cancer years after transplant. With the achievement of 3 months of an uncomplicated postoperative course with favorable renal function, the recipient reaches a milestone. Patients who have not experienced an episode of rejection can be expected to have a favorable prognosis. During the second 3 months, there still needs to be the constant vigilance for an episode of rejection, but a greater emphasis is then placed on the long-term consequences of immunosuppression. The potential hazards include infection, liver disease, malignancy (especially skin, cervical and lymphoid neoplasms), and steroid-induced complications.

THE FUTURE

The body of knowledge in the field of immunology and the HLA system has grown greatly in the last 10 years. This knowledge will be the basis of renal transplantation research into the next century. Questions yet to be answered include: What roles do the yet unidentified HLA loci play? Is HLA matching the answer to improved short- and long-term graft and patient survival in cadaveric transplantation? Will the primary match prove to be the HLA-B and -DR combination? What about the minor antibodies such as endothelial antibodies, idiotypic antibodies, minor HLA system antigens, and red cell antigens? One of the unanswered immunologic mysteries continues to be why in identical HLA transplants do 10% of the recipients reject the grafts within the first year? Answers to these questions are essential as we look to transplantation as a long-term management therapy and not merely a stop-gap between illness and death.

Over 14% of the persons on the UNOS waiting list are highly sensitized individuals.[82] What immune modification techniques will facilitate successful transplantation with this group of individuals? Will the imminent arrival of human recombinant erythropoietin (r-Hu EPO) for the treatment of anemia in ESRD aid this group of patients?[83] Will the successful treatment of anemia in ESRD with r-Hu EPO improve the quality of life of individuals to such a degree that transplantation will be a less appealing option to those who have a higher incidence of morbidity after transplant, such as sensitized patients or the older dialysis population?

What will the role of the living donor be in renal transplantation in the future? Trends indicate that the percentage of living donors is diminishing rather than increasing. What are the factors leading to this phenomenon? Can this trend be reversed? Should this trend be reversed?

Today more than 92% of the renal transplants are covered by Medicare.[6] As the federal government further regulates health care costs, what impact will this have on renal transplantation in the future? What proactive strategies will hospital administration, nursing, and transplant programs implement to ensure the viability of renal transplantation programs in such an environment?

As one looks to the next decade there are several unknowns. However, one need only review all the advances made over the last 50 years to see that "the now" and "the future" are indeed exciting times. The future is filled with questions, but those in the transplant field are open to the quest.

REFERENCES

1. The National Kidney Foundation, Inc. (1989). *The kidneys, kidney disease and related conditions.* (Campaign Series, Public Education Kit). New York: Author.
2. United Network of Organ Sharing (1989). *UNOS Update, 5*(5). Richmond, Va: Author.
3. Health Care Financing Administration (1986). *End-stage renal disease facility survey tables 1986.* Baltimore: Author.
4. Held PJ, Pauly MV and Diamond L (1987). Survival analysis of patients undergoing dialysis. *Journal of the American Medical Association, 257,* 645-650.
5. Task Force on Organ Transplantation (1985). *Report to the Secretary and Congress on immunosuppressive therapies.* Rockville, Md: Health Resources and Services Administration (NTIS N. HRP-0906975).
6. Eggers PW (1988). Effect of transplantation on the Medicare end-stage renal disease program. *New England Journal of Medicine, 318*(4), 223-229.
7. Murray J, Barnes BA and Atkinson JC (1971). Eighth report of the Human Kidney Transplant Registry. *Transplantation, 11,* 328-337.
8. Fox RC and Swazey JP (1974). *The courage to fail,* (2nd ed, rev). Chicago: The University of Chicago Press.
9. Ghose MK (1979). Histocompatibility. In Hekelman FP and Ostendarp CA (eds). *Nephrology nursing: perspectives of care* (pp 213-233). New York: McGraw-Hill Book Co.
10. Tilney NL and Kirkman RL (1986). Surgical aspects of kidney transplantation. In Garovoy MR and Guttmann RD (eds). *Renal transplantation* (pp 93-124). New York: Churchill Livingstone.
11. Sutherland DE, Fryd DS and So SKS (1985). The long-term effect of splenectomy versus no splenectomy on renal allograft survival: reanalysis of a randomized prospective study. *Transplantation Proceedings, 27,* 136-137.
12. Opelz G and Terasaki PI (1976). Prolongation effect of blood transfusions on kidney graft survival. *Transplantation, 22,* 380-383.
13. Rodey GE (1986). Blood transfusions and their influence on renal allograft survival. *Progress in Hematology, 14,* 99-121.
14. Solheim BG, Flatmark A, Halvorsen S, Jerwell J, Pape J and Thorsby E (1980). Effect of blood transfusions on renal transplantation. *Transplantation, 30,* 281-284.
15. Opelz G, Mickey MR and Terasaki PI (1981). Blood transfusions and kidney transplants: remaining controversies. *Transplantation Proceedings, 13,* 136-141.
16. Terasaki PI, Perdue S, Ayoub G, Iwaki Y, Park MS and Mickey MR (1982). Reduction of accelerated failures by transfusions. *Transplantation Proceedings, 14,* 251-259.
17. Opelz G, Grover B and Terasaki PI (1981). Induction of high kidney graft survival rate by multiple transfusions. *Lancet, 1,* 1223-1225.
18. Salvatierra O, Vincenti F, Amend W, Potter D, Iwaki Y, Opelz G, Terasaki P, Duca R, Cochrun K, Hones D, Stoney RJ and Feduska NJ (1980). Deliberate donor-specific transfusions prior to living related renal transplantation: a new approach. *Annals of Surgery, 192,* 543-552.
19. Whelchel JD, Shaw JF, Curtis JJ, Luke RG and Diethelm AG (1982). Effect of pretransplant stored donor-specific blood transfusions in early renal allograft survival in one-haplotype living related transplants. *Transplantation, 34*(6), 326-329.
20. Whelchel JD, Curtis JJ, Barger BO, Luke RG and Diethelm AG (1984). The effect of pre-transplant stored donor-specific blood transfusions on renal allograft survival in one-haplotype living-related transplant recipients. *Transplantation, 38*(6), 654-656.
21. Anderson CB, Sicard A and Ethredge EE (1982). Pretreatment of renal allograft recipients with azathiaprine and donor-specific blood products. *Surgery, 92,* 315-321.
22. Kahan BD, Van Buren CT, Flechner SM (1985). Clinical and experimental studies with cyclosporine in renal transplantation. *Surgery, 97,* 125-130.
23. Hardy MA, Chabot J and Tannenbaum G (1988). The biology of transfusion-induced immunosuppression: meeting highlights. *Literature Scan: Transplantation, 4*(1), 31-32.
24. Johnson JP, McCauley CR and Copley JB (1982). The quality of life of hemodialysis and transplant patients. *Kidney International, 22,* 286-291.
25. Flechner SM, Novick AC, Braun WE, Popowniak KL and Steinmuller D (1983). Functional capacity and

rehabilitation or recipients with a functioning renal allograft for ten years or more. *Transplantation, 35*(6), 572-576.

26. Evans RW, Manninen DL, Garrison LP, Hart LG, Blagg CR, Gutman RA, Hull AR and Lowrie EG (1985). The quality of life of patients with end-stage renal disease. *New England Journal of Medicine, 312*(9), 553-559.

27. Evans RW, Manninen DL, Maier A, Garrison LP and Hart LG (1985). The quality of life of kidney and heart transplant recipients. *Transplantation Proceedings, 17* (1), 1579-1582.

28. Simmons RG and Abress L (1988). Quality of life and rehabilitation differences among alternate end-stage renal disease therapies. *Transplantation Proceedings, 20*(1) (Suppl 1), 379-380.

29. Kjellstrand CM, Simmons RL, Buselmeier TJ and Najarian JS (1972). Kidney: Section I. Recipient selection, medical management, and dialysis. In Najarian JS and Simmons RL (eds). *Transplantation* (pp 3-25). Philadelphia: Lea & Febiger.

30. American Society of Transplant Physicians (1988). *Statement of criteria for selection of ESRD patients for renal transplantation*. Alexandria, Va: American Council on Transplantation.

31. United Network for Organ Sharing (1988). *UNOS policies*, 4.2. Screening potential transplant recipients for HIV antibody. Richmond, Va: Author.

32. Rubin RH (1988). Infection in the renal and liver transplant patient. In Rubin RH and Young LS (eds). *Clinical approach to infection in the compromised host* (2nd ed, pp 557-621). New York: Plenum Medical Book Co.

33. Helderman JH (1986). The role of cardiovascular disease in renal transplantation. In Garovoy MR and Guttmann RD (eds). *Renal transplantation* (pp 209-232). New York: Churchill Livingstone.

34. Najarian JS, Sutherland DER and Morrow CE (1983). Kidney transplants for high-risk patients. *Kidney International, 23*, S10.

35. Khauli RB, Novick AC and Braun WE (1983). Improved results of cadaver renal transplantation in the diabetic patient. *Journal of Urology, 130*, 867-870.

36. Delia JA, Weintach LA and Kaldany A (1981). Improving survival after renal transplantation for diabetic patients with severe coronary artery disease. *Diabetes Care, 4*, 380-384.

37. Whelchel JD (1987). Overview of renal transplantation. *Emory University Journal of Medicine, 1*(2), 89-105.

38. United Network for Organ Sharing (1988). *UNOS policies*, 3.4 ABO "O" kidneys into ABO "O" recipients. Richmond, Va: Author.

39. Hunsicker LG (1986). Histocompatibility testing. Part 2: Place of HLA matching in clinical renal transplantation. In Garovoy MR and Guttmann RD (eds). *Renal transplantation* (pp 28-48). New York: Churchill Livingstone.

40. Singal DP, Mickey MR and Terasaki PI (1969). Serotyping for homotransplantation. XXIII. Analysis of kidney transplants from parental versus sibling donors. *Transplantation, 7*, 246-250.

41. Opelz G, Mickey MR and Terasaki PI (1977). Calculation on long-term graft and patient survival in human kidney transplantation. *Transplantation Proceedings, 9*, 27-30.

42. Diethelm AG, Barger BO, Whelchel JD and Barber WH (1987). Organ transplantation. In Davis JH (ed). *Clinical surgery* (pp 3172-3209). St Louis: The CV Mosby Co.

43. Terasaki P, Mickey MR, Iwaki Y, Cicciarelli J, Cecka M, Cook D and Yuge J (1989). Long term survival of kidney grafts. *Transplantation Proceedings, 21*(1), 615-617.

44. Opelz G and Terasaki P (1977). Significance of mixed leukocyte culture testing in cadaver kidney transplantation. *Transplantation, 23*, 375-379.

45. Jensen EB and Lamm LO (1978). Renal transplantation and HLA-A, B matching: theoretical considerations concerning pool size. *Transplantation, 25*, 265-268.

46. United Network for Organ Sharing (1988). *UNOS Update, 4*(12). Richmond, Va: Author.

47. Task Force on Organ Transplantation (April 1986). *Organ transplantation: issues and recommendations: report of the Task Force on Organ Transplantation*. Rockville, Md: Health Resources and Services Administration (NTIS No. HRP-0906976).

48. Marchioro TL, Brittain RS, Hermann G, Holmes J, Waddell WR and Starzl TE (1964). Live donors in renal homotransplantation. *Archives of Surgery, 88*, 711-720.

49. Health Care Financing Administration (1988). The fifty largest kidney transplant programs for 1987; final official totals from the Health Care Financing Administration. *Nephrology News and Issues*, Clinical Bulletins, *9*, 37.

50. United Network for Organ Sharing (1988). *UNOS Annual Report 1987*. Richmond, Va: Author.

51. Spital A, Spital M and Spital R (1986). The living kidney donor: alive and well. *Archives of Internal Medicine, 146*, 1993-1996.

52. Keown RA and Stiller CR (1986). Kidney transplantation. *Surgical Clinics of North America, 66*(3), 517-539.

53. Spital A and Spital M (1988). Kidney donation: attitude findings. *Transplantation Proceedings, 20*(1) (Suppl 1), 383-384.

54. Velosa JA, Anderson VE and Torres PP (1985). Long-term renal status of kidney donors: calculated small risk of kidney donors. *Transplantation Proceedings, 17*, 100-103.

55. Hakim RM, Goldszer RC and Brenner BM (1984). Hypertension and proteinuria: long-term sequellae of uninephrectomy in humans. *Kidney International, 25*, 930-934.

56. Penn I, Halgrimson CG, Ogden D and Starzl TE (1970). Use of living donors in kidney transplantation in man. *Archives of Surgery, 101*, 226-231.

57. Dunn JF, Nylander WA, Richie RE, Johnson HK, MacDonnell RC and Sawyers JL (1986). Living related kidney donors. A 14-year experience. *Annals of Surgery, 203*, 637-643.

58. Bay WH and Herbert LA (1987). The living donor in kidney transplantation in man. *Annals of Internal Medicine, 106*, 719-727.

59. Brown CJ and Sussman M (1982). A transplant donor follow-up study. *Dialysis and Transplantation, 11*(10), 897-898.

60. Barry JM, Hefty T, Fisher SM and Norman DJ (1985). Donor specific blood transfusions and successful spousal kidney transplantation. *Journal of Urology, 133*, 1024-1025.

61. Ploeg RH, Goosens D, McAnulty JF, Southard JH and Belzer FO (1988). Successful 72-hour cold storage of dog kidneys with UW solution. *Transplantation, 46*, 191-196.

62. United Network for Organ Sharing (1988). *UNOS policies*, 3.3. Mandatory sharing for six antigen matched kidneys. Richmond, Va: Author.

63. Gittes RF and Waters WB (1979). Sexual impotence: the overlooked complication of a second renal transplant. *Journal of Urology, 83*, 240-245.

64. Lancaster LE (ed) (1984). *The patient with end stage renal disease* (2nd ed). New York: John Wiley & Sons.

65. Stark JL (1984). The renal system. In AACN: *Core Curriculum for Critical Care Nursing* (pp 347-450).

66. Conway PM and Davis CP (1987). The diabetic transplant patient: nursing considerations. *ANA Journal, 14*(6), 379-383, 410.

67. Otwell JA and Leidigh JC (1988). Teaching renal transplant patients with steroid-induced diabetes mellitus. *ANNA Journal, 15*(5), 295-300.

68. Guyton AC (1986). *Textbook of medical physiology*. Philadelphia: WB Saunders Co.

69. Gunnarsson R, Arner P, Lundgren G, Magnusson G, Ostman J and Groth CG (1979). Diabetes mellitus — A more-common-than-believed complication of renal transplantation. *Transplantation Proceedings, 11*, 1280-1281.

70. Kahan BD, Flechner SM, Lorber MI, Golden D, Conley S and Van Buren CT (1987). Complications of cyclosporine prednisone immunosuppression in 402 renal allograft recipients exclusively followed at a single center from one to five years. *Transplantation, 43*, 197-204.

71. Whitehouse FW (1986). Diabetes mellitus: current concepts of proper management. *Hospital Medicine, 22*, 231-251.

72. Peterson PK and Anderson RC (1906). Infection in renal transplant recipients: current approaches to diagnosis, therapy, and prevention. *American Journal of Medicine, 81*(1A), 2-10.

73. European Multicentre Trial Group (1980). Cyclosporin in cadaveric renal transplantation: one-year follow-up of a multicentre trial. *Lancet, 2*, 986-989.

74. Canadian Multicentre Transplant Study Group (1986). A randomized clinical trial of cyclosporin in cadaveric renal transplantation. *New England Journal of Medicine, 314*, 1219-1225.

75. Sutherland DER, Strand M, Fryd DA, Ferguson RM, Simmons RL, Ascher NL and Najarian JS (1984). Comparison of azathioprine anti-lymphocyte globulin versus cyclosporine in renal transplantation. *American Journal of Kidney Disease, 60*, 456-461.

76. Van Dorp WT, Koote AMM, Van Gernert GW, Van Es LA and Paul LC (1989). Infections in renal transplant patients treated with cyclosporine or azathioprine. *Scandinavian Journal of Infectious Diseases, 21*, 75-80.

77. Chmielwski C (1987). Early recognition of infection after renal transplantation. *ANNA Journal, 14*(6), 389-391.

78. Rubin RH, Wolfson JS, Cosimi AB and Tolkoff-Rubin NE (1981). Infection in the renal transplant recipient. *American Journal of Medicine, 70*, 405-411.

79. Tilney NL (1988). The early course of a patient with a kidney transplant. In Morris PJ (ed). *Kidney transplantation principles and practice* (pp 263-283). Philadelphia: WB Saunders Co.

80. Ortho Multicenter Transplant Study Group (1985). A randomized clinical trial of OKT3 monoclonal antibody for acute rejection of cadaveric renal transplants. *New England Journal of Medicine, 313*, 337-342.

81. Department of Health and Human Services/Health Care Financing Administration (1989). *Catastrophic protection and other new benefits: an unofficial notice to Medicare beneficiaries explaining benefits under the Medicare Catastrophic Act of 1988*, pp 7-8. Washington, DC: Author.

82. US Department of Health and Human Services (1988). *Report of the scientific and clinical status of organ transplantation*. Rockville, Md: Division of Organ Transplantation.

83. Paganini E (1988). The treatment of anemias in dialysis patients: present and future potentials of erythropoietin therapy, *Nephrology News and Issues, 10*, 36-39.

12

Heart Transplantation

Part I *Suzanne Nicholson Macdonald*
Part II *Nancy Allen Naucke*

Part I

Heart transplantation has advanced dramatically in the past two decades. It has evolved from an experimental therapy to a successful treatment modality, offering survival and enhanced quality of life to patients with end-stage heart disease.

HISTORICAL PERSPECTIVE

Heart transplantation began with experimental work by Carrel and Guthrie, who performed canine cervical heart transplantation in 1905.[1,2] Continuing laboratory efforts were enhanced by the advent of cardiopulmonary bypass in the 1950s. In 1960 a series of experiments was performed by Lower and Shumway using orthotopic canine transplants. These operative procedures provided the foundation for the clinical application of human heart transplantation.[3,4]

The first human heart transplant was performed by Dr. Christiaan Barnard in South Africa in 1967.[5,6] Early enthusiasm for the procedure, in many centers worldwide, decreased abruptly as a result of poor survival rates. Only a few centers continued research and clinical efforts, most notably Stanford University, in addition to University of Capetown, South Africa, the Medical College of Virginia, and Hôpital de la Pitie, Paris.[7] The pioneering efforts of these centers resulted in a renewal of activity and interest in heart transplantation by the late 1970s. Patient survival has been enhanced by improved diagnosis and treatment of rejection and infection, immunosuppressive therapy and improved donor and recipient selection criteria.[8,9]

As of March 1989, 9139 orthotopic heart transplants had been performed worldwide, with the majority of transplant activity since 1984 (Fig. 12-1). Heart transplants are being performed in 204 centers worldwide and in 118 centers in the United States alone.[10] The cost of a cardiac transplant ranges between $50,000 and $150,000 in the first year (including hospitalization and outpatient costs) and varies between institutions.[11] The cost of transplantation at the time of transplant, including hospital charges, organ acquisition charges, and transplant team charges, averaged $115,000 in 1987.[12]

Since cardiac transplantation is no longer considered experimental, the majority of third-party insurance companies, Medicare, and some state Medicaid programs cover the cost of transplantation.

INDICATIONS FOR CARDIAC TRANSPLANTATION

The primary indications for transplant candidates are cardiomyopathy and coronary artery disease, according to the Registry of the International Society for Heart Transplantation (ISHT). Less common indications include valvular heart disease, congenital heart disease, myocarditis, and graft rejection (Fig. 12-2). Specific etiologic groups may vary between institutions. The average age of heart transplant

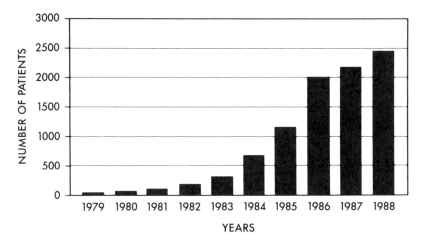

Fig. 12-1 Number of heart transplants performed by year. (From The Registry of the International Society for Heart Transplantation: Sixth Official Report – 1989 by Heck CF, Shumway SJ and Kay MP [1989]. *Journal of Heart Transplantation, 8*[4], 271. Copyright 1989 by the International Society for Heart Transplantation. Reprinted by permission.)

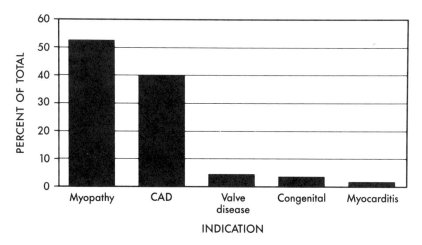

Fig. 12-2 Indications for orthotopic heart transplantation. (From The Registry of the International Society for Heart Transplantation: Sixth Official Report – 1989 by Heck CF, Shumway SJ and Kaye MP [1989]. *Journal of Heart Transplantation, 8*[4], 272. Copyright 1989 by the International Society for Heart Transplantation. Reprinted by permission.)

SELECTION CRITERIA

End-stage heart disease — prognosis of less than 6
  to 12 months
New York Heart Association class III or IV
Unable to be treated by conventional medical or
  surgical therapy
Age criteria flexible — based on "physiologic age"
  rather than absolute chronologic age
Psychosocial stability

recipients is 43.8 years, with a range from newborn to 70 years.[10] In addition, the majority of patients undergoing heart transplant are men.

Since the introduction of triple-drug therapy in 1985 at the University of Arizona, actuarial survival rates at 1 and 2 years are 93% and at 3 years 91%.[13]

SELECTION CRITERIA

Careful selection of transplant recipients has been a major factor in the current success of heart transplantation. Conservative selection criteria have resulted in increased long-term postoperative survival. In experienced transplant programs with established long-term success, selection criteria are being expanded (see the box at left). Most transplant candidates have end-stage heart disease, with a limited prognosis of less than 6 to 12 months' survival. Transplant candidates meet New York Heart Association class III or IV criteria (see the box below) and are unable to be successfully treated by other forms of conventional surgical or medical therapy. Patients undergoing transplant evaluation generally have one or more of the following: decreased functional ability, severe left ventricular dysfunction associated with a left ventricular ejection fraction of less than 20%, and life-threatening dysrhythmias.[8,11]

There are no absolute age limitations for heart transplant. Careful selection of patients over 50 years of age has resulted in increased success in this age group. There appear to be no significant differences in short- and long-term survival between patients over 50 when compared with patients under 50.[14,15] The impressive survival rates found in the older age-group are influenced by the use of strict selection criteria in this patient population. Selection is often based on the "physiologic age" of the patient instead of the absolute chronologic age.[9]

NEW YORK HEART ASSOCIATION CLASSIFICATION

Class	Functional Classification
I	Patients with cardiac disease but without resulting limitations of physical activity. Ordinary physical activity does not cause undue fatigue, palpitation, dyspnea, or anginal pain.
II	Patients with cardiac disease resulting in slight limitation of physical activity. They are comfortable at rest. Ordinary physical activity results in fatigue, palpitation, dyspnea, or anginal pain.
III	Patients with cardiac disease resulting in marked limitation of physical activity. They are comfortable at rest. Less than ordinary physical activity causes fatigue, palpitation, dyspnea, or anginal pain.
IV	Patient with cardiac disease resulting in inability to carry on any physical activity without discomfort. Symptoms of cardiac insufficiency or of the anginal syndrome may be present even at rest. If any physical activity is undertaken, discomfort is increased.

From Underhill SL (1982). *Cardiac nursing* (p 152). Philadelphia, Pennsylvania: JB Lippincott Co; by permission of the American Heart Association, Inc.

With the current imbalance in the potential recipient–donor ratio, however, there is ethical debate about the use of scarce donor hearts for older patients whose natural life span is nearing completion. The extended long-term survival (greater than 5 years) is not well established for older patients. Since non-transplant-related medical complications increase with age and the normal life span is approximately 75 years,[16] these issues affect this potential recipient population and require careful consideration.

Cardiac transplants are also performed with success in children. However, experience with neonates and with children less than 2 years of age is limited. This age-group represents a challenging new area of growth in transplantation.

A successful heart transplant requires psychologic stability and a supportive social environment for the recipient.[17,18] The posttransplant period is marked by physical and psychologic stresses unique to the recipient and family. Problems may include the ongoing threat of medical complications (e.g., rejection or infection), medication side effects, financial difficulties (e.g., cost of medication, health care follow-up), loss of insurance coverage, problems returning to work, and uncertainty about long-term survival.

CONTRAINDICATIONS TO CARDIAC TRANSPLANTATION

There are several contraindications to cardiac transplant (see the box at top, right). These include pulmonary hypertension, irreversible organ dysfunction, active infection or unresolved pulmonary infarctions, active peptic ulcer disease, severe vascular disease, insulin-dependent diabetes with secondary complications, systemic disease or malignancy, and psychosocial problems.

Fixed pulmonary vascular resistance (PVR) greater than 6 to 8 Wood units (480 to 640 dynes/sec/cm^{-5}) remains an absolute contraindication for orthotopic heart transplant.[1,6,7] Pulmonary hypertension places too great a burden on the donor heart's normal right ventricle, resulting in right-sided heart failure. Vasodilator agents (nitroprusside, nitroglycerin, or prostacyclin) or oxygen may be admin-

---

CONTRAINDICATIONS TO CARDIAC TRANSPLANTATION

Pulmonary hypertension (fixed pulmonary vascular resistance $\geq$ 6-8 Wood units (480-640 dynes/sec/cm^{-5})
Irreversible organ dysfunction
Active infection
Unresolved pulmonary infarction
Active peptic ulcer disease
Insulin dependent diabetes with secondary complications
Systemic disease or malignancy
Psychosocial contraindications

---

istered in an attempt to reduce the PVR in patients with less severe pulmonary hypertension (4 to 6 Wood units). In addition, an oversized donor heart may be used to enhance the work capacity of the donor right ventricle.[7,9,15] In patients with a PVR greater than 8 Wood units, heterotopic transplantation may be considered.

Irreversible organ dysfunction, such as renal or hepatic failure, is a contraindication to cardiac transplantation.[11,18] Organ dysfunction would be worsened by the nephrotoxic and hepatotoxic effects of cyclosporine and azathioprine. Patients with reversible renal or liver dysfunction secondary to decreased cardiac output, however, may be considered for transplant.

Active infection or unresolved pulmonary infarctions are absolute contraindications to transplant. Active infection is a contraindication because of the threat of exacerbation of the infection or sepsis with immunosuppressive therapy. Recent and unresolved pulmonary infarctions predispose the patient to pulmonary abscesses.[1,15,19] Pulmonary infarctions should be healed and other unclear pulmonary x-ray findings identified and resolved before transplant.[20]

Active peptic ulcer disease (PUD) predisposes the patient to bleeding, perforation, and sepsis. Gastric or duodenal ulcers are exacerbated by steroid and aspirin therapy used postoperatively.[6] Ulcers should be healed before transplant. Transplant recipients with a history of PUD should be treated routinely with antacids and H_2 inhibitors in addition to aggressive endoscopic follow-up if indicated.[9]

Severe cerebrovascular or peripheral vascular disease is an absolute contraindication to transplant. If surgical correction is feasible, patients may be considered for transplant.[1,11]

Insulin-dependent diabetic patients are felt to be acceptable transplant candidates by many centers, except in the presence of secondary complications, such as diabetic retinopathy, nephropathy, and vascular disease.[2,7-9,15,20] In the past, with the use of high-dose steroid therapy, the patient with insulin-dependent diabetes was at high risk for the development of secondary diabetic complications, including infection. Immunosuppression with cyclosporine and azathioprine, however, allows the reduction or elimination of prednisone, enabling selective transplantation in this population.

Serious diseases that would limit survival after transplant are considered contraindications to transplant. This is a broad category that includes illnesses such as severe systemic lupus erythematosis, cystic fibrosis, amyloidosis, and malignancy. Transplants have been performed in patients with malignancies considered "cured" or in mild systemic diseases; however, experience is limited and transplants under such circumstances should be considered experimental at this time.

Active alcohol or drug abuse is likely to seriously jeopardize the recipient's health and survival. Severe psychiatric disorders or mental deficiencies that would limit the ability of the recipient to comply with the medical regimen are also contraindications to transplant.

THE OPERATIVE PROCEDURE

Orthotopic transplantation, originally described by Lower and Shumway in 1960, is the favored and most frequently used surgical technique for heart transplantation.[21-23] Orthotopic transplantation involves excision of the recipient's heart and replacement with the donor heart in a relatively normal anatomic position. Heterotopic (piggyback) transplantation, less commonly used, is reserved for cases of elevated PVR or when the donor's heart size is significantly smaller than the recipient's.

In heterotopic transplantation, the donor heart is placed in the right side of the chest, parallel to the native heart. The donor heart acts as an auxiliary pump to the native heart, with

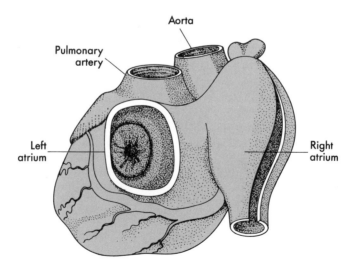

Fig. 12-3 Completed atriotomies of donor heart. (From Copeland JG [1984]. *Modern technics in surgery—cardiac thoracic surgery* [p 66-6]. New York: Futura Publishing Company, Inc. Copyright 1984 by Futura Publishing Company, Inc. Reprinted by permission.)

blood flow through both hearts or either heart.[1,4] Limitations of heterotopic transplantation include thromboembolism from the native heart and subsequent need for anticoagulation; space limitation; mechanical difficulty performing cardiac procedures, such as cardiac catheterization or biopsy; ongoing postoperative angina in ischemic heart disease patients; and the use of prosthetic graft material for the pulmonary artery anastomosis.[21,23]

The donor cardiectomy is performed through a median sternotomy. The heart is removed by transection of the superior and inferior vena cavae, pulmonary veins and artery, and aorta (Fig. 12-3). The sinus node is preserved by careful suture ligation and division of the superior vena cava cephalad to the superior vena caval right atrial junction.[20] Crystalloid cardioplegia solution and topical cooling with

cold saline at 4° C is used for cardiac preservation.[8]

Because orthotopic transplantation is the most widely used technique, this surgical procedure will be described.[1,6,21,23] The chest is opened through a median sternotomy. Cannulation of the aorta and both vena cavae is performed, and cardiopulmonary bypass is initiated (Fig. 12-4). Excision of the native heart is begun with an incision made along the atrioventricular groove. Transection of the great vessels is made at the valvular level, preserving as much usable aorta and main pulmonary artery as possible. The recipient's heart is excised at the mid-atrial level, leaving the atrial cuffs intact above the atrioventricular groove (Fig. 12-5).

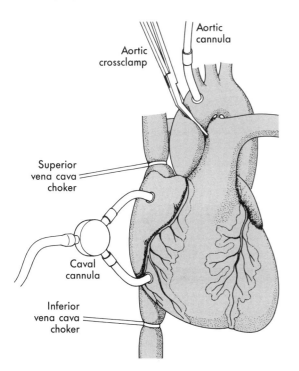

Fig. 12-4 Recipient heart at start of cardiopulmonary bypass. (From Copeland JG [1984]. *Modern technics in surgery—cardiac thoracic surgery* [p 66-7]. New York: Futura Publishing Company, Inc. Copyright 1984 by Futura Publishing Company, Inc. Reprinted by permission.)

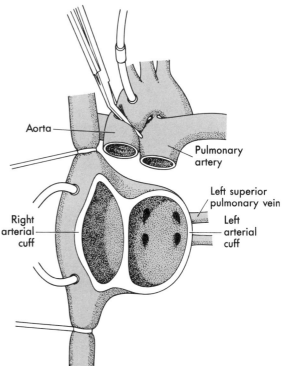

Fig. 12-5 Recipient atrial cuffs and great vessels after cardiectomy. (From Copeland JG [1984]. *Modern technics in surgery—cardiac thoracic surgery* [p 66-10]. New York: Futura Publishing Company, Inc. Copyright 1984 by Futura Publishing Company, Inc. Reprinted by permission.)

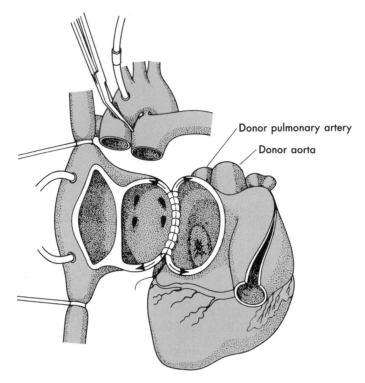

Donor pulmonary artery

Donor aorta

Fig. 12-6 Beginning of left atrial suture line. Arrows indicate direction of suture line. (From Copeland JG [1984]. *Modern technics in surgery — cardiac thoracic surgery* [p 66-11]. New York: Futura Publishing Company, Inc. Copyright 1984 by Futura Publishing Company, Inc. Reprinted by permission.)

The donor heart's anastomotic sites are trimmed to approximate the recipient's atrial cuffs. Anastomoses are then made between the donor atria and the recipient atrial cuffs, respectively, in addition to the interatrial septum (Fig. 12-6). As the atrial anastomoses are completed, the atria are filled with saline to minimize air collection and to cool the heart. Topical cooling is performed with saline (4° C) flushed into the pericardial wall. After completion of the left atrial suture line, saline is also flushed continuously through a left atrial line to provide further cooling, until completion of the aortic anastomosis.[9] The aortic and pulmonary anastomoses are then performed.

The caval (umbilical choker) tapes are removed and the cardiac chambers are filled, removing air from the heart. Remaining air is carefully evacuated by aortic venting, gentle agitation, and aspiration from the cardiac chambers. Cardiac circulation is restored by releasing the aortic cross-clamp, and the patient is slowly weaned from cardiopulmonary bypass.

Spontaneous defibrillation of the heart may occur; however, electrical defibrillation may be necessary. A resuscitation period of between 30 and 60 minutes is generally required to establish optimal cardiac function.[21] During this period cardiopulmonary bypass is discontinued if (1) a sinus rhythm is established and maintained, (2) remaining air is removed, (3) the heart exhibits normal contractility, (4) and hemostasis is ensured (Fig. 12-7). Inotropic agents are often necessary during the immediate postoperative period. A pulmonary artery catheter may be placed for postoperative cardiac output moni-

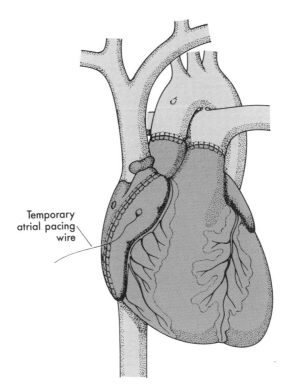

Temporary
atrial pacing
wire

Fig. 12-7 Completed cardiac transplant. (From Copeland JG [1984]. *Modern technics in surgery—cardiac thoracic surgery* [66-15]. New York: Futura Publishing Company, Inc. Copyright 1984 by Futura Publishing Company, Inc. Reprinted by permission.)

toring. In addition, epicardial pacing wires and anterior mediastinal chest tubes are placed before the patient leaves the operating room.

POSTOPERATIVE NURSING CARE

A cardiac transplant recipient, having received a new heart, generally recovers more rapidly than does a patient who has undergone conventional open heart surgery. The immediate postoperative care of the transplant recipient is similar to the open heart surgery patient, with the additional concerns of rejection and increased susceptibility to infection.

Rejection

Optimal care of the cardiac transplant recipient involves a collaborative approach between nurse and physician colleagues. The major problems encountered after cardiac transplant are discussed in terms of causes, assessment, and interventions. Although the etiologic factors are fairly straightforward, the assessments are often complex, and the interventions are frequently interdependent in nature.

Cardiac rejection, an immunologic response directed against the donor heart, remains a major cause of transplant mortality. There are three types of cardiac rejection: hyperacute, acute, and chronic. Hyperacute and chronic rejection will be briefly described; acute rejection, because of its occurrence in the early postoperative period and nursing care considerations, will be the focus of this section.

Hyperacute rejection. Hyperacute rejection occurs immediately after transplant, generally in the operating room. Although hyperacute rejection is rare, it is life threatening. Prompt retransplantation must be performed; however, mechanical assist device support (usually replacement with an artificial heart) may be used until a suitable donor is found. Hyperacute rejection is a humoral response, mediated by B lymphocytes. It is caused by an ABO blood group incompatibility or reactive lymphocyte cross-match between recipient and donor.[20,24]

This type of rejection may be prevented by ensuring ABO blood group compatibility and establishing a negative lymphocyte cytotoxic antibody screen against a panel of donor antigens before the transplant procedure. If the transplant candidate has a positive cytotoxic antibody screen, indicating the presence of preformed antibodies, a negative lymphocyte cross-match must be established with the donor before transplant.

Pathologic manifestation of hyperacute rejection includes deposition of platelet thrombi throughout the coronary vessels, endothelial damage, and interstitial hemorrhage. This results in generalized myocardial ischemia and cardiac collapse.[25,26]

Chronic rejection. Chronic rejection, or graft atherosclerosis, refers to the insidious process of accelerated graft atherosclerosis in the transplanted heart. Chronic rejection generally occurs after the first 3 months. Accelerated graft atherosclerosis involves diffuse disease marked by concentric narrowing throughout the coronary arteries.[20] The diffuse nature of the disease usually makes treatment alternatives such as percutaneous transluminal angioplasty or coronary artery bypass grafting useless. The cause of chronic rejection is unknown, but it is felt to be an ongoing, low-grade, immunologically mediated injury that damages the coronary intima.[8,23,27] Chronic rejection may cause myocardial infarction or death or may necessitate retransplant.[20] An incidence of graft atherosclerosis of between 40% and 50% at 5 years has been reported in some transplant centers.[23] Accelerated graft atherosclerosis presents a major problem with an impact on long-term survival for this population.

The transplant recipient does not have chest pain or pressure related to myocardial ischemia because the donor heart is denervated. Because of this "silent ischemia," the transplant recipient and health care providers must monitor for signs of cardiac failure that may be associated with myocardial ischemia. As part of routine posttransplant follow-up, yearly cardiac catheterization with coronary arteriography is performed to monitor for graft atherosclerosis.

Acute rejection. Acute rejection occurs most frequently in the first 3 months after transplant, lessening in severity and incidence thereafter.[28]

Cause. Acute rejection is a cell-mediated response activated by T lymphocytes.[24,25] Acute rejection is histologically characterized by cardiac interstitial and perivascular mononuclear cell infiltration that can progress to cellular necrosis if untreated.[1,11,24,29]

Assessment. Endomyocardial biopsy remains the gold standard for medical detection and definitive diagnosis of cardiac rejection.[11,20] Interpretation of cardiac biopsies is often based on a classification system developed by Billingham.[29] Using this system, the degree of cardiac rejection can be separated into four major categories: mild, moderate, severe, and resolving or resolved. Mild rejection is characterized by early perivascular and endocardial infiltrates. In moderate rejection there are increased interstitial, perivascular, and endocardial infiltrates. Focal myocyte damage may also be present. Severe rejection is manifested by increased inflammatory infiltrates including neutrophils, interstitial hemorrhage, and myocyte necrosis. Resolving or resolved rejection is characterized by active fibrosis and scar formation with decreased or absent infiltrate.

Postoperative endomyocardial biopsies are done routinely for early detection of cardiac rejection, often before clinical symptoms are present. Cardiac biopsies are performed at decreasing intervals for the first 3 months postoperatively. After 3 to 6 months, biopsies may be done approximately every 3 months until 1 year and then one to four times yearly thereafter. Endomyocardial biopsy protocols vary among institutions.

The transvenous biopsy technique was adapted for use in cardiac transplantation by Caves and Billingham in 1972.[30] The approach

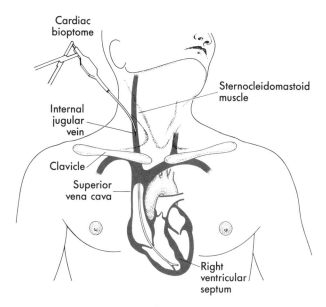

Fig. 12-8 Endomyocardial biopsy technique; transvenous biopsy approach through the right internal jugular vein.

used for the endomyocardial biopsy is through the right internal jugular vein, using local anesthesia (Fig. 12-8). A bioptome catheter is advanced into the right ventricle under fluoroscopy. Three to five tissue samples are obtained for analysis.[6,7]

The procedure takes approximately 15 minutes. The risk of complication is less than 0.5%, with pneumothorax being the most frequent complication.[7] Vital signs are monitored during the procedure and for approximately 15 minutes after completion of the biopsy. Chest x-ray evaluation is also performed in some centers after the procedure to rule out complications such as pneumothorax or cardiac tamponade.[24] The insertion site, generally requiring only a light pressure dressing or small bandage, should be monitored for bleeding.

There are several noninvasive methods for diagnosing rejection that are currently being investigated as an alternative or adjunct to the endomyocardial biopsy. These include echocardiography, urine polyamine levels, cytoimmunologic monitoring, serum prolactin levels, and nuclear medicine techniques.[20,23,31,32] These techniques, although promising, are not yet reliable enough to replace the endomyocardial biopsy.

Since the advent of cyclosporine therapy, the character and presentation of cardiac rejection has changed. Cardiac rejection in cyclosporine-treated patients appears to be less severe yet more indolent in nature[7,20] and associated with less intramyocardial edema.[7,11] Clinical indicators of rejection, although useful, are less reliable than in patients treated with conventional therapy (azathioprine and prednisone only). Some patients may remain asymptomatic during mild cases of acute rejection, with clinical signs and symptoms of rejection seen only when cardiac rejection has progressed.

Assessment for subjective and objective signs and symptoms (defining characteristics) of acute rejection is an ongoing nursing responsibility. Clinical indicators of rejection should be monitored closely. Subjectively, the patient may report a decrease in exercise tolerance, fatigue, lethargy or dyspnea. Objectively, signs of cardiac failure such as peripheral edema and jugular venous distention may be present. Auscultation of the lungs and heart is performed routinely to monitor for crackles, pericardial friction rub, S3 gallop and an irregular cardiac rhythm. Continuous or 12-lead ECG monitoring for dysrhythmias (primarily atrial) is done. A decrease in electrical voltage may signify rejection in conventionally (azathioprine and prednisone) treated patients.

Vital signs are monitored as ordered and needed. If a central venous or pulmonary artery catheter is in place the patient should be monitored for unexplained elevations in cardiac pressures or decreased cardiac output. Decreased cardiac output and hypotension are usually seen only in advanced cases of cardiac rejection where myocyte necrosis has occurred.[7,20,25]

Cardiac enlargement, as determined by chest x-ray examination, may also be associated with rejection. Intake and output is monitored and the patient is weighed daily.

Interventions. Patients undergoing endomyocardial biopsy for the first time should be taught about the purpose and procedural technique. In addition, the nurse may accompany the patient or assist during the biopsy procedure. The first cardiac biopsy is performed 5 to 10 days after surgery.

Treatment of moderate to severe rejection requires hospitalization. Moderate to severe rejection is initially treated with methylprednisolone pulsed therapy (e.g., 1 g/day for 3 days). For cases of severe rejection that are resistant to pulsed corticosteroids, OKT-3 may be used. An increase in cyclosporine or prednisone dosages may also be necessary to treat resistant rejection.

Mild rejection episodes may be treated or monitored on an outpatient basis. Mild or resolving rejection episodes may require additional corticosteroids or no treatment.[4,20,33]

Treatment regimens vary significantly among institutions. Cardiac biopsy is repeated 4 to 7 days after treatment is instituted to assess for the resolution of rejection.

The presence of clinical indicators suggestive of cardiac rejection should be reported to the

ACUTE REJECTION

Assessment
Defining characteristics

Positive cardiac biopsy—specific degree is variable
  SUBJECTIVE
    Decreased exercise tolerance
    Fatigue
    Lethargy
    Dyspnea
  OBJECTIVE
    Peripheral edema
    Crackles
    Jugular venous distention
    S3 gallop
    Pericardial friction rub
    Dysrhythmias (primarily atrial)
    Decreased ECG voltage (conventional treatment)
    Decreased cardiac output
    Hypotension
    Cardiac enlargement on x-ray studies

Assessment techniques

Check biopsy insertion site for bleeding or infection.
Monitor for signs of cardiac failure:
  Skin turgor for edema
  Jugular venous distention
  Auscultate lung sounds for crackles
  Auscultate heart for S3 or irregular rhythm
Monitor cardiac rhythm and obtain 12-lead ECG once daily.
Measure for drop in QRS voltage on 12-lead ECG once daily (conventional immunosuppressed patients).
Monitor patient's vital signs or mental status as ordered or indicated by patient's condition.
Monitor for increased CVP/cardiac pressures or drop in cardiac output.
Assess chest x-ray studies for cardiac enlargement.
Monitor intake and output.
Weigh patient daily.

Interventions
Prepare and teach patient regarding the biopsy procedure.
Administer immunosuppressive medications.
Report clinical indicators suggestive of cardiac rejection.
Provide emotional support.

physician immediately. Emotional support and explanations about treatment and procedures will decrease the patient's anxiety and fear during diagnosis and treatment of rejection.

The box on p. 220 summarizes the assessment parameters and interventions relevant to acute rejection in the heart transplant patient.

Infection

Infection is the major cause of morbidity and mortality for cardiac transplant recipients.[11,23,34] The incidence of infection has decreased and is easier to treat in patients receiving cyclosporine-based immunosuppression (triple- or quadruple-drug therapy) compared with conventional immunosuppression (azathioprine and prednisone alone).[20]

Cause. The cardiac transplant recipient receives long-term immunosuppressive therapy to prevent rejection. Immunosuppression in turn predisposes the patient to infection. Infection episodes are more common during the first 3 postoperative months, when immunosuppression is greatest.[24] In addition to long-term immunosuppressive therapy, the patient is predisposed to further infection by the following related risk factors; inadequate primary defenses such as disruption of skin integrity through surgery and placement of invasive lines and tubes, decreased ciliary action from general anesthesia and intubation, malnutrition, extremes in age, and increased immunosuppressive therapy for the treatment of rejection.[24,34,35]

The most common site of infection is the lungs.[36,37] Infections, however, can occur elsewhere, such as in the central nervous system; ears, eyes, nose and throat; gastrointestinal tract; genitourinary tract; or skin or other organs, such as the pancreas and gallbladder.

Cardiac transplant recipients are at risk for a wide range of opportunistic infections. Infectious organisms can be divided into four main categories—bacterial, viral, fungal, and protozoal[8,20,24] (see Chapter 3). Bacterial infections are the most common infections seen in the transplant population[4,5]; the incidence of viral infections, however, has increased with the use of cyclosporine.

Assessment. Prevention, detection, and early treatment of infection are primary challenges to the critical care nurse caring for the cardiac transplant patient. Infection in the cardiac transplant patient is considered life threatening until proven otherwise.[36] The presence of etiologic risk factors is assessed during all phases of the transplant process, including the preoperative period.

Preoperative evaluation of both donor and recipient blood serologies and cultures is performed (e.g., for cytomegalovirus antibody titer) to identify patients at risk for primary infections and aid in later diagnosis of infections.[20] Abnormal laboratory values, specifically an elevated white blood cell count with a left shift in the differential count, or leukopenia may predispose or signal an episode of infection. Cultures should also be monitored for positive results.

Assessment techniques may reveal the following defining characteristics of infection. Subjectively, the patient may report lethargy, weakness, chills, dyspnea, pain, or a history of fevers. Because pulmonary infections are the most common infections seen in this population, the patient may exhibit shortness of breath, cough (with or without sputum production), and localized crackles or wheezes.[36]

In the immediate postoperative period, and if a pulmonary infection is suspected, the lungs are auscultated frequently. A chest x-ray examination is done daily. If a pulmonary infiltrate or nodule is noted, a transtracheal aspirate (TTA) for Gram stain and culture will be obtained. If diagnosis is still uncertain, the TTA may be followed by fine-needle aspirate, bronchial biopsy, bronchiole alveolar lavage, or computed tomography.

The presence and condition of surgical or traumatic wounds and insertion sites of invasive tubes and lines are assessed for signs of infection, such as delayed healing, redness, swelling, or drainage. Vital signs, particularly temperature, are monitored frequently.

The level of knowledge by the patient and significant others should be assessed. This assessment should include knowledge of the prevention, transmission, and signs and symptoms of infection.

Interventions. Broad-spectrum prophylactic antibiotics are usually administered preoperatively and for approximately 48 hours postoperatively. In addition, specific antibacterial or antiviral prophylaxis may also be given for 1 to 2 months postoperatively. Antibacterial and antifungal mouthwashes may be used to prevent oral infections. Additional antibiotics are generally not instituted until a specific organism is identified by culture.

Infection control precautions are instituted immediately after surgery. Isolation precautions vary among institutions and are the responsibility of all health care personnel. The extremes in isolation precautions, from specially adapted rooms with positive-negative air flow systems to regular private rooms, remains controversial. During the immediate postoperative period, while immunosuppression is greatest, strict isolation may be instituted. For the remainder of the initial hospitalization, mask and handwashing precautions are usually sufficient, and the patient may be kept in a private room. Readmissions require a private room, with handwashing as a minimum isolation protocol.

The patient is generally weaned from mechanical ventilation and extubated within 24 hours. Invasive lines and tubes are discontinued

---

INFECTION

Assessment

Defining characteristics

Presence of etiologic risk factors increasing patient's susceptibility to infection

SUBJECTIVE
   Lethargy
   Weakness
   Chills
   Dyspnea
   Pain
   History of fevers

OBJECTIVE
   Shortness of breath
   Cough/sputum production
   Crackles or wheezes
   Fever
   Abnormal laboratory values — elevated WBC, leukopenia
   Positive culture results
   Presence of lesions, invasive lines or tubes

Assessment techniques

Assess wounds and line/tube insertion sites for signs or symptoms of infection: redness, swelling, drainage.

Obtain vital signs every 4 hours, particularly temperature.

Auscultate lungs for crackles/wheezes every 4 hours.

Obtain chest x-ray studies daily.

Monitor laboratory abnormalities.

Obtain cultures per order.

Interventions

Administer antimicrobial therapy as prescribed.

Institute protective isolation precautions.

Use good handwashing technique.

Discontinue invasive lines and tubes as soon as possible.

Maintain aseptic wound and invasive line care.

Report infection around wounds or lines.

Limit unnecessary procedures.

Report temperature elevations above 38° C or per specified parameters.

Employ aggressive pulmonary therapy as ordered.

Report laboratory abnormalities.

Report positive culture results.

Restrict visitors and health professionals with known infection or exposure to communicable disease.

Maintain optimal nutrition and hydration.

Teach patient and significant others: prevention, transmission, signs and symptoms of infection.

as soon as possible or changed frequently to decrease risk of infection. Strict aseptic wound and line care is performed. Aggressive pulmonary therapy, including coughing and deep breathing, incentive spirometry, and percussion and drainage should be performed.

Visitors and health care professionals with colds or infectious diseases are not allowed contact with the patient. If a knowledge deficit exists in the family or significant other regarding infection, teaching is indicated. Teaching should include infection prevention techniques and modes of infection transmission. In addition, the patient is taught to identify and report signs and symptoms of infection.

The box on p. 222 summarizes the assessment parameters and interventions relevant to infection in the heart transplant patient.

DECREASED CARDIAC OUTPUT

Decreased cardiac output (< 2.0 L/min) refers to a decrease in the amount of blood ejected by the heart, as measured in liters per minute. Significantly decreased cardiac output will result in compromised circulation and tissue perfusion.

Cause

There are several potential causes for decreased cardiac output during the early postoperative period. Primary factors that may be related to a decreased cardiac output are cardiac rejection, preservation injury, hemorrhage, cardiac tamponade, hypovolemia, hypothermia and dysrhythmias. These etiologic factors may be distinctly separate or can be interrelated. Cardiac rejection, a significant factor potentially resulting in decreased cardiac output, was described earlier in this chapter and will not be covered in this section.

Preservation injury, resulting in myocardial depression and decreased cardiac output, may occur during organ retrieval, the cold ischemic period, or implantation of the donor heart.[24,25]

Hemorrhage, intraoperatively or in the immediate postoperative period, is a serious complication. This risk of bleeding may be increased by preoperative anticoagulation therapy and adhesions from previous surgery.

Cardiac tamponade may result from hemorrhage into the pericardial space or as a result of occlusion of mediastinal chest tubes.[38] The pericardial space in patients with long-standing cardiomyopathy is usually significantly enlarged, which increases the risk of tamponade.[1]

Hypovolemia may result from hemorrhage, aggressive diuresis, or sepsis.[25] Surgically induced hypothermia, resulting in peripheral vasoconstriction and increased afterload, can also decrease cardiac output until the patient is sufficiently rewarmed.[24]

Dysrhythmias, if severe, can compromise cardiac hemodynamics, resulting in decreased cardiac output. The causes of atrial and ventricular dysrhythmias in the immediate postoperative period are numerous, including rejection, electrolyte imbalances, acidosis, and medications.[25] Atrial dysrhythmias in particular may be related to rejection.

Assessment

Nursing assessment to identify decreased cardiac output is critical for timely nursing and medical intervention. Because decreased cardiac output is a broad nursing diagnosis with multiple etiologic factors, it is important to fully assess the problem and determine appropriate interventions based on the correct cause. As suggested by Carpenito,[35] the nurse may need to break down the diagnosis into more specific nursing diagnoses based on the specific cause.

To decrease the risk of infection in the immunosuppressed transplant patient, the use of invasive hemodynamic monitoring lines, such as Swan-Ganz catheters to measure cardiac output, may be restricted. A pulmonary artery catheter for measuring cardiac output may be positioned during surgery, exiting through a mediastinal stab wound; it can be easily removed in the early postoperative period. Central venous pressure (CVP) and arterial lines are routinely used, but are withdrawn as soon as possible. Then the use of clinical indicators to determine decreases in cardiac output is essential.

Subjectively, the patient may express symptoms of weakness, restlessness, vertigo, dyspnea, or fatigue. Objectively, the patient may exhibit decreased tissue perfusion manifested by cold, clammy skin, cyanosis of the mucous membranes, and mental status changes. Peripheral pulses may be diminished or absent. Other assessment parameters include peripheral or sacral edema, jugular venous distention, and oliguria. A cardiac gallop and dysrhythmias may be present. The patient may develop pulmonary crackles and orthopnea. Hemodynamic changes include a decreased blood pressure (mean arterial pressure <60), tachycardia (>110 beats/min), and increased filling pressures (increased CVP, PCWP). Low filling pressures may be associated with hypovolemia or hemorrhage.

Vital signs and hemodynamic parameters are monitored frequently and abnormalities reported. The cardiac rhythm is monitored continuously. Chest tube output is measured and recorded every 2 hours, monitoring for abrupt decreases in chest tube drainage. Intake and output is recorded, specifically noting decreased urinary output. The chest x-ray studies are monitored for mediastinal widening.

Changes in skin and mucous membrane color, such as mottling or cyanosis, are monitored. In addition, skin temperature changes (e.g., cool or clammy skin) and decreased peripheral pulses are noted. Cardiac and pulmonary auscultation is performed every 4 hours or as needed. Abnormalities in laboratory blood tests are monitored, specifically hemoglobin and hematocrit values and electrolyte levels.

Interventions

Medications are administered as ordered. Myocardial depression generally responds to intravenous inotropic or chronotropic support (i.e., isoproterenol, dobutamine, epinephrine) in the immediate postoperative period, which is prescribed to maintain optimal heart rate and contractility. Inotropic support is titrated according to hemodynamic parameters and discontinued within approximately 4 to 5 days after transplant.[20]

Dysrhythmias may be successfully treated with pharmacologic therapy, cardioversion, and temporary or permanent pacing. Bradycardia and junctional rhythms, possibly related to preservation injury, are not uncommon. Temporary epicardial pacing may be required in addition to inotropic support immediately after surgery. Supraventricular and ventricular dysrhythmias may require antidysrhythmic therapy or cardioversion.

Because the donor heart is denervated, autonomic nervous system innervation no longer exists. Medications whose primary effects are mediated through the autonomic nervous system, such as digoxin and atropine, will have little effect on heart rate. Likewise, carotid sinus massage or the Valsalva maneuver, mediated through the parasympathetic nervous system, will also be ineffective.[1] Because of the lack of parasympathetic neural control, the resting heart rate is higher, approximately 90 to 110 beats/min.

An ECG may reveal a second p wave originating from the remaining atrial cuff in the recipients native SA node (Fig. 12-9). This impulse, however, does not cross the donor suture line. The SA node in the donor heart initiates the electrical impulse that results in ventricular contraction.

Clotting factors are normalized during surgery with medications (e.g., phytonadione [Aquamephyton]) to reduce bleeding. Optimal surgical hemostasis is also critical to reduce the risk of postoperative bleeding. In addition,

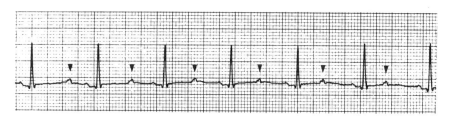

Fig. 12-9 Electrocardiogram tracing revealing a second p wave originating from the recipient's native SA node.

blood product replacement is given during surgery and in the immediate postoperative period.

Adequate rewarming of the patient must be ensured on return from the operating room. Chest tube drainage is maintained by turning and repositioning the patient every 2 hours. The chest tubes are stripped as necessary to maintain patency. Changes in skin and mucous membrane temperature and color are reported; in addition, changes in the patient's sensorium must be reported immediately.

In serious cases of decreased cardiac output, mechanical assistance may be required when inotopic or chronotropic support, in addition to atrial pacing, are inadequate to maintain adequate circulation. The nurse assists in the preparation for mechanical assistance support (intraaortic balloon pump or ventricular assist device) if necessary. The patient should be reassured and given explanations as appropriate.

The box below summarizes assessments and interventions relevant to the heart transplant patient with decreased cardiac output.

CARE OF THE PATIENT WITH DECREASED CARDIAC OUTPUT

Assessment

*Defining characteristics**

SUBJECTIVE
  Weakness
  Restlessness
  Vertigo
  Dyspnea
  Fatigue
OBJECTIVE
  Decreased tissue perfusion (e.g., cool clammy skin or changes in skin and mucous mem branes)
  Diminished or absent peripheral pulses
  Peripheral or sacral edema
  Jugular venous distention
  Oliguria
  Cardiac gallop
  Dysrhythmias
  Pulmonary crackles
  Orthopnea or shortness of breath
  Mental status changes
  Decreased blood pressure (MAP < 60)
  Tachycardia (>110 beats/min)
  Alteration in filling pressures

Assessment techniques

Monitor vital signs as ordered or indicated; note decreases in BP, pulsus alternans, and increased or thready heart rate.
Monitor hemodynamic readings as ordered, noting alteration in CVP, PAW, and CO.
Monitor cardiac rhythm continuously.
Measure and record chest tube (CT) output every 2 hours.
Record intake and output.
Monitor chest x-ray studies for mediastinal widening.
Monitor for changes in skin temperature or skin/mucous membrane color.
Perform cardiac/pulmonary auscultation every 4 hours.
Monitor blood test abnormalities.

Interventions

Administer medications as ordered.
Report dysrhythmias per protocol.
Ensure normothermia after return from operating room.
Turn and reposition patient every 2 hours.
Strip chest tubes as ordered and needed.
Report abrupt decreases in CT drainage.
Report urine output <30 ml/hr.
Report changes in mental status.
Report blood test abnormalities.
Assist in preparation for surgical mechanical assist support if necessary.
Provide assurance and explanations as appropriate.

---

*References 1, 24, 39, 40.

HYPERVOLEMIA
Cause

Excessive total body water is a common problem for cardiac transplant patients postoperatively.[25] Excessive fluid volume can be related to treatments such as fluid replacement during and immediately after surgery and corticosteroid therapy. Fluid excess can also be exacerbated by excessive sodium intake.

Assessment

Subjective assessment may reveal complaints of dyspnea, fatigue, or restlessness. Objective assessment includes identification of edema, weight gain, jugular venous distention, and oliguria. Pulmonary examination may reveal crackles and wheezes, in addition to changes in the respiratory pattern. Alteration in hemodynamic and cardiac rhythm may occur. Blood tests may indicate dilutional abnormalities.

The patient should be monitored for peripheral or centralized edema and jugular venous distention. The patient is weighed daily; a weight gain of greater than 2 pounds per day should be noted. Intake and output is totaled every 8 hours, noting whether the intake is greater than the output.

Pulmonary and cardiac assessments should be performed every 4 hours, noting a new onset of crackles, wheezes, or an S3 gallop. The patient is monitored for tachypnea, shortness of breath, restlessness, and anxiety. The chest x-ray studies

---

HYPERVOLEMIA

Assessment
Defining characteristics*
SUBJECTIVE
  Dyspnea
  Fatigue
  Anxiety
  Restlessness
OBJECTIVE
  Weight gain
  Jugular venous distention
  Oliguria
  Intake greater than output
  Pulmonary crackles or wheezes
  Changes in respiratory rate or pattern
  Chest x-ray studies indicating pulmonary congestion
  S3 gallop
  Elevated hemodynamic readings: BP, CVP, PAP, PAWP
  Laboratory blood test abnormalities

Assessment techniques
Monitor patient for edema (peripheral or centralized).
Monitor for jugular venous distention.
Weigh daily—note weight gain greater than 2 lb/day.
Record intake and output every 8 hours, noting input greater than output.
Perform pulmonary and cardiac auscultation every 4 hours.
Monitor chest x-ray films daily for pulmonary congestion.
Monitor hemodynamic pressures.
Monitor blood tests for abnormalities.

Interventions
Administer diuretic therapy as ordered.
Administer inotropic support (e.g., dopamine or dobutamine) or vasodilator therapy (nitroprusside) as ordered.
Report abnormal hemodynamic changes.
Report abnormal blood test findings, specifically: Hgb, Hct, electrolytes, BUN, creatinine.
Restrict fluid intake as ordered.
Coordinate dietary assessment and teaching with dietitian.
Institute low-sodium diet as ordered.
Reposition every 2 hours.
Support and elevate edematous areas.

---

*References 35, 39, 40.

should be monitored daily for pulmonary congestion. Hemodynamic pressures (mean arterial pressure, central venous pressure, pulmonary artery pressure, and pulmonary artery wedge pressure) are evaluated as ordered.

Interventions

Inotropes (e.g., dopamine or dobutamine) or vasodilators (nitroprusside or nitroglycerin) are administered as ordered. Abnormal hemodynamic pressure changes or laboratory blood test abnormalities must be reported. Fluid intake is restricted as ordered. Dietary assessment and teaching is coordinated with the dietitian. A low-sodium diet is instituted if indicated. Positional changes should be made a minimum of every 2 hours, while supporting and elevating edematous areas.

The box on p. 226 summarizes assessments and interventions relevant to the heart transplant patient with hypervolemia.

KNOWLEDGE DEFICIT

There is a great deal for the patient and family to know about heart transplantation and how it will change their lives. Providing the appropriate information and ensuring an adequate level of understanding are perhaps the most difficult challenges to the transplant team.

Cause

Knowledge deficits occur in five areas: medications, diet, exercise, psychosocial changes, and health monitoring for the prevention of rejection and infection. Patient and family information that is necessary for optimal postoperative survival is in most cases new information. Other factors that may complicate the educational process include lack of recall, lack of interest, cognitive limitations, information misinterpretation, unfamiliarity with available resources, and the patient's refusal of further education.[40] The patient's knowledge base will be influenced by educational and socioeconomic background, medical history, and cognitive ability.

Assessment

Assessment for a knowledge deficit begins during the evaluation and waiting phases, when the patient is a candidate for transplantation. Assessment focuses on the current level of knowledge in each of the five identified areas.

Assessment of educational and socioeconomic background will aid in providing appropriate teaching. The patient's medical history will also influence the knowledge level and need for additional life-style changes. An older patient, for example, with a 10-year history of ischemic heart disease may have already made significant life-style changes involving diet and exercise, in addition to having maintained a detailed medication regimen. On the other hand, a 30-year-old patient with a recent onset of viral cardiomyopathy may have little knowledge about optimal health maintenance.

Cognitive ability will also determine learning ability. In severe cases, cognitive function may be adversely affected in the preoperative period by low cardiac output and decreased cerebral perfusion.

Interventions

Patient education is a primary nursing responsibility in all phases of cardiac transplantation. Interventions are multidisciplinary in nature. The nurse is responsible for assessing teaching needs, which may require consultants from dietary, cardiac rehabilitation, and social services departments.

Medication teaching. Patient survival depends on compliance with the immunosuppressive regimen, which requires knowledge of the purpose, dosage, route of administration, and side effects of drugs. Formal medication teaching begins when the patient is extubated and able to participate.

Teaching goals include (1) patient demonstration of correct administration of medications and (2) verbalization of medication names, dosages, routes of administration, action, and side effects. Independence in medication administration should proceed from supervised medication administration while in the intensive care unit or intermediate care unit to safe, independent administration at the time of discharge. It is imperative that the patient and family fully understand the importance of taking prescribed medications as scheduled — and the life-threatening implications of not taking them.

Exercise and cardiac rehabilitation. Formal cardiac rehabilitation begins on postoperative day 3 or 4, when invasive lines are removed. Exercise for the cardiac transplant recipient includes walking, bicycling, treadmill, weights, and strengthening exercises. Exercise is progressive and based on the patient's activity tolerance. The patient should be monitored before, during, and immediately after exercise. After hospital discharge the patient should ideally continue aerobic exercise through an outpatient rehabilitation and exercise program three to five times per week.

Psychosocial changes. Allender et al[41] described the following six psychologic stages associated with heart transplantation: evaluation period, waiting period, immediate postsurgical period, first rejection episode, recovery period, and hospital discharge. The following stages have been expanded but are similar to those described by Allender et al.

Evaluation period. Because of the terminal condition of the patient undergoing transplant evaluation, transplantation offers a chance for survival. Generally, by the time a patient undergoes transplant evaluation he understands the severity of his disease and limited prognosis.

During this stressful period, a full physical and psychologic evaluation of the patient is often made by the transplant team. Psychologic evaluation consists of interview by the psychologist or psychiatrist and social worker. In addition, the patient undergoes testing of intellectual capacity, memory, and personality as well as a neuropsychologic screening examination.[41] These tests provide information on the psychologic stability of the patient. If the patient is accepted for transplant, these tests provide information about educational needs and baseline intellectual and personality functioning. While the transplant team is evaluating the patient, the patient and family also evaluate the transplant program and staff. The patient and family should receive verbal and written explanations of the program's survival statistics, team composition, evaluation procedures, and description of the phases of the transplant process.

The serious nature of the transplant process needs to be clearly explained to the patient and family. The potential benefits as well as the problems associated with a transplant must be described. Information about transplantation, however, is often poorly understood by the patient and family during this period, because of the patient's critical condition. Patients may minimize their problems in an attempt to enhance acceptance.[41] Most patients "prefer the uncertainty of transplantation to the certainty of death."[42]

Waiting period. The waiting period is probably the most stressful time for the patient and family. The waiting and associated anxiety is especially prolonged now because of the donor shortage. This period is commonly described as the patient "waiting to live or waiting to die." The family members attempt to maintain hope but are often plagued by fear and worry that the patient will die before a donor heart is found.

With counseling and support the patient and family can find a balance between accepting the possibility of death while maintaining hope for survival through transplant.[43] Support groups for the patient and family (combined or separate) are helpful. Counseling may be needed during this period and should be tailored to the patient's and family's needs. In addition, a preoperative tour of the hospital is beneficial.

Hospitalization period. During hospitalization there is generally a sense of relief that the transplant has occurred. The patient's mood can vary between euphoria and depression, enhanced by high doses of steroid therapy. The patient and family focus on recovery and education begins. The patient may experience his first rejection or infection episode, often shattering the belief that he will not have any complications. In addition, the patient begins to incorporate the acceptance of the new heart. Nursing care consists of providing physical care, education, and support.

Hospital discharge through the first 3 months. The patient may begin to assume some duties he performed before the onset of illness. Thus it is often a period of readjustment for the family to "let go" and allow the patient to reestablish a certain degree of independence. Role reversal often occurs during this period.

Clinic follow-up appointments to assess physical and psychologic condition are frequent and tapered gradually. Education continues, and the patient and family are encouraged to gain independence as they wean from the security of the transplant team's care. Support groups and supportive networks formed between transplant families are helpful during this period.

Long-term follow-up. The patient must often remain near the transplant center for follow-up for 2 to 3 months; however, this period will vary among institutions. At that time, if the patient lives at a distance from the transplant center, the patient and family return home. The patient generally resumes work if able. Role redefinition is usually still occurring during this period. The patient may begin to face significant obstacles, such as employment difficulty and financial problems. In addition, the patient must perform health monitoring activities and undergo routine medical appointments. The effects of chronic immunosuppressive therapy (e.g., weight gain and hypertension) can also become problematic. The patient and family begin to adjust to the uncertainty of their future and are aided by periodic phone calls from the transplant coordinator and medical follow-up.

Health monitoring. Health monitoring refers to the patient's responsibility for self-care in the prevention and detection of infection or rejection. Discharge teaching should highlight the following patient responsibilities: attend clinic appointments as scheduled; undergo biopsy procedures as scheduled; obtain routine blood tests, including cyclosporine levels at periodic intervals as requested; administer medication independently and as directed; identify and report signs and symptoms of rejection; and identify and report signs and symptoms of infection. The importance of health care monitoring is critical to the transplant recipient's long-term survival.

DISTURBANCE IN SELF-CONCEPT: PSYCHOLOGIC ISSUES

Transplanting a healthy organ in place of a terminally diseased heart promises the potential for a new lease on life. The recipient, however, deals with many changes in addition to the mere acquisition of a new organ. These changes are often difficult, requiring major life-style alterations.

Cause

Three dominant areas affecting the patient's psychologic status after transplant are health status (physical and psychologic), family and marital status, and employment and financial status. Problems in any of these areas can result in a disturbance in the patient's self-concept.

Assessment

Health status. Physical rehabilitation is significantly improved after cardiac transplant, when compared with pretransplant physical functioning. Functional rehabilitation, broadly defined—primarily relating to physical functioning—ranges from 85% to 91% after transplant.[43-45]

Infection and rejection remain the most common complications during the first 2 years.[6] Accelerated graft atherosclerosis (AGAS) or chronic rejection, however, is a major factor limiting long-term survival.[8,11,22,25] The incidence can reach 40% to 50% at 5 years, in the experience of some transplant centers.[11,25] Since without retransplantation AGAS leads to death, this complication clearly results in uncertainty for the transplant patient's survival.

The majority of the remaining physical complications are the result of long-term immunosuppressive therapy.[46] Cyclosporine-related complications include nephrotoxicity, hypertension, gingival hyperplasia, tremors, hirsutism, seizures, and malignancies, particularly lymphoproliferative disease. Complications primarily related to prednisone include osteoporosis, resulting in compression fractures; aseptic necrosis of the joints; steroid-induced diabetes; obesity; cushingoid facies; and mood alterations.[8,11,25] Other complications include hepatic dysfunction and impotence.

In a study conducted by Lough et al comparing symptom frequency and symptom distress from medication side effects, symptoms occurring most frequently were not necessarily perceived as the most upsetting. The most frequently described symptoms included skin fragility and bruising, hirsutism, and changed facial and body image. These symptoms, however, were not the most distressing. Impotence was the most distressing symptom described by patients; the occurrence was 28% in men receiving azathioprine-prednisone therapy and 11% in men receiving cyclosporine-prednisone therapy. The second most upsetting symptom for both treatment groups was decreased interest in sex.[47,48]

Physical symptoms affect the patients' psychologic status and in turn their self-concept. Long-term immunosuppression resulting in changes in physical appearance will have a significant effect on body image. Body image changes include weight gain, redistribution of weight, skin bruising and fragility, acne, and hirsutism. Mood alterations, including depression, are also common. Medication-related symptoms change over time, varying in occurrence and severity for each transplant recipient.[49] The psychologic health of the patient is also integrally related to family and marital status and employment and financial status.

Family and marital status. Family and marital stability positively influence the transplant patient's well-being. The patient's significant others are also critical participants in the transplant process. Family members' roles include caregiver, support person, and patient advocate. These roles and their significance vary with the transplant period and the patient's individual needs.

In an exploratory study examining family adjustment to heart transplant, Mishel and Murdaugh[50] described family adjustment as an adaptive process. This process requires a redefinition of reality described as "redesigning the dream." The authors described three periods: immersion (waiting period), passage (surgical and immediate postsurgical period), and negotiation (recovery phase after discharge).

Immersion refers to the partner's heightened vigilance, protective behaviors, and role reversal that occur while the patient is waiting for a donor heart. *Passage* involves the emotional release and expression of the stressful events encountered during immersion. Family members vacillate between feeling life will return to normal and the possibility of complications. This results in the realization that life has changed and the patient is vulnerable. The final period, *negotiation,* is characterized by role

realignment, with the integration of the patient's vulnerability and unpredictable future.

Employment and financial status. The patient's employment status and financial status are generally worsened after transplant. The ability to return to work is an important factor affecting the patient's self-concept. Lough et al[47] found a higher quality of life reported by recipients who were employed compared with nonemployed recipients. The majority of transplant recipients are physically able to work, but some are unable to do so as a result of financial or insurance-related limitations.

A study by Meister et al[51] reported four major variables that affect recipients' ability to return to work: age, length of disability before transplant, control over working conditions, and insurance coverage. Patients were grouped into four categories: 32% had returned to work; 25% were retired; 7.5% were medically disabled; and 36% were insurance disabled. The "insurance disabled" group were those patients able to work but not working because of financial limitations. Unfortunately, this large group of patients are dependent on disability incomes or government-subsidized health care to cover the cost of medical expenses. If they were to return to work they would lose their benefits and are generally considered medically uninsurable.[51]

In addition to the problem of unemployment, financial problems are further complicated by the high cost of medications and health care follow-up. The cost of medications average approximately $6000 per year using triple-drug therapy, including cyclosporine.[12]

Interventions

The patient and family should receive clear explanations about health problems encountered after transplant. In particular, medication side effects and possible treatment should be addressed. Teaching and counseling should be adapted to the specific needs and concerns of each patient.

Support groups are helpful in all phases of transplant. Specific phases can be combined or separated (e.g., the waiting period versus the posttransplant period). Group focus can be educational (structured) or therapeutic (unstructured). Group composition can combine or separate the patient and significant others. The specific type of support group will depend on the patient's needs and available support staff. One-on-one psychologic counseling may be necessary for difficult problems.

Currently, Medicare covers 1 year of post-transplant immunosuppressive therapy costs for eligible recipients. An extension of Medicare coverage would ease the financial burden of medication costs. The Medicare Catastrophic Coverage Act of 1988 will provide continual reimbursement for medication costs for those eligible, beginning in 1990. A nationally based government insurance program to assist in medical costs for transplant recipients should also be considered. Vocational rehabilitation should be implemented for work reentry when appropriate. Federal and state agencies cannot discriminate against people with preexisting conditions and thus provide a potential employment source. In addition, increased employer assistance and community support would enhance a recipient's ability to return to work.[51]

SUMMARY

Heart transplantation has become a successful and progressive treatment alternative for patients with end-stage heart disease. With increasing knowledge and experience, recipient selection criteria are being refined. Although the number of potential cardiac transplant candidates is increasing, the cardiac donor population has remained constant. The future of cardiac transplantation will be affected by the severe recipient-donor imbalance.

A heart transplant recipient presents challenging acute care needs to the critical care nurse. Postoperative nursing diagnoses frequently seen in the heart transplant population include potential for acute cardiac rejection; potential for infection; alteration in cardiac output; alteration of fluid volume (excess); knowledge deficit of medications, diet, exercise, psychosocial changes, and health monitoring for the prevention of infection and rejection; and disturbance in self-concept. Appropriate assessment of nursing diagnoses forms an essential basis for an optimal long-term outcome.

Part II

MECHANICAL CIRCULATORY ASSISTANCE AS A BRIDGE TO TRANSPLANT

There are currently 1324 individuals awaiting heart transplants today in the United States at 147 centers across the country.[52] Because of the shortage of suitable heart donors, it is estimated that 20% to 40% of heart transplant candidates will die before a donor can be found.[53]

Although many of these potential recipients die suddenly at home while on a waiting list, a number of individuals die from progressive heart failure while in the hospital, despite maximal pharmacologic support and intraaortic balloon counterpulsation. It is these patients who might benefit from more sophisticated mechanical circulatory assistance before heart transplant. This section outlines the development of mechanical assistance for the heart, discusses patient selection criteria, types of devices, nursing care, results, and ethical considerations.

Historical development of mechanical assistance

In 1927 Charles Lindbergh demonstrated interest in the development of a cardiac support system, supposedly because his sister-in-law suffered from severe valvular heart disease. Working with Dr. Alexis Carrell of the Rockefeller Institute, they developed a pump oxygenator in 1935 and called it the "robot heart."[54]

The heart-lung machine was first used clinically in 1953 by John Gibbon for repair of an atrial septal defect.[55] In 1957 Stuckey et al used the heart-lung machine to support a patient with cardiogenic shock following acute myocardial infarction[56]; the patient lived another 23 years. This was the first successful use of mechanical circulatory assistance for postinfarction cardiogenic shock. The first use of the heart-lung machine for postcardiotomy cardiogenic shock was by Spencer et al[57] in 1963; they supported a patient after repair of an aortic–left atrial fistula and mitral annuloplasty. From the early 1960s until recently, the most common indication for mechanical circulatory assistance has been for patients with postcardiotomy failure. Currently, the most common use of mechanical circulatory assistance has been as a "bridge" to cardiac transplant.

The first mechanical bridge to transplant occurred on April 4, 1969, when a 47-year-old man with ischemic cardiomyopathy at the Texas Heart Institute could not be weaned from cardiopulmonary bypass after an infarctectomy.[58] Dr. Denton Cooley et al replaced the patient's heart with a Liotta total artificial heart. Circulation was supported for 64 hours until a donor heart became available. The patient died of pneumonia 32 hours after transplant.

Reemtsma et al[59] reported in 1978 the successful use of the intraaortic balloon to support three patients with hemodynamic deterioration before cardiac transplant. All three patients survived hospitalization. These three patients represent the first successful cases of bridging to transplant with the use of mechanical assistance.

On December 2, 1982, a new era of total artificial heart implantation began when a 61-year-old man suffering from chronic congestive cardiomyopathy and chronic obstructive pulmonary disease at the University of Utah survived 112 days after the implantation of the Jarvik-7 total artificial heart.[60] Although many problems were encountered, this case demonstrated that the total artificial heart could provide circulatory support for extended periods of time. The original concept of the Jarvik-7 was as a permanent "solution" to end-stage heart failure. The dismal results with the permanent total artificial heart caused abandonment of this program. However, these cases, in conjunction with tremendous improvements in patient survival after heart transplant, were instrumental in reviving the concept of temporary mechanical support of a transplant candidate with a total artificial heart.[61]

The first successful artificial heart bridge to transplant was performed at the University of Arizona in 1985.[62] A 27-year-old man with viral cardiomyopathy was supported on a Jarvik-7 device for 9 days before transplant. His recovery was complete, and he was discharged from the hospital and continues to do well 5 years after transplant.

The first long-term survivor of cardiac transplant after support with a ventricular assist device was on September 5, 1984, when a 51-year-old man with ischemic cardiomyopathy was supported for 9 days with a Novacor electrical, implantable, left ventricular assist device inserted by Oyer et al[63] at Stanford University. Almost simultaneously, Hill et al[64] implanted a Pierce-Donachy left ventricular assist device as a bridge to transplant in a patient with profound heart failure.

These landmark cases established the short-term efficacy of mechanical circulatory support. The results published in a series of patients bridged to transplant between 1984 through 1988 demonstrated that mechanical circulatory support effectively maintained vital organ functions for up to 90 days while a suitable donor was sought. After transplant, the patients had good cardiac function without long-term sequelae from the period of mechanical support.[65]

Patient selection for mechanical assistance

There are currently three categories of potential candidates for mechanical assistance: (1) patients suffering profound acute cardiogenic shock from myocardial infarction, (2) patients on cardiopulmonary bypass who have undergone successful cardiac surgical repair but are unable to wean from bypass, and (3) patients with end-stage cardiomyopathy awaiting transplant whose condition deteriorates before a suitable donor can be found. The individual who is a candidate for a mechanical assist device as a bridge to transplant must first meet the criteria for heart transplant. To ensure that scarce donor hearts are not implanted in patients with minimal chance for survival, patients must be selected very carefully. The inclusion and exclusion criteria are the same as for any other heart transplant candidate and are shown in the box on p. 233.

The guidelines for exclusion by age are no longer confined strictly to individuals under 50 years of age. Physiologic age is considered, and candidates up to the age of 60 may be selected if no other health problems prevail. In addition, the National Institutes of Health Study Group has outlined the exclusion of patients who have incurred central nervous system damage as a

CRITERIA FOR PATIENT SELECTION FOR MECHANICAL ASSISTANCE AS A BRIDGE TO HEART TRANSPLANT

Inclusion criteria

End-stage cardiac failure not amenable to other
  conventional medical or surgical modalities
Supportive family structure

Exclusion criteria

End-organ damage to liver or kidneys
Active malignancy
Recent gastrointestinal bleeding
Recent cerebrovascular accident
Recent pulmonary embolus or severe pulmonary
  disease
Previous alcohol or other drug abuse problems
Irreversible pulmonary hypertension ($\geq$ 6-8 pulmo-
  nary Wood units)
Active infection unresponsive to antibiotic therapy
Preformed circulating cytotoxic antibodies (per-
  cent of reactive antibodies)
Blood dyscrasia
Diffuse peripheral vascular disease

result of hypoperfusion before assist device insertion.[66] The goal of careful selection and screening of potential assist device candidates is to prevent complications and increase survival. The rigorous postinsertion care places great emotional strain on both the patient and the family; therefore psychologic evaluation before insertion and psychologic support after insertion are necessary components to the care of the patient who requires a mechanical assist device.

Hemodynamic criteria. The hemodynamic criteria for initiating mechanical assistance in patients with cardiogenic shock unresponsive to conventional therapy including maximum pharmacologic intervention and the intraaortic balloon pump are fairly widely accepted. These criteria are as follows:

Mean arterial pressure < 60 mm Hg
Left or right atrial pressure > 20 mm Hg
Cardiac index of < 2 L/m^2

Systemic vascular resistance > 2100 dynes/
  sec/cm^5
Urine output < 20 ml/hr

Types of mechanical assistance

Intraaortic balloon pump. Currently the most widely used form of left ventricular assistance is intraaortic balloon pumping (IABP). The preoperative, intraoperative, and postoperative use of IABP has gained widespread acceptance in the management of high-risk patients with low cardiac output states caused by reversible ventricular dysfunction. It has also proved to be a useful method to support the patient who develops hemodynamic deterioration while awaiting cardiac transplant. The effectiveness of IABP is based on an instantaneous decrease in systolic arterial pressure (afterload), left ventricular end-diastolic pressure (preload), mean left atrial and pulmonary capillary wedge pressures, and modest increases in cardiac output. The IABP augments existing circulation. The balloon is computer programmed to be synchronized with the R wave of the ECG or aortic pressure tracing. During diastole the balloon inflates and propels blood to the coronary arteries. During systole the balloon deflates and reduces myocardial oxygen consumption by decreasing left ventricular afterload. Advantages of the IABP counterpulsation include the following: (1) percutaneous insertion can be done at the bedside, (2) equipment is widely available (it is not an investigational device), (3) IABP is reliable, (4) it is not as expensive as other mechanical assist devices, and (5) the patient is not totally dependent on the device.

Disadvantages of the IABP include the following: (1) effectiveness is limited during tachycardia and dysrhythmias, (2) increase in cardiac output is limited, (3) insertion can be difficult and it cannot be inserted in someone with obstructive aortic–femoral vascular lesions, (4) thromboembolic complications may occur, (5) vascular injury may occur, and (6) there is a risk of infection, thrombocytopenia, and mesenteric ischemia.[67]

Although of proven clinical benefit in a wide range of cardiac disorders, the IABP is capable of only modest increases in cardiac output and has no primary effect on preload reduction.

Generally the degree of augmentation of the cardiac output is approximately 500 to 800 ml/min, or a 10% increase in cardiac output.[68]

In contrast, intracorporeal left ventricular assist devices are true blood pumps designed to maintain adequate systemic perfusion. Although they are more invasive, comparisons of their effectiveness for the clinical reversal of profound left ventricular failure show that the left ventricular assist device is capable of delivery of 6 to 7 L/min. The ventricular assist device can capture the entire cardiac output by diversion of oxygenated blood from either the left atrium or the left ventricle to the artificial pump. Reperfusion occurs via an arterial cannula placed into the aorta or femoral artery.

Ventricular assist devices. There are four basic types of ventricular assist devices: (1) the roller pump, (2) the centrifugal pump, (3) the pneumatic pump, and (4) the electrical pump. Currently, certain ventricular assist devices are available for bridge to transplant on an investigational basis only. Selected institutions have been granted approval based on their transplant history and on completion of appropriate training programs by the surgeons, nursing staff, and biomedical engineering support team. Each device has specific advantages and disadvantages. Device selection depends on institutional availability, size of the potential recipient, and the clinical situation at the time of insertion (in the ICU, catheterization lab, or operating room).

Roller pump. The roller pump diverts blood to the external pump via an external cannula. An example of a roller pump is the extracorporeal membranous oxygenation (ECMO) system, which is essentially a means of providing portable cardiopulmonary bypass for temporary emergency support (Fig. 12-10). A withdrawal cannula is placed in the right atrium, and the infusion cannula is placed in the aorta. Groin cannulation may be used as an alternative. The system requires a membrane oxygenator, and the patient must have continuous heparin therapy. The introduction of a commercially available bypass system (Cardiopulmonary System, Bard, Inc.) allows rapid percutaneous groin cannulation. This can provide rapid circulatory support under emergency conditions, thus pro-

viding support until definitive therapy can be undertaken.

The advantages of the ECMO system include the following: (1) it is a portable system that can be inserted in the ICU or catheterization lab; (2) an IABP can be left in place in the uncannulated groin to provide pulsatile flow; (3) it can support flows greater than 2 L/m^2/min; and (4) since a thoracotomy is not necessary, increased bleeding may not be as much of a problem, although bleeding as a result of coagulopathy and heparinization is common. In addition, ECMO is not an investigational modality and is readily available at centers where thoracic surgery is performed. The ECMO system provides both cardiac and respiratory support and is useful in patients with biventricular failure.

The disadvantages of the roller pump system are (1) the increased risk for bleeding and thrombotic complications, (2) the potential for pulmonary complications resulting from low perfusion, (3) limited mobility of the patient because of the required femoral cannulation site, and (4) the limitation of the device for short-term use only. Because of these disadvantages, it is best suited for potential heart transplant recipients if there is a reasonable hope of obtaining a donor within 48 hours or if rapid reversal of cardiogenic shock is required to maintain vital organ perfusion.

Centrifugal pump. Centrifugal pumps have for the most part displaced roller pumps as circulatory assist devices, because they are safer for long-term pumping.[69] The centrifugal pump device is a kinetic energy pump (centrifugal force) constructed from smooth rotary cones that are mounted and sealed as one (vortex housing). When the cones rotate together, they create a vortex or whirlpool effect and accelerate the blood during its course between the inlet and outlet ports of the pump head. Rotational energy is recovered in the form of pressure-flow work. The pump operates at a constant speed and generates a nearly constant pressure over a wide range of flow rates. The housing for the pump is sealed at the bottom with a magnet. The magnet on the cone is driven by the magnet on the console motor. The higher the speed in revolutions per minute, the greater the centrif-

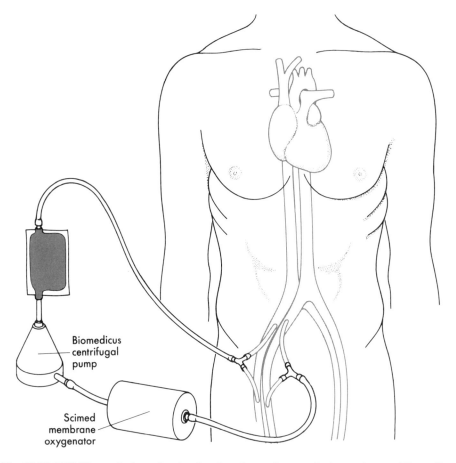

Biomedicus
centrifugal
pump

Scimed
membrane
oxygenator

Fig. 12-10 ECMO perfusion circuit showing femoral cannulation using a Biomedicus centrifugal pump and a Scimed membrane oxygenator.

ugal force inside the cone and the greater the output of the device. Examples of centrifugal pumps include the Biomedicus, the Medtronic, and the Centrimed pumps.

The advantages of the centrifugal pump are that it is a simpler pump, so there is (1) less damage to formed blood elements, (2) decreased risk of air entrapment, and (3) the design of the pump minimizes build-up of outflow pressure because it is a pressure-dependent device. The greatest disadvantage of centrifugal pumps is the nonphysiologic nature provided by the nonpulsatile flow. In addition, other disadvantages include the following: (1)

the pump may be prone to overheating, (2) with extended use, fibrin deposits may develop in the plastic cone and baseplate of the pumping chamber, and (3) anticoagulation is necessary at low flow rates of the device.

Pneumatic pumps. The pneumatic ventricular assist device consists of a polyurethane blood sac that provides a smooth surface to inhibit blood coagulation, inflow and outflow mechanical valves, and a sensing instrument that provides information to the pump for regulation of flow. The control console for the pneumatic device is electrically powered and allows for three different modes of operation: (1) fixed

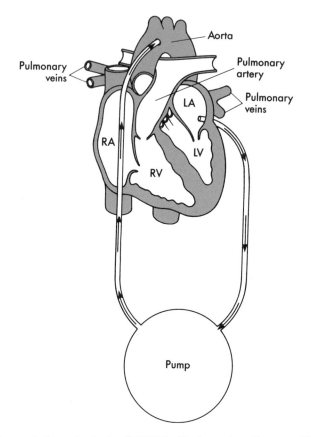

Fig. 12-11. Left ventricular assist device (L-VAD). (Redrawn from Brannon PHB and Towner SB (1986). Ventricular failure: new therapy using the mechanical assist device. *Critical Care Nurse, 6*(2), 70-84.)

rate mode, (2) fill-to-empty volume mode, and (3) ECG synchronization.

EXTERNAL PNEUMATIC PUMPS. The externally driven pneumatic device has a sac-type pump that rests on the abdominal wall with inlet and outflow cannulas traversing the abdominal wall below the costal margin. The venous return of blood is through the pump inflow cannula to the device and may be via cannulation of either the atrium or the left ventricular apex. The arterial flow of the device is via the pump outflow cannula, which contains a woven Dacron graft sewn either to the ascending aorta (for left ventricular support) or to the pulmonary trunk (for right ventricular support).

Examples of external pneumatic devices include the Pierce-Donachy device (Thoratec Laboratories Corporation, Berkeley, Calif.), the Sarns assist device, and the Symbion assist device. The advantages of the external pneumatic device include (1) capability of either right or left (Fig. 12-11) ventricular support or biventricular support (Fig. 12-12), (2) external positioning so that the device may be placed in smaller individuals, and (3) the option of either atrial cannulation or ventricular cannulation.[70]

Atrial cannulation of the external device is preferred if the heart is expected to recover, because it is technically simpler and less injurious to the myocardium. However, when the

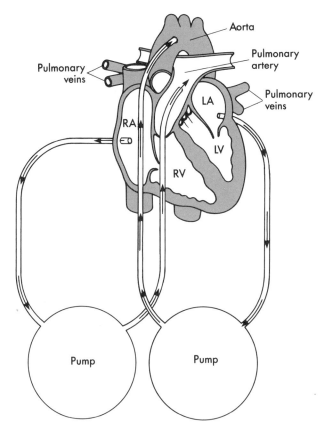

Fig. 12-12. Right and left ventricular assist device (Bi-VAD). (Redrawn from Brannon PHB and Towner SB (1986). Ventricular failure: new therapy using the mechanical assist device. *Critical Care Nurse,* 6(2), 70-84.)

ventricular assist device is intended as a bridge to transplant, ventricular cannulation is acceptable.

INTERNAL PNEUMATIC ASSIST DEVICE. An example of an internal pneumatic ventricular assist device is the Thermedics Model 14 ventricular assist device. It is a pusher plate blood pump that is pneumatically driven by an external console and has a maximum stroke volume of 85 ml. It is inserted into the left ventricular apex and a silicone rubber ring is sewn into the ventricular apex, permitting insertion of the metal inflow tube. The disadvantages of the Thermedics internal ventricular assist device are related to the size of the device. If the

patient is small (less than 120 pounds), it may not be feasible to position the device within the abdominal cavity below the ventricular apex. In addition, the Thermedic device can only assist the left ventricle and is not appropriate for right ventricle support. If right ventricular support is required, pharmacologic stimulation of the right ventricle or another assist device for support would be necessary.[71]

Electrical pumps

NOVACOR. The Novacor Model 100 left ventricular assist device (Fig. 12-13) consists of a balanced solenoid converter, dual pusher plate, sac-type blood pump, and a microprocessor-based control and monitoring console.[72] The

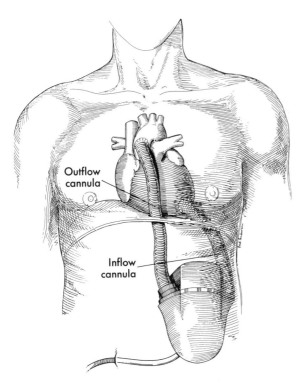

Fig. 12-13. Novacor ventricular assist device in place.

can be made to operate asynchronously during periods of ventricular fibrillation to provide adequate pump stroke volume, and (4) the patient can be ambulatory and exercising once other methods of support are weaned. The disadvantages of the Novacor electrical device include the following: (1) it can only be used for isolated left ventricular dysfunction, (2) the size of the device is such that it allows for implantation in an individual who weighs 120 pounds or more, and (3) the only method for cannulation is through the ventricular apex. Also important to consider when using an isolated left ventricular assist device is the fact that a significant percentage of patients have a patent foramen ovale,[73] which is not clinically significant when right and left atrial pressures are nearly equal. After placement of a left ventricular assist device, the left atrial pressure decreases, but in the presence of right ventricular dysfunction, the right atrial pressure can remain elevated. The difference in atrial pressures can result in right-to-left shunting across a patent foramen ovale. To prevent this problem, the atrial septum should be inspected for patent foramen ovale and if present, should be oversewn before initiation of left ventricular assistance.[74]

Total artificial heart

Currently, pneumatically powered hearts are under development at the University of Utah, the Cleveland Clinic Foundation, the Free University of Berlin, the University of Tokyo, the National Research Center (Osaka), the University of Kyoto, the Institute for Transplantation and Artificial Organs (Moscow), the University of Purkinje (Brno), and the University of Vienna. Clinical use of the total artificial heart as a bridge to transplant began with the 1985 implantation of the Jarvik-7 into a 27-year-old male with viral myocarditis at the University of Arizona. Since this historic operation, many centers have implanted temporary artificial hearts as bridge to transplant. There are currently three devices approved by the FDA and in use at selected centers for temporary support for patients awaiting cardiac transplant.

Penn State heart. One device is the Penn State heart, developed and used at the Pennsylvania State University. It is pneumatically powered

device is implanted in the anterior left upper quadrant of the abdomen so that the pump inflow conduit pierces the pericardial portion of the diaphragm to receive blood from a rigid cannula inserted into the left ventricular apex. The outflow conduit takes the blood from the blood pump to the aorta, where it is anastomosed to either the thoracic or abdominal aorta.

The control console is located externally and is connected to the implanted energy converter via an extension cable and the percutaneous leads. The device effectively decompresses the left ventricle, allowing for resting of the left ventricular wall; it operates in synchronous counterpulsation to the left ventricle. The advantages of the Novacor implantable assist device include the following: (1) it can generate flow outputs of 2 to 8 L/min for total cardiac support of the patient, (2) the operational modes can be adjusted and timed to allow for weaning of the device and loading the ventricle if there is ventricular recovery, (3) the device

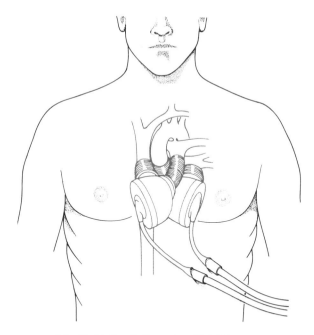

Fig. 12-14 Jarvik-7 total artificial heart.

and consists of two separate ventricles, each with a polyurethane blood sac and a rigid polysulfone case. The ventricles can deliver a 70 ml stroke volume and are driven by compressed carbon dioxide that reaches the heart through externalized drive lines. Each ventricle works independently: The left ventricle is programmed to maintain a predetermined arterial pressure and the right ventricle is regulated by the left atrial pressure. The Penn State heart was implanted in two patients: the first patient died of fungal sepsis 17 days after insertion; the second patient died 13 months after insertion — it was not possible to obtain a suitable donor for him because of the presence of preformed antibodies.[75]

Jarvik-7 and Jarvik 7-70. The two most commonly used artificial hearts are the Jarvik-7 total artificial heart and the Jarvik-7-70 or "mini-Jarvik" (manufactured by Symbion, Inc.) (Fig. 12-14). The Jarvik-7 is a pneumatically powered device that consists of two separate prosthetic ventricles connected to an external drive unit by percutaneous tubes.[76] The ventricles are roughly spherical in shape and are made of

segmented polyurethane. Pulses of compressed air displace a flexible diaphragm that is composed of Biomer. Movement of the diaphragm empties the ventricles. The control of cardiac output with the Jarvik-7 device is based on a variable stroke volume; pumping parameters are set so that there is incomplete filling of the ventricles with each beat, but complete emptying occurs. The major determinant of pump filling is atrial pressure; increased cardiac preload will result in increased cardiac output.

The maximum stroke volume of the Jarvik-7 heart is 100 ml, but the smaller scale device (Jarvik-7-70) has been used, and it delivers a 70 ml stroke volume. The advantages of the total artificial heart are (1) physiologic circulatory control, (2) potential flow volumes of 12 L/min, and (3) complete cardiac replacement that does not interfere with the anastomoses of the donor heart. The disadvantages of the total artificial heart are (1) expense, (2) availability limited to selected centers, (3) a required high dose of anticoagulation medication, (4) risk of thromboembolism, and (5) size of the device not suited for all candidates.

NURSING CARE OF THE PATIENT WITH MECHANICAL CIRCULATORY SUPPORT

The patient with a mechanical assist device who is awaiting cardiac transplant offers a unique challenge to the critical care nurse. The goals of care are to prevent thromboembolism, infection, and pulmonary complications; provide adequate nutrition for tissue healing; assess neurologic status; and offer emotional support to the patient and family. In addition, measures must be taken to prevent the formation of cytotoxic antibodies with the administration of blood products to maintain the patient's candidacy for heart transplant.

Anticoagulation

The anticoagulation regimens used in patients with mechanical assist devices implanted vary among institutions. Most patients who are in the operating room are fully heparinized at the time of insertion, with reversal of anticoagulation with protamine sulfate (while still in the operating room). Prolonged cardiopulmonary bypass time and multiple cannulation sites in the heart and great vessels make bleeding a common complication.[77] Ventricular assist systems that are designed to require little or no anticoagulation, such as Novacor and Thoratec, are advantageous; however, thromboembolism remains a potential problem because of the large artificial surface (blood sac) that comes into contact with blood. Coagulation studies (including partial thromboplastin time, prothrombin time, and fibrinogen and platelet count) should be monitored every 6 hours for the first 24 hours and then daily. At least 2 units of whole blood should be in the blood bank at all times in case of bleeding complications. Blood product replacement should be with either washed cells or leukopore-filtered cells to prevent the formation of antibodies that could complicate finding a suitable donor. In addition, if a decrease in platelet count occurs, necessitating platelet transfusion, only HLA-type specific platelets should be used. Some centers currently have available special platelet filters that prevent antibody formation. The use of cryoprecipitate and vitamin K should be avoided because of the risk of clot formation in the ventricular assist devices. Typically, patients receive no anticoag-ulants for at least 48 hours postoperatively to allow postoperative bleeding to subside. Thereafter some patients receive low-molecular-weight dextran at 25 ml/hr to prevent blood stasis, whereas others receive continuous intravenous heparin infusions. If the patient is able to be extubated and is taking oral medication, he may be switched to warfarin at a dosage that maintains a prothrombin time of 1.5 times preoperative baseline levels. Currently improved anticoagulation regimens have been under investigation, and therapy varies among centers and types of devices.

Infection

Potential infection is a great concern in bridging the patient to transplant, because an infection could preclude transplantation.[78] Some centers use protective isolation techniques with the patient and use the circulatory air flow ICU rooms normally designated for transplant patients. Strict aseptic techniques are used during all dressing changes, frequent handwashing with bactericidal solution is recommended, and visitors and traffic in and out of the patient's room are minimized. Daily leukocyte count is checked, temperature is monitored every 2 hours, and cultures are done (blood, urine and sputum) for a patient with a temperature of 38.3° C. Prophylactic antibiotic coverage is usually given for the first 3 days. Additional antibiotic coverage is considered if the patient has had a prolonged hospitalization or required surgical reexploration. Prevention is the best way to minimize or avoid infection and presents a daily challenge to the ICU nurse.

Nutrition

It has been demonstrated that nutrition plays a vital role in the acutely ill patient both in wound healing and the reduction of potential infection.[79] At some centers, total parenteral nutrition is begun within 48 hours after the insertion of the device. Tube feedings in the immediate postoperative phase are not recommended, because gastric absorption is questionable. Once the patient is extubated, a full liquid diet is started and progressed as tolerated. Total parenteral nutritional support may be discontinued once oral caloric intake is adequate.

Additional snacks and high-calorie protein drinks may be helpful.

Pulmonary care

The postoperative goal after a mechanical assist device is implanted is early extubation. Once the patient is hemodynamically stable and postoperative bleeding has stabilized, efforts are made to extubate the patient. Once spontaneous respiratory parameters and adequate arterial blood gases are achieved, the patient can be extubated. Close attention to breath sounds at regular monitoring intervals should be made by the ICU nurse. Changes in condition that could indicate atelectasis, pulmonary emboli, early congestive heart failure, or pulmonary edema may be indicative of potential alteration in cardiac output related to the device parameters. Once extubated, the patient can be turned, and deep breathing every 1 to 2 hours should be encouraged. Care must be taken to splint the chest to prevent discomfort and dislodging the cannulas of the assist device.

Neurologic assessment

Because of the problems with thromboembolic strokes with total heart implantation, frequent neurologic checks (using the Glasgow Coma Scale) are continual nursing observations that should be made at least every 2 hours. Level of consciousness may be impaired by sedation, hypoxia, decreased cardiac output, or cerebral emboli. The nurse's careful observations are important for detecting early changes in cerebral function.[80]

Patient and family support

Dependency on a mechanical assist device places great emotional strain on the patient and family members. The critical needs for stabilization of bleeding, adequate oxygenation, pain relief, and device monitoring in the immediate postoperative period are often replaced by feelings of frustration and helplessness by the patient and team members if the patient requires assistance for prolonged periods while awaiting transplant. The presence of a large console and other support equipment in the patient's room can be frightening and intimidating to family members as well as the patient.

Incisional pain and immobility can contribute to the patient's frustrations. The relationship between the nurse and the patient and family can contribute positively to emotional well-being. Therapeutic communication, opportunities for family visits, and minimalization of noise and distraction can contribute to a positive environment for the assist device patient. Friends, as well as representatives of chaplain services and psychiatry and social services may also provide needed support for the patient and family.

RESULTS AND FUTURE DIRECTIONS

One of the largest experiences using ventricular assist devices for bridge procedures has been with the Pierce-Donachy pump. Early results have been excellent.[70] As of December 1988, 75 patients had received a Pierce-Donachy assist device; 54 of these had received transplants and 45 of these had survived.[81] As of December 1989, 59 patients had received the Novacor left ventricular assist device; 33 of these patients were bridged to transplant and 28 are currently alive. The longest bridge to transplant was 163 days, and the longest survivor after transplantation is 64 months.[82] The clinical updates (as of December 1989) of the Jarvik-7 and the Jarvik 7-70 total artificial heart revealed 155 patients had received a Jarvik total artificial heart; 111 of these had been bridged to transplant. There are 80 patients who were bridged to transplant who have survived 30 days after transplant.[83] The Thermedics and Biomedicus devices have also been used successfully in bridge to transplant procedures.[81,84]

Animal trials of permanent implantable ventricular assist devices are underway at several centers. Clinical trials of implantable ventricular assist devices will probably be undertaken within the next 5 years. In addition to being used for bridge procedures, they will also be used as permanent implantable support systems.[84]

SUMMARY

Mechanical circulatory assistance before cardiac transplantation is still considered a new clinical field. It is too soon to draw definitive conclusions; however, early results are encouraging for bridge to transplant procedures using ventricular assist devices and the total artificial heart. Results of bridge to transplant procedures must be carefully studied, and justification for the required cost, personnel hours, research efforts, and institutional commitment can only be made after careful examination of the data. Review of results of bridge to transplant compared with results of transplant achieved for those individuals not requiring mechanical assistance will ultimately be the justification for continued endeavors in the mechanical circulatory assist field.

REFERENCES

1. Funk M (1986). Heart transplantation: postoperative care during the acute period. *Critical Care Nurse, 6*(2), 27-44.
2. Myerowitz PD (1987). The history of heart transplantation. In Myerowitz PD (ed). *Heart transplantation* (p 1-18). New York: Futura Publishing Co, Inc.
3. McGregor C, Oyer P and Shumway N (1986). *Heart and heart-lung transplantation. Progress in Allergy, 38,* 346-365.
4. Frazier O and Cooley D (1986). Cardiac transplantation. *Surgical Clinics of North America, 66*(3), 477-489.
5. Levett J and Karp R (1985). Heart transplantation. *Surgical Clinics of North America, 65*(3), 613-635.
6. Slater AD, Klein J and Gray L (1987). Clinical orthotopic cardiac transplantation. *American Journal of Surgery, 153,* 582-593.
7. Firth B (1987). Southwestern Internal Medicine Conference: Replacement of the failing heart. *American Journal of the Medical Sciences, 293*(1), 50-65.
8. Andreone P, Olivari M and Ring W (1987). Clinical considerations of cardiac transplantation in organ transplantation. *Radiologic Clinics of North America, 25*(2), 357-366.
9. Copeland J, Emery R, Levinson M, Icenogle T, Carrier M, Ott R, Copeland J, Rhenman M and Nicholson S (1987). Selection of patients for cardiac transplantation. *Circulation, 75*(1), 2-9.
10. Heck C, Shumway S and Kaye M (1989). The Registry of the International Society for Heart Transplantation: Sixth Official Report – 1989. *Journal of Heart Transplantation, 8*(4), 271-256.
11. Schroeder J and Hunt S (1987). Cardiac transplantation: update 1987. *Journal of the American Medical Association, 258*(21), 3142-3145.
12. US General Accounting Office: Shikles J, Schnupp A and Hogberg R (1989). Heart transplants – concerns about cost, access, and availability of donor organs. *Report to the Chairman, Subcommittee on Health, Committee on Ways and Means, House of Representatives,* 1-44.
13. Copeland JG. Personal communication. November 10, 1988.
14. Carrier M, Emery R, Riley J, Levinson M and Copeland J (1986). Cardiac transplantation in patients over 50 years of age. *Journal of the American College of Cardiology, 8*(2), 285-288.
15. Hardesty R (1988). Heart transplantation at the University of Pittsburgh: 1980 to 1987. *Transplantation Proceedings, 20*(1) Suppl 1:737-740.
16. US Senate Special Committee on Aging (1987-1988). *Aging America – trends and projections.* US Department of Health and Human Services.
17. Nicholson S (1987). Uncertainty in cardiac transplant recipients prior to and after cardiac catheterization. Unpublished master's thesis, University of Arizona, 1-76.
18. Myerowitz PD (1987). Selection and management of the heart transplant recipient. In Myerowitz PD (ed). *Heart transplantation* (pp 73-88). New York: Futura Publishing Co, Inc.
19. Hunt SA (1987). Selection, evaluation and preoperative management of heart and heart-lung recipients. In Gullucci V et al (eds). *Heart and heart-lung transplantation update* (pp 27-31). Italy: Uses Edizioni Scientifiche Firenze.
20. Copeland J (1988). Cardiac transplantation. *Current Problems in Cardiology, 13*(3), 163-224.
21. Copeland J (1984). Heart transplantation: modern techniques in surgery – cardiac thoracic surgery. New York: Futura Publishing Company, Inc., 66, 1-18.
22. Goldstein J (1985). Heart transplantation. *Investigative Radiology, 20*(5), 446-454.
23. McGregor C (1987). Current state of heart transplantation. *British Journal of Hospital Medicine,* April, 310-318.
24. Whitman G and Hicks L (1988). Major nursing diagnoses following cardiac transplantation. *Journal of Cardiovascular Nursing, 2*(2), 1-10.
25. Murray K and Howanitz EP (1987). Perioperative and postoperative management of the heart transplant patient. In Myerowitz PD (ed). *Heart transplantation* (pp 169-218). New York: Futura Publishing Co, Inc.
26. Billingham ME (1987). Histological monitoring of acute rejection and other pathological aspects of the transplanted heart. In Gullucci V et al (eds). *Heart and heart-lung transplantation update* (pp 123-131). Italy: Uses Edizioni Scientifiche Firenze.
27. Murdock D, Collins E, Lawless C, Molnar Z, Scanlon P and Pifarre R (1987). Rejection of the transplanted heart. *Heart and Lung, 16*(3), 237-245.
28. Copeland JG, Emery R, Levinson M, Icenogle R, Riley J, McAleer M, Copeland J and Dietz R (1986). Cyclosporine: an immunosuppressive panacea? *Journal of Cardiovascular Surgery, 91,* 26.
29. Billingham MD (1981). Diagnosis of cardiac rejection by endomyocardial biopsy. *Heart Transplantation, 1*(1), 25-30.
30. Caves P, Stinson Billingham M and Shumway N (1974). Serial transvenous biopsy of the transplanted human heart. *Lancet,* May, 821-826.
31. Carrier M, Russell D, Wild J, Emery R and Copeland J (1987). Prolactin as a marker of rejection in human heart transplantation. *Journal of Heart Transplantation, 6*(5), 290.

32. Guthaner D, Schnittger I, Wright A and Wexler L (1987). Diagnostic challenges following cardiac transplantation. *Radiologic Clinics of North America, 25*(2), 367-376.

33. Myerowitz PD and Gilbert E (1987). Myocardial biopsy following heart transplantation. In Myerowitz PD (ed). *Heart transplantation* (pp 219-238). New York: Futura Publishing Co, Inc.

34. Hamill R and Maki D (1987). Infectious complications of heart transplantation. In Myerowitz PD (ed). *Heart Transplantation* (pp 309-338). New York: Futura Publishing Co, Inc.

35. Carpenito L (1987). Nursing diagnosis – application to clinical practice. Philadelphia: JB Lippincott Co.

36. Icenogle T and Copeland J (1987). Emergency evaluation of the acutely ill heart transplant patient. *Boswell Hospital Proceedings, XIII*(1), 10-16.

37. Losman J (1983). Heart transplantation: a challenge for the eighties. *Acta Cardiologica, 38*(3), 163-182.

38. Wulff K and Hong P (1982). Surgical intervention for coronary artery disease. In Underhill S et al (eds). *Cardiac nursing* (pp 338-354). Philadelphia: JB Lippincott Co.

39. Gordon M (1987). Manual of nursing diagnosis. New York: McGraw-Hill Book Co.

40. Kim M, McFarland G and McLane A (1989). Nursing diagnoses. St. Louis: The CV Mosby Co.

41. Allender J, Shisslak C, Kaszniak A and Copeland J (1983). Stages of psychological adjustment associated with heart transplantation. *Heart Transplantation, 2*(3), 228-231.

42. Christopherson L (1976). Cardiac transplant: preparation for dying or for living. *Health and Social Work, 1*(1), 58-72.

43. Christopherson L (1987). Cardiac transplantation: a psychological perspective. *Circulation, 75*(1), 57-62.

44. Baldwin J and Stinson E (1985). Quality of life after cardiac transplantation. *Quality of Life and Cardiovascular Care, 1*(7), 332-335.

45. Gaudiani V, Stinson E, Alderman E, Hunt S, Schroeder J, Perlroth M, Bieber C, Oyer P, Reitz D, Jamieson S, Christopherson L and Shumway N (1981). Long-term survival and function after cardiac transplantation. *Annals of Surgery, 194*(4), 381-385.

46. Lough M (1988). Quality of life for heart transplant recipients. *Journal of Cardiovascular Nursing, 2*(2), 11-22.

47. Lough M, Lindsey A, Shinn J and Stotts N (1985). Life satisfaction following heart transplantation. *Heart Transplantation, 4*(4), 446-449.

48. Lough M, Lindsey A, Shinn J and Stotts N (1987). Impact of symptom frequence and symptom distress on self-reported quality of life in heart transplant recipients. *Heart and Lung, 16*(2), 193-200.

49. Lough M (1986). Quality of life issues following heart transplantation. *Progress in Cardiovascular Nursing, 1,* 17-23.

50. Mishel M and Murdaugh C (1987). Family adjustment to heart transplantation: redesigning the dream. *Nursing Research, 36*(6), 332-38.

51. Meister N, McAleer MJ, Meister J, Riley J and Copeland J (1986). Returning to work after heart transplantation. *Journal of Heart Transplantation, 5*(2), 154-161.

52. United Network for Organ Sharing (1990). *UNOS Update, 6*(1), 11.

53. Swerdlow JL (1989). *Matching needs, saving lives.* Washington, DC: The Annenberg Washington Program.

54. Lindbergh C (1976). *History of medicine.* New York: Simon & Schuster, Inc.

55. Gibbon HJ, Jr (1954). Application of a mechanical heart and lung apparatus to cardiac surgery. *Minnesota Medicine, 37,* 171.

56. Stuckey JH, Newman MN, Dennis C et al (1957). The use of the heart-lung machine in selected cases of acute myocardial infarction. *Surgical Forum, 8,* 342-344.

57. Spencer FC, Eisman B, Trinkle JK and Rossi NP (1965). Assisted circulation for cardiac failure following intra-cardiac surgery with cardiopulmonary bypass. *Journal of Thoracic and Cardiovascular Surgery, 49,* 56-73.

58. Cooley DA, Liotta D, Hollman GL, Bloodwell RD, Leachman RD and Milam JD (1978). First human implantation of a cardiac prosthesis for staged total replacement of the heart. *Transplantation American Society of Artificial Internal Organs, 24,* 252-259.

59. Reemtsma K, Drusin R, Edie R, Bregman D, Dobelle W and Hardy M (1978). Cardiac transplantation for patients requiring mechanical circulatory support. *New England Journal of Medicine, 298,* 670-671.

60. DeVries WC, Anderson JL, Joyce LD, Anderson SL, Hammond EH, Jarvik RK and Kolff WJ (1984). Clinical use of the total artificial heart. *New England Journal of Medicine, 310,* 273-278.

61. Magovern JA and Pierce WS (1990). Mechanical circulatory assistance before heart transplantation. In Baumgartner WA, Reitz BA and Achuff S (eds). *Heart and heart-lung transplantation.* Philadelphia: WB Saunders Co.

62. Copeland JG, Levinson MM, Smith R et al (1986). The total artificial heart as a bridge to transplantation: a report of two cases. *Journal of the American Medical Association, 256,* 2991-2998.

63. Portner PM, Oyer PE, McGregor CG, Baldwin JC, Ream AK, Wyner J, Zusman DR and Shumway YE (1985). First human use of an electrically powered implantable ventricular assist system. *Artificial Organs 9*(A), 36.

64. Hill JD, Farrar DJ, Hershon JJ, Compton TG, Avery GJ, Levin BS and Brent BN (1986). Use of a prosthetic ventricle as a bridge to cardiac transplantation for post-infarction cardiogenic shock. *New England Journal of Medicine, 314,* 626-628.

65. Kanter KR, Ruzevich SA, Pennington DG, McBride LR, Swartz BA and Willman VL (1988). Follow-up of survivors of mechanical circulatory support. *Journal of Thoracic and Cardiovascular Surgery, 96*(1), 72-80.

66. National Heart, Lung and Blood Institute (1980). Mechanical assisted circulation: report of the NHLBI Advisory Council working on organ circulatory assistance and artificial heart. Bethesda MD: Author.

67. Pelletier LC, Pomar JC, Bosch Y, Galinanes M and Hebert Y (1986). Complications of circulatory assistance with intra-aortic balloon pumping: a comparison of surgical and percutaneous techniques. *Heart Transplantation, 5,* 138-142.

68. Weintraum RM and Thurer RL (1983). The intra-aortic balloon pump — a ten year experience. *Heart Transplantation, 3,* 8-15.

69. Olivier Jr JF, Maher TD, Liebler GA, Park SB, Burkholder JA and Magovern GJ (1984). The use of the Biomedicus centrifugal pump in traumatic tears of the thoracic aorta. *Annals of Thoracic Surgery, 38,* 586-591.

70. Pennington DG, Samuals LD, Williams G, Palmer D, Swartz MT, Codd JE, Merjavy JP, Langunulf D and Joist JH (1985). Experience with the Pierce-Donachy ventricular assist device in postcardiotomy patients with cardiogenic shock. *World Journal of Surgery, 9,* 37-46.

71. Farrar DJ, Hill JD, Gray LA Jr, Pennington DG, McBride LR, Pierce WS, Pae WE, Glenville BF, Russ DF, Galbraith TA and Zumbro GL (1988). Heterotopic prostatic ventricles as a bridge to cardiac transplantation: A multicenter trial in 29 patients. *New England Journal of Medicine 318,* 333-340.

72. Novacor 100A left ventricular assist system operator's manual. 7799 Paradee Lane, Oakland, CA 1983.

73. Magovern JA, Pae WE, Richenbacher WE and Pierce WS (1986). The importance of a patent foramen ovale in left ventricular assist pumping. *Transplantation: American Society of Artificial Internal Organs, 32,* 449-453.

74. Pierce WS, Gray LA Jr, McBride LR and Fraier OH (1989). Other postoperative complications (Panel 4). *Annals of Thoracic Surgery, 47,* 96-102.

75. Magovern JA and Pierce WS (1990). Mechanical circulatory assistance before heart transplantation. In Baumgartner WA, Reitz BA and Achuff S (eds). *Heart and heart-lung transplantation* (p 76). Philadelphia: WB Saunders Co.

76. DeVries WC and Joyce LD (1983). The artificial heart. *Clinical Symposia, 35*(6), 4-32.

77. Reedy JE, Ruzevich SA, Swartz MT, Termulen DF and Pennington DG (1989). Nursing care of a patient receiving prolonged mechanical circulatory support. *Progress in Cardiovascular Nursing, 4,* 1-9.

78. McBride LR, Ruzevich SA, Pennington DG, Kennedy DJ, Kanter KR, Miller LW, Swartz MT and Termulen DF (1987). Infectious complications associated with ventricular assist device support. *American Society for Artificial Internal Organs and Transplantation, 33,* 201-202.

79. Heart diseases (1988). In Kinney JM, Jeejeehboy KN, Hill GL and Owen OE (eds). *Nutrition and metabolism in patient care* (pp 477-509). Philadelphia: WB Saunders Co.

80. Mulford E (1987). Nursing perspectives for the patient receiving postoperative ventricular assistance in the critical care unit. *Heart and Lung, 16,* 246-255.

81. Farrar DJ, Lawson JH, Litwak P and Lederwall G (1989). The thoracic VAD system as a bridge to transplantation. *Journal of Heart Transplantation, 8*(A), 86.

82. Novacor Annual Report: *Clinical update.* January 2, 1990, Oakland, CA.

83. Symbion Clinical Update: *A current report on use of the Symbion J7-100 and J7-70 (TAH) as a bridge to transplant.* December 1, 1989. Tempe, AZ.

84. Hill JD. Bridging to cardiac transplant (1989). *Annals of Thoracic Surgery, 47,* 167-171.

13

Heart-Lung Transplantation

Thomas S. Ahrens and Catherine Powers

The chronic diseases disturbing lung function have remained, despite impressive medical advances, some of the most difficult diseases to treat. Diagnosis of many chronic diseases of the lung are frequently synonymous with progressive, debilitating prognoses. Current treatments are almost exclusively palliative. At the center of these types of pulmonary diseases are diseases of the parenchyma (e.g., chronic obstructive diseases such as chronic bronchitis, emphysema, and various types of fibrotic conditions, including cystic and interstitial fibrosis). In addition to the parenchymal diseases, disturbances of the pulmonary vasculature exist (e.g., primary and secondary pulmonary hypertension). No available curative treatment exists for persons with these conditions. Frequent exacerbations of the primary problem, eventually resulting in a terminal event, results in a difficult life for people unfortunate enough to have one of these conditions.

Complicating the pulmonary problem is the resultant effect of the lung condition on the right side of the heart. Most persons with one of the conditions cited will develop, to some extent, right ventricular dysfunction. Although more will be presented on the cardiac problems associated with pulmonary dysfunction, it is important to consider that many patients with lung disease may die of complications of right-sided heart failure. By the time many of these patients develop symptoms, right-sided heart dysfunction may be beyond treatment. The net effect is a condition that has two organ systems failing—the heart and lungs. Definitive treatment at this point requires both heart and lung interventions.

The advent of heart-lung transplantation has offered a glimmer of hope to some of these patients.[1] At this time and for the immediate future, it will be the only definitive therapy for patients with severe pulmonary disease that has also produced right-sided heart failure.[2] Although not without problems, heart-lung transplantation has the potential to significantly improve the quality of life of persons previously severely limited in both physical and psychologic fulfillment.

To present how heart-lung transplantation plays a role in treatment of pulmonary disturbances, five aspects associated with heart-lung transplantation will be addressed. These aspects include an introduction to the pathophysiology of the origins of heart-lung dysfunction, an introduction to the reasons for heart-lung transplantation, the perioperative nursing implications of lung-heart transplantation, major technical/surgical aspects of the procedure, and future trends in heart-lung transplantation.

Considering that the primary problem requiring heart-lung transplant usually involves a pulmonary disturbance (an exception would be Eisenmenger's syndrome), the surgical procedure would more accurately be referred to as lung-heart transplant. Although this point is minor, it is more accurate in the sense of indicating that the primary pulmonary disturbance is usually the reason for the transplant procedure. For the sake of being consistent with general terminology, however, the term heart-lung transplantation will be used.

Cardiopulmonary relationships

The human cardiopulmonary system is typical of mammalian evolutionary development, which separated the left- and right-sided heart function. Reasons for the separation of the right- and left-sided heart function become obvious when considering the advantages of a dual cardiovascular system. To allow the two key gas exchange processes in human physiology, (i.e., the entrance of oxygen and elimination of carbon dioxide), the alveolar-capillary membrane had to remain thin. This kept the distance between the alveoli and capillaries short, facilitating the transfer of gases. The result of the short distance and thin alveolar capillary structures was a relatively fragile membrane. Typically, the capillaries are capable of transporting blood and keeping vascular volume inside the capillaries if excessive hydrostatic pressures are not present and osmotic pressures are normal. If pressures in the capillaries start to rise, or if osmotic pressures fall, the fragile pulmonary capillary starts to leak. The resulting leak of plasma into the interstitial pulmonary spaces increases the amount of extravascular lung water (EVLW). The elevation in EVLW results in an increase in intrapulmonary shunting, effectively making gas exchange (specifically oxygen) more difficult.

To keep pressures in the pulmonary circuit low, the cardiovascular system could have developed in one of two ways—either by keeping the pressure necessary to perfuse all organs very low or developing a circulation that would allow high pressures in some organs but keep the pulmonary pressures low. Mammalian development opted for the latter through the development of separate heart-lung circulations. The left side of the heart is capable of generating the high pressures necessary to perfuse all organs, with venous blood from these organs returning to the right side of heart. The right side pumps blood into a highly compliant pulmonary circulation and keeps pressures low enough to avoid increases in EVLW.

An interesting example of animals that have not adapted a separate right- and left-sided heart system are reptiles (Fig. 13-1). It is interesting to note that reptiles do not grow tall; they can grow long but not tall. For example,

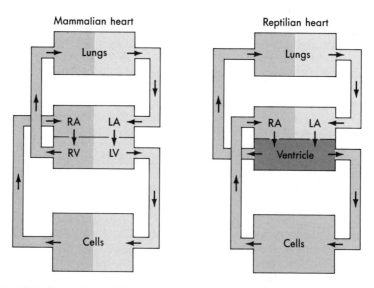

Fig. 13-1 Comparison of heart systems in mammals, *left,* and reptiles, *right.*

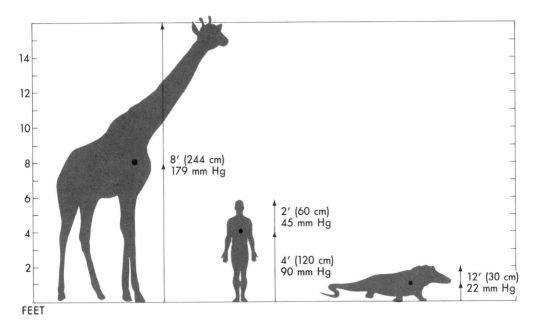

Fig. 13-2 Pressure required to overcome hydrostatic pressure and perfuse organs. • indicates position of heart.

snakes and crocodiles or alligators can achieve lengths of over 20 feet. Yet they do not grow to a height of over a few feet because of their cardiovascular systems. With some variations, reptiles generally have a common ventricular chamber.[3] The common ventricular chamber produces the same pressures in the systemic circulation as in the pulmonary circulation. This is tolerable as long as pressures in the system remain low, to avoid increasing hydrostatic pressure and increasing lung water. The common ventricular chamber of the reptile requires a small height to avoid the need to pump blood upward. If the reptile was tall, a pressure necessary to perfuse the head of the reptile would have to be generated. Such a situation would produce excessively high pressures in the lung, increasing EVLW and causing pulmonary edema. Reptiles can avoid pulmonary edema only by keeping the lung pressure low through maintaining most of the organs on a similar plane as the heart (Fig. 13-2). This allows low pressures to adequately perfuse the body while keeping low pressures in the pulmonary vasculature as well. The comparison of reptilian physiology is one way of illustrating the key advantages to the separation of the heart and lung circulations. It also allows for a good introduction to the difference between the pulmonary circulation and right-sided heart function from the systemic circulation and left-sided heart function.

EFFECTS OF LUNG DYSFUNCTION ON THE RIGHT SIDE OF THE HEART

Several circumstances will cause the pulmonary circulation to become altered. Pulmonary hypertension (including primary and secondary types as well as variations such as the Eisenmenger complex), chronic lung disease (e.g., emphysema, alpha-1-antitrypsin deficiency, chronic bronchitis, pulmonary fibrosis), patent foramen ovale, and cystic fibrosis all produce changes in pulmonary pressures, although for various reasons. A brief review of each will illustrate the deterioration of both the heart and lungs that accompanies these conditions.

The important concept to bear in mind during this review is the similarities between all problems of pulmonary induced right ventricular failure. The primary similarity is the high pressure (resistance) faced by the right ventricle as it tries to eject blood into the pulmonary circulation. The high pulmonary pressure causes right ventricular compensation by hypertrophy and dilation. Eventually, however, right ventricular failure results. Manifestations of right ventricular failure include systemic venous engorgement, including hepatic and renal congestion and dependent edema.[4] As the right side of the heart continues to fail, less blood will be ejected to the left side of the heart. The result will be left ventricular hypovolemia, eventually leading to hypovolemic hypotension. As each of the primary conditions amenable to heart-lung transplantation is reviewed, keep in mind the similarity in all clinical presentations.

Pulmonary hypertension

Pulmonary hypertension can be categorized into three types: primary, secondary active, and secondary passive.[5] Primary pulmonary hypertension has no known cause. Secondary pulmonary hypertension has a probable origin. Secondary active pulmonary hypertension is associated with known problems of pulmonary circulation (i.e., hypoxic alveolar vasoconstriction or obstruction of blood flow [pulmonary emboli]). Secondary passive pulmonary hypertension differs from the other two forms of hypertension in that it is in response to left ventricular failure. Both primary and secondary active pulmonary hypertension produce elevated pulmonary pressures as a result of loss of vascular distensibility (for reasons largely unclear at present) and space (as a result of destruction of capillaries). Pulmonary hypertension, while some differences in the literature exist, is generally defined as a mean pulmonary artery pressure (PAP) greater than 25 mm Hg. In addition to the pulmonary artery pressure, the pulmonary resistance may also be used in the definition of pulmonary hypertension. The most common measurement is the pulmonary vascular resistance (PVR). Normal values are

40 to 150 dynes/sec/cm^5. Two other forms of resistance measurement may be used—the pulmonary vascular resistance index (PVRI) and Wood units. PVRI uses cardiac index instead of cardiac output in the PVR calculation. The normal PVRI is between 200 and 300 dynes/sec/cm^5. Wood units, a value obtained by not multiplying by 80 in the PVR formula to convert to dynes, may be used with a normal value between 0.5 and 2.0. Methods for computing measurements of pulmonary vascular resistance can be found in the box below.

In secondary passive pulmonary hypertension the pulmonary pressures elevate in an attempt to overcome the increasing pressure in the left ventricle as the left ventricle fails. To continue to push blood forward, the pulmonary artery mean pressure elevates just high enough to overcome the resistance of the diastolic pressure in the left ventricle. This is one of the most commonly seen hemodynamic disturbances, associated with virtually all types of left ventricular failure. Three characteristics are present with this type of pulmonary hypertension: (1) the pulmonary arterial diastolic (PAD) pressure is closely associated with the left ventricu-

---

MEASUREMENT OF PULMONARY RESISTANCE

Pulmonary vascular resistance formula

$$\frac{\text{Mean pulmonary artery pressure} - \text{Right atrial pressure}}{\text{Cardiac output}} \times 80$$

Normal: 40 to 150 dynes/sec/cm^5

Pulmonary vascular resistance index formula

$$\frac{\text{Mean pulmonary artery pressure} - \text{Right atrial pressure}}{\text{Cardiac index}} \times 80$$

Normal: 200 to 300 dynes/sec/cm^5

Wood units

$$\frac{\text{Mean pulmonary artery pressure} - \text{Right atrial pressure}}{\text{Cardiac output}}$$

Normal: 0.5 to 2.0 Wood units

---

lar end-diastolic pressure (LVEDP) and therefore the pulmonary capillary wedge pressure (PCWP); (2) the pulmonary arterial pressures tend to be lower than those associated with the other forms of pulmonary hypertension, because the pressure elevates just high enough to overcome the resistance provided by the LVEDP; (3) this type of pulmonary hypertension can be associated with both left- and right-sided heart failure.

Primary and secondary active pulmonary hypertension are both associated with poor outcomes with present medical treatment.[6] Pressures seen in these types are typically very high, with systolic pressures frequently exceeding 50 mm Hg and diastolic pressures over 30 mm Hg. The causes of these two types differ but the net effect on the pulmonary pressures is similar.

Primary pulmonary hypertension is a manifestation of the loss of vascular compliance. Secondary active produces hypertension from loss of compliance as well, but also from the loss of vascular space. The loss of compliance is potentially caused by hypoxic vasoconstriction secondary to low alveolar oxygen (PaO_2) levels. As alveolar air flow is diminished as a result of obstruction from secretions or collapse of airways, more oxygen is removed from the alveoli than is replaced. The PaO_2 decrease is followed by a compensatory vasoconstriction in an attempt to divert blood flow away from impaired alveoli. The result is more blood flow being forced through the rest of the lung, basically causing the same blood volume to be distributed to a smaller area. The net effect is the placing of a constant volume in a smaller space, causing an increase in pressure. This type of hypertension may respond favorably to oxygen therapy, through elevating the PaO_2.[7]

Loss of vascular space can occur in some types of chronic lung disease when alveoli become overdistended. The overdistention results in destruction of the capillaries perfusing the region. This has the same effect as mentioned earlier: forcing of the same blood volume through a smaller area. There currently is no treatment for this type of disturbance.

Primary pulmonary hypertension results in loss of compliance, making the blood vessels more resistive to flow. The resulting increase in pressure necessary to overcome the resistance is provided by the right ventricle. Regardless of the cause of the hypertension, the right ventricle must generate higher pressures to continue to move blood forward. The right side of the heart will handle this increased resistance in a manner similar to that of the left ventricle in responding to systemic hypertension. The right ventricle will hypertrophy and dilate, then eventually fail. Right ventricular stroke volume is maintained until the heart can no longer hypertrophy and dilate. Right ventricular stroke work index elevates markedly as the resistance increases. Right ventricular end-diastolic pressures elevate, producing an elevation in right atrial (and central venous) pressures. As the right ventricular stroke volume decreases, failure is manifested by the inability to move blood forward to the left ventricle. The clinical result is a loss of cardiac output from left ventricular hypovolemia secondary to the right side of the heart's inability to move blood forward.

Clinically, the patient has various degrees of respiratory distress and venous hypertension. Engorgement of the venous system results in distention of visible veins such as neck veins, peripheral and dependent edema, and weight gain secondary to venous congestion. The origin of the problem is difficult to identify—left ventricular failure producing right ventricular failure or some form of pulmonary hypertension—based on clinical signs. Cardiac catheterization is necessary to determine whether the right side of the heart alone is involved or whether biventricular failure exists.

In addition to the physical signs of right ventricular failure, exercise tolerance falls significantly. The reasons for exercise intolerance are probably related to the inability of the right side of the heart to move large enough volumes of blood into the lungs for adequate oxygenation. To maintain normal exercise tolerance, alveolar ventilation (Va), the amount of air exchanged at the alveolar level per minute, must be matched by an equal increase in right ventricular cardiac output. If either minute ventilation or cardiac output fails to keep pace with the other, inadequate oxygen transport will result and exercise intolerance will occur. Patients with pulmonary parenchymal disease (COPD) will have difficulty meeting the increased alveolar ventilation requirement. Patients with pulmonary hypertension or septal defects will have difficulty matching a Va increase with a comparable cardiac output increase.

Other diseases associated with the need for heart-lung transplantation will produce the same problems as just described. Cystic fibrosis, for example, another entity producing right-sided heart failure, does so by increasing resistance to blood flow. The increased resistance to blood flow is caused by the loss of blood vessels as airways dilate as a result of airway obstruction. In this respect cystic fibrosis is similar to chronic lung disease. The resulting right ventricular failure secondary to the increased resistance results in right-sided heart dysfunction similar to pulmonary hypertension. Although symptoms may be present before the development of right-sided heart failure, primarily as a result of the initial pulmonary problem, any condition associated with high pulmonary resistance can lead to right-sided heart failure. Symptomatology of right ventricular failure associated with pulmonary disease includes central vein distention, cyanosis, dysrhythmias, chest pain, and syncope. All these symptoms are related to intrapulmonary shunting and right-sided heart failure.

If the patient is initially seen without irreversible right ventricular failure, lung transplant alone may suffice. Whether single or double lung transplantation will be performed depends on the pulmonary disturbance.

The point at which heart-lung transplantation becomes the treatment of choice can be identified by response to medical therapy and organ function. As the patient becomes unresponsive to medical therapy and organ function is failing, heart-lung transplantation becomes the only therapeutic option.

HISTORICAL ASPECTS

The history of human organ transplantation was presented in Chapter 2; however, some aspects related to heart-lung transplantation are interesting to review. The feasibility of cardiopulmonary transplantation was explored by Demikhov in the late 1940s.[8] Demikhov was active in many types of transplants, ranging from half-body (Fig. 13-3) to heart-lung transplants. His earliest successful investigation of heart-lung transplan-

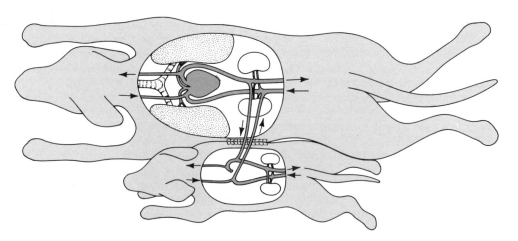

Fig. 13-3 Scheme for joining a puppy to an adult dog. After removal of its heart and lungs, the puppy is sutured to the vessels of a large dog. (Redrawn from Demikhov VP (1962). Experimental transplantation of vital organs. New York: Plenum Publishing Co.)

tation was in canine subjects. Demikhov achieved survival rates of greater than 5 days in 2 of 67 animals. Other early studies in the 1950s and early 1960s employed different airway anastomosis sites (tracheal instead of bronchial) but attained similar survival rates. These early attempts in the canine population were hampered by the disruption of the normal respiratory pattern once the lungs were denervated. This was manifested by a slow respiratory rate with an increased tidal volume and insufficient minute ventilation. There was concern that the same response would occur in human transplantation.

Later in the 1960s, Nakae et al[9] demonstrated in primates an ability to maintain a normal breathing pattern despite pulmonary denervation and the absence of an intact Hering-Breuer inflation reflex. This reflex in primates appeared to serve as a protective mechanism for preventing excess lung inflation rather than a control of normal ventilation. The regulation of spontaneous respiration in primates (baboons), though, is similar to that in humans (i.e., in the mid-brain region). By 1972 the 2-year survival rate in baboons had reached 20% (5 of 25 baboons).[10] This further demonstrated the ability of primates to withstand cardiopulmonary denervation. In 1980 longer survival rates in primates were reported at Stanford than had previously been reported.[11] The improved success rates were attributed largely to the use of postoperative cyclosporine to aid immunosuppression.

Jamieson et al[12] reviewed the brief history of human heart-lung transplantation and illustrated the current improvements from these early efforts. They reported on the first human transplant, initially reported in 1968 by Cooley on a 2-month-old infant with complete atrioventricular canal defect. The patient died 14 days after surgery as a result of respiratory insufficiency. The following year, Lillehei performed a heart-lung transplant on a 43-year-old man with emphysema and pulmonary hypertension. The patient died of pneumonia 8 days after transplant. Barnard performed a transplant in a 49-year-old patient with chronic obstructive pulmonary disease. This patient survived 23 days and died of pneumonia and necrosis of the bronchial anastomoses.

During the next decade several key developments aided in the feasibility of long-term survival of cardiopulmonary transplantation in humans. These included the use of Cyclosporin A, introduction of rabbit antithymocyte globulin, and endomyocardial biopsy techniques for diagnosis of cardiac rejection. These events, plus better patient selection techniques, improved perioperative management, and closer immunologic monitoring, have all contributed to increased human survival rates.

In 1981 Stanford University initiated a heart-lung transplant program that has since served as the most active heart-lung transplant program in the United States. The first procedure was performed on a 46-year-old woman with primary pulmonary hypertension. While this patient did well postoperatively, early survival rates were encouraging but relatively low: 5 of the first 17 died (29%). Survival rates are rapidly improving, however—from 1986 through 1987, survival was 62% at 1 year after transplant and 61% and 2 years.[13] Reasons for death are primarily infections, rejection, and heart failure.

The number of heart-lung transplants has rapidly increased since the early 1980s. From 1981 to 1989, 501 transplants were performed.[14] Major centers include Stanford, Pittsburgh, and London. However, many centers will now perform heart-lung transplants given the appropriate circumstances. Technical and medical support is available at several centers, although the majority of transplants are still performed at the major centers.

PERIOPERATIVE PERIOD
Preoperative management

A preoperative rehabilitation program can be used to increase the patient's strength and endurance. A typical preoperative exercise program includes treadmill walking, stationary bicycling, light weight-training, and calisthenics. At some centers preoperative exercise training is encouraged to optimize the patient's functional ability, physical exercise tolerance, and emotional well-being during a difficult waiting period. The potential for improvement in overall function by participating in an individually tailored exercise program may enable the patient to handle the actual surgery and the immediate postoperative period with less difficulty.

Psychosocial support group meetings can also be of value during this difficult waiting period. These meetings are generally coordinated by a team consisting of physicians, nurses, social worker, physical therapist, dietitian, and transplant coordinator. Potential recipients and their families can meet to discuss common concerns, ask questions, and explore feelings about their future.

Medical clinic visits are also an important component of preoperative management of patients awaiting heart-lung transplantation. The recipient must be brought to optimal medical condition in the preoperative period to aid in postoperative recovery. The medical management team generally consists of a cardiologist, pulmonologist, psychiatrist, and the cardiothoracic transplant surgeon. Medical clinic visits are usually conducted bimonthly or more often if the patient's condition warrants closer supervision.

Another method to assist in preparing the patient and family for transplantation is educational sessions on concepts of immunosuppression and the importance of compliance to the medical regimen, relaxation techniques, the need for organ donation awareness in the general public, and alterations in life-style that the transplant recipient faces postoperatively. Tours of the intensive care unit and nursing divisions can be helpful by increasing the patient's familiarity with the transplant area and health care team members.

The preoperative period can be extremely difficult for patients and their families. Candidates may feel they are "working against the clock" as their disease further incapacitates them. This is one reason that physiologic and psychosocial support must be an integral part of their preoperative care.

Donor criteria: selection of the donor

Many of the criteria for heart-lung donors are similar to those for any transplant donor.

SPECIFIC DONOR CRITERIA FOR HEART-LUNG TRANSPLANTS

No thoracic trauma (penetrating chest injury or lung contusion)
No history of pulmonary or cardiac disease (ECG normal)
No evidence of pulmonary or systemic infection
Insignificant smoking history
Pao_2 more than 90 mm Hg with Fio_2 0.40 and PEEP <5 cm H_2O
Pao_2 more than 350 mm Hg with Fio_2 1.0 and PEEP 0
Peak inspiratory pressure <20 cm H_2O with tidal volume 15 ml/kg and normal blood gases
Sputum negative for gram stain and culture
Fiberoptic bronchoscopy (optional)
Chest measurements compatible with potential recipient
    Sternal notch to xiphoid
    Sternal notch to acromial process
    Chest circumference at fourth intercostal space (expiration)
    Chest circumference in maximum arch (expiration)
    Axilla to costal arch in midaxillary line
    Clavicle to costal arch in midclavicular line

However, some exeptions exist in the case of heart-lung transplant patients. These are listed in the box above.

In addition to the aforementioned criteria, successful matching between donor and recipient includes ABO blood group compatibility and, at times, a negative lymphocyte crossmatch.

The principal limiting factor to expanding the number of heart-lung transplants is the scarcity of donors. Even when a potential donor meets the criteria, brain death is frequently associated with complicating factors such as neurogenic pulmonary edema, thoracic trauma, gastric aspiration, and pulmonary infection. Therefore the donor must be managed carefully to protect the lungs from infection, atelectasis, aspiration of gatric contents, and the resulting complications of neurogenic pulmonary edema.

Surgical considerations for the donor

Based on the findings of the early investigators of cardiopulmonary transplantation, cardiopulmonary evisceration must be accomplished without damaging the phrenic, recurrent laryngeal, and vagus nerves. Meticulous attention must also be paid to hemostatic control of the enlarged bronchial and mediastinal collateral vessels in the recipient.

The donor operation may or may not be carried out in the same institution as the recipient operation.[15] Initial attempts at pulmonary artery flushing were not successful, limiting transplants to regional donors.[16] Cooling of the heart-lung bloc was the primary method of organ recovery at this time, although some success was achieved with autoperfusion and ventilation while the heart-lung bloc was immersed in ice water. Recent advances have allowed for long-distance organ recovery to become possible. Primary among these techniques is the pulmonary artery flush technique with greater emphasis on achieving adequate cooling of the bloc.[15]

The donor is premedicated with steroids and broad-spectrum antibiotics. A median sternotomy is performed, followed by an anterior pericardiectomy. The donor is then heparinized and cannulation of the right atrial appendage and the transverse aorta takes place. The donor is then cooled by perfusate. If the heart fibrillates, a left ventricular apical vent is placed. The innominate artery, the ascending aorta, the inferior vena cava (IVC), and the superior vena cava (SVC) are isolated. The trachea is isolated and encircled high, between the SVC and the aorta. The pleural cavities are opened and the inferior pulmonary ligaments and the mediastinal pleura are divided over the esophagus on the right and the aorta on the left. The SVC is doubly ligated and divided. The IVC is also divided. The aorta is then cross-clamped and 500 ml of cardioplegic solution is infused. The aorta is divided above the cross clamp. The trachea is clamped and divided at least five rings above the carina, and the heart-lung bloc is removed. The heart-lung bloc is then immersed in cold (4° C) solution and transported to the recipient institution.

Surgical considerations for the recipient

According to those experienced in the recipient operation, the most technically challenging aspect is the excision of the recipient's heart and lungs.[17] To aid in visualization of the nerves and vessels that must remain intact, the heart is excised first, followed by each lung separately.

Preparation for the recipient operation generally includes a routine shave and prep with betadine and premedication with azathioprine, cyclosporine, antilymphoblast globulin (MALG), and broad-spectrum antibiotics. This routine varies from institution to institution, depending on physician preference and/or protocol. The patient is intubated under sterile conditions and a PA catheter, if it is to be used, is placed. All blood products to be administered during the operation should go through a warmer on a 20-micron filter.

During the operative procedure a median sternotomy and pericardectomy are performed. The thymic fat is removed and the pleural spaces are opened and pleural adhesions divided. The ascending aorta and both cavae are cannulated through the right atrium. The heart is then removed. A left phrenic pedicle is created and the left lung is removed. Creation of a right phrenic pedicle and removal of the right lung follows. The trachea is then exposed and transected just above the carina. The donor heart-lung bloc is sewn in with three anastomoses: the trachea, the right atrium, and the aorta. Some surgeons prefer at this point to draw the omentum up into the chest and completely wrap it around the tracheal anastomosis to protect and revascularize the area (Fig. 13-4).

The patient is then ventilated gently with a low FiO_2 and is weaned from cardiopulmonary bypass using isoproterenol (Isuprel) to maintain a heart rate of 100 beats per minute. Drainage tubes are placed in the pericardial and pleural cavities, and the chest is closed.

One of the major intraoperative complications during the recipient operation has been bleeding, because these patients are fully heparinized and on bypass. In addition, some patients (e.g., those with Eisenmenger's syndrome) have greatly enlarged bronchial arteries

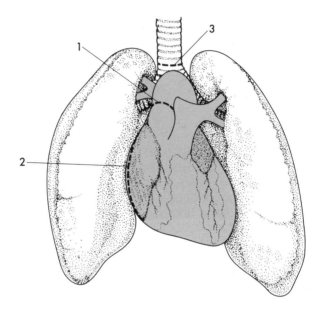

Fig. 13-4 Anastomotic sites in heart-lung transplantation. *1,* Aorta; *2,* right atria; and *3,* trachea.

that tend to bleed profusely when the lungs are removed. These arteries need to be carefully secured before the donor organs are implanted. In addition, patients with pleural or pericardial adhesions are prone to bleeding when scar tissue has to be removed. As scar tissue is excised, a raw and bleeding surface is exposed. Because of problems with bleeding, it is prudent to ensure absolute hemostasis before implanting the donor organs.

POSTOPERATIVE MANAGEMENT
General principles

Postoperative care of the heart-lung transplant recipient incorporates various aspects of critical care management, including hemodynamic monitoring and support, continuance of immunosuppression, chest physiotherapy (e.g., pulmonary toilet), fiberoptic bronchoscopy, and patient education (including discharge planning).

After stabilization in the operating room, the heart-lung transplant recipient is moved directly to the intensive care unit (ICU). A 2:1 nurse-patient ratio for the first 12 to 16 hours is often

necessary because of the need for frequent measurement of vital signs, hemodynamic monitoring, initiation of chest physiotherapy, and the complexity of medication administration in the immediate postoperative period. The nurse-patient ratio is reassessed after the first 12 to 16 hours and then can often be reduced to a 1:1 ratio.

Reverse isolation may be instituted on the patient's arrival in the ICU. Reverse isolation, while not universally accepted, is designed to prevent infection with opportunistic organisms. Specific procedures vary from institution to institution, but generally personnel entering the room should adhere to strict handwashing and wear gloves and a mask. Use of reverse isolation, while perhaps not preventing organism transmission to the degree desirable, may be of value simply by having all personnel use good handwashing techniques.

Once the patient is in the ICU, the electrocardiogram and hemodynamic pressures are monitored and the patient is supported with mechanical ventilation. The use of PA catheters is not universal and depends on institutional or physician preference. The use of PA catheters is included here to present a more comprehensive postoperative picture.

A head-to-toe nursing assessment is performed after the patient enters the ICU. Baseline vital signs (heart rate, arterial blood pressure, temperature, pulmonary artery pressure, central venous pressure, and pulmonary capillary wedge pressure) and cardiac outputs are obtained. SaO_2 and SvO_2 monitoring, if used, are instituted at this point. After stabilization of the patient a 12-lead ECG, a portable chest x-ray film, and postoperative blood work are obtained. Blood work typically includes assessment of complete blood count (CBC), prothrombin time (PT), partial thromboplastin time (PTT), thrombin time, arterial blood gases (ABGs), blood urea nitrogen (BUN), SMA6, calcium, magnesium, and phosphorus values.

Mediastinal and bilateral pleural chest tubes are attached to water seal and low suction. The patient is covered with warm blankets to aid in rewarming and to prevent additional heat loss. Upper extremities are loosely restrained to prevent any movement, which may dislocate lines and tubes as the patient awakens from anesthesia.

Medications

Medication administration in the postoperative period falls into five basic pharmacologic categories: vasodilators, inotropic agents, diuretics, antibiotics, and immunosuppressive agents.

Vasodilators. Vasodilators commonly employed postoperatively for the heart-lung transplant recipient include intravenous nitroglycerine, sodium nitroprusside, and, more recently, prostaglandin E. Nitroglycerin is used at a low dose (generally 0.5 to 1.0 µg/kg/min) to prevent coronary vasospasm. Sodium nitroprusside is used to maintain an approximately normal systemic vascular resistance. Prostaglandin E may be used to titrate pulmonary vascular resistance and pulmonary artery pressures close to normal limits.

Inotropic and chronotropic support. Inotropic support is provided by dopamine, dobutamine, or isoproterenol. Dopamine is often administered at low doses (1 to 5 µg/kg/min) to improve blood flow to the kidneys and increase the glomerular filtration rate and to increase cardiac contractility to improve cardiac output. Dobutamine is primarily employed to increase the stroke volume through increasing contractility. Isoproterenol is used to maintain the patient's heart rate above 100 beats per minute and serves to support the denervated heart.[17] The denervated heart may be prone to bradycardia because of myocardial sensitivity to ischemia and because the heart is no longer responsive to direct autonomic nervous system stimulation. Epicardial pacemaker wires, placed during surgery, may be attached to a temporary pacemaker to aid in maintenance of a regular cardiac rhythm.

Diuretics. Diuretics may include furosemide (Lasix) and/or mannitol by continuous intravenous infusion. The dosage is titrated to provide for a urine output of generally greater than 50 to 100 ml per hour. Strict intake and output measurements and daily weights aid in the measurement of diuretic effectiveness. Lymphatic drainage is absent in the transplanted lungs; therefore hydration is kept as low as possible to minimize leakage of fluid into the lungs.[18] The patient's weight is often kept 3 to 5 kg below normal preoperative weight. Careful diuresis and fluid management are also used to minimize or reverse a reimplantation response of the pulmonary tissue to transplantation. Reimplantation response occurs as the result of removal, manipulation, and reimplantation of the lungs. The response causes disruption of the pulmonary lymphatic system (usually lasting 7 to 21 days), an increase in alveolar permeability, and a decrease in serum oncotic pressure. Interstitial pulmonary edema and a decrease in lung compliance are noted. Diuresis and fluid restriction for the first 2 to 3 weeks postoperatively will minimize and reverse this condition. After weaning from the furosemide and/or mannitol intravenous infusion, the patient may be given intermittent prn doses of various diuretics to maintain an adequate urine output.

Antibiotics. Broad-spectrum intravenous antibiotics are used prophylactically in the heart-lung transplant recipient and are continued until the mediastinal and pleural chest tubes are discontinued. Chest tube removal usually occurs after 48 to 72 hours, depending on whether pleural effusions or pneumothoraces develop. A variety of agents may be used to prevent opportunistic infections. These agents include sulfa drugs, antifungal agents, and acyclovir to prevent herpes virus infections.

Immunosuppressants.   Immunosuppressive agents used for these patients include cyclosporine (CSA), azathioprine (Imuran), Orthoclone monoclonal antibody (OKT-3), and either Minnesota antilymphoblast globulin (MALG) or rabbit antithymocyte globulin (RATG). Corticosteroids are generally not used initially to allow for tracheal healing. The adequacy of immunosuppression is monitored indirectly by daily measurement of cyclosporine levels, complete blood counts, chest x-ray films, and ABGs. Endomyocardial and transbronchial biopsies also serve as measurements of immunosuppression effectiveness. Corticosteroids such as prednisone may be started after 14 days.

Pulmonary management

The goals for ventilation of the heart-lung transplant recipient are to maintain the lowest peak airway pressure, and to maintain the lowest possible FiO_2 while maintaining a normal PaO_2 (between 80 and 100 mm Hg). Early extubation is a goal in the initial postoperative period. ABGs are obtained 20 minutes after the patient is placed on the ventilator and after any subsequent ventilatory changes. Continuous SaO_2 monitoring by pulse oximetry and SvO_2 monitoring by the PA catheter may also be employed.

Secretions are mobilized and removed from the tracheobronchial tree by chest physiotherapy, postural drainage, manual and mechanical vibrations, endotracheal suctioning, humidification, and frequent turning, coughing, and deep-breathing exercises. To aid safe suctioning techniques and prevent damage to the tracheal anastomosis site, a sample suction catheter is marked at a level designated by the surgeon after the first bronchoscopy. This level indicates the point to insert the catheter during suctioning.

The importance of vigorous chest physiotherapy and coughing and deep breathing exercises to aid in the removal of secretions lies in the fact that the entire heart-lung bloc is without any type of neural connection, and the direct bronchial arterial blood supply and lymphatic drainage has been interrupted.[17] The patient requires frequent encouragement to cough and take deep breaths because the denervated lung has no sensory afferent pathway to signal the need for coughing.[19] Tracheal irritation may, however, induce coughing. Turning the patient from side to side and gradually elevating the head of the bed should be initiated as early and as frequently as possible to encourage spontaneous ventilation and to reduce dependent edema in the transplanted lungs.

Fiberoptic bronchoscopy is generally performed in the operating room before the chest is closed. The bronchoscope is moved to the intensive care unit with the patient and kept at the bedside. Bronchoscopies are performed as warranted to view the healing process at the tracheal anastomosis, to remove mucous plugs, to obtain specimens for culture and sensitivity, and for transbronchial biopsies.

Patient education

Patient education is an important aspect of the postoperative pulmonary management. Patients need to be reminded to cough and incorporate this into their daily routine. The patient does not feel irritation or the need to cough below the level of the tracheal suture line.

Explaining all procedures and the plan of care is a top priority in reducing postoperative fear and anxiety. Teaching about the medical regimen, precautions necessary because of immunosuppression, exercise programs (light weight-training, walking, calisthenics, bicycling) and diets directed toward reduction of risk factors are also an integral part of patient care.

Other important aspects of nursing care include monitoring for signs or symptoms of infection, psychologic support, and encouragement in the difficult transitional period.

ASSESSMENT OF TRANSPLANT FUNCTION

Because there are no definitive clinical signs and symptoms of cardiac transplant rejection, the endomyocardial biopsy is used to obtain data for identification of cardiac rejection. Biopsies may be performed weekly for approximately 2 to 3 months after surgery. For 3 to 6 months biopsies are done once or twice a month as the patient's clinical picture warrants. After 6 months biopsies may be required every 4 to 6 months. These biopsies can be done by the patient's referring cardiologist if the physician is skilled in the technique. The biopsy specimens can then be sent to the transplant center for evaluation.

Patients are routinely discharged after 4 to 8 weeks of hospitalization. Initially outpatient evaluation takes place approximately twice a week. Routine monitoring includes chest x-ray evaluation, ECGs, serial pulmonary function studies (PFTs), ABGs, blood work (including cyclosporine levels), and the endomyocardial biopsy.

Assessment of pulmonary transplant function and detection of acute lung rejection can be obtained by PFT and transbronchial lung biopsies (TBBs). TBBs may be obtained at 3 months and annually. Biopsies may also be warranted when a reduction in spirometric measurements in lung function occurs (decrease in forced expiratory volume, i.e., FEV_1 and FVC). Biopsy specimens may be taken from the region of maximal abnormalities as determined by x-ray evaluation, or, when x-ray findings are normal, from basal segments of a lower lobe.[20]

Annual return visits are done to evaluate the patient's overall functional status. Invasive cardiac evaluation (cardiac catheterization) and pulmonary function evaluation are done during this visit. It has been documented that early and rapid development of diffuse atherosclerotic heart disease in the donor heart does occasionally occur in heart transplant patients.[21] Unfortunately, these patients will not experience the early warning signs of angina because of the denervated heart. The lack of warning signs warrants the need for yearly cardiac catheterizations.[22] Deterioration of results on PFTs may be an indication of lung rejection. Serial monitoring by the patient at home is the best way to identify trends in posttransplant pulmonary function. Regular measurement of pulmonary function, in particular FEV_1, allows early detection of acute lung rejection and monitoring efficacy of augmented immunosuppression.[23] Home pulmonary function testing spirometers can measure FEV_1 and FVC. Patients are educated to measure PFTs, generally about twice daily, and average their results. A significant decrease in PFTs may warrant further exploration by complete PFTs and/or transbronchial biopsy.

COMPLICATIONS

Potential complications for the heart-lung transplant recipient include rejection, infection, reimplantation response, hemorrhage, tracheal anastomotic necrosis, bronchiolitis obliterans (progressive airway damage), and the potentially harmful side effects of immunosuppressive therapy (e.g., systemic arterial hypertension, nephrotoxicity, hirsutism, and lymphoproliferative disease).

Rejection

Cardiac rejection and pulmonary rejection are separate and distinct entities. Cardiac rejection is diagnosed definitively by endomyocardial biopsy. Unfortunately, there are currently no reliable techniques to identify pulmonary rejection. The lungs may reject when the endomyocardial biopsy findings are negative. Biopsies of the lung (either transbronchial or open lung) may be warranted to aid in identification of pulmonary rejection. Instead, diagnosis of pulmonary rejection is based on clinical status. Manifestations of rejection are evidenced by worsening infiltrates on the chest x-ray films, deteriorating ABGs, a low-grade fever (often only 0.5° C elevation), bronchiole alveolar lavage (BAL), a sudden deterioration of PFTs and an elevated WBC count.[17] Suspected episodes of acute pulmonary rejection are treated with intravenous doses of methylprednisolone. Differentiation of rejection from an infectious state or the reimplantation response is vital in the care and treatment of these patients.

Infection

Infection remains a major source of morbidity and mortality for transplant recipients. Primary infections include cytomegalovirus (CMV) and various other pneumonias, including pneumocystis and *Pseudomonas*. Fungal infections such as aspergillosis are also potential infections.[20] Infections are primarily caused by the suppression of the immune system. Diagnosis is based on careful surveillance of the patient's condition, chest x-ray evaluation, BAL, bronchoscopy with specimens sent for cultures, and, if necessary, an open lung biopsy. Infections are caused by common bacterial and viral organisms as well as opportunistic organisms; therefore any infection is treated aggressively and vigorously.

Reimplantation response

The reimplantation response is a phenomenon noted in the transplantation of pulmonary tissue. Signs and symptoms of this response include fever, tachypnea, and diffuse pulmonary infiltrates and/or pulmonary edema noted on chest x-ray evaluation. A ventilation-perfusion mismatch may also be detected by a $\dot{V}Q$ scan. Arterial blood gases may also deteriorate (decrease in Pao_2). The reimplantation response is generally transient and often occurs in the immediate or early postoperative period, lasting an average of 7 days. Vigorous chest physiotherapy and diuresis are the appropriate modes of treatment for the reimplantation response. Occasional reintubation and mechanical ventilation with PEEP are necessary for a short time while lung function recovers.

Hemorrhage

Hemorrhage may be a postoperative complication related to the patient's preoperative condition. As mentioned before, pleural adhesions or scarring, enlarged bronchial vessels, and the use of cardiopulmonary bypass make the patient prone to postoperative bleeding and/or tamponade. Treatment involves the administration of blood products (packed red blood cells, platelets, and fresh frozen plasma) and at times synthetic vasopressin (DDAVP). Additional protamine sulfate may be given to reverse the effects of heparin used during cardiopulmonary bypass.

Tracheal anastomotic necrosis

Tracheal anastomotic necrosis is diagnosed by visualization during bronchoscopy. Necrosis may be accompanied by hemoptysis. Presence of necrosis may postpone the use of steroids postoperatively, since the sequelae to tracheal necrosis (rupture of tracheal suture site) can be fatal. Tracheal anastomotic necrosis is less likely to occur after the first 3 to 4 weeks after transplantation.

Bronchiolitis obliterans

Bronchiolitis obliterans is a late complication of heart-lung transplantation. It is often accompanied by pulmonary vascular intimal thickening and bronchiectasis.[17] Airway disease associated with bronchiolitis obliterans has become the most important long-term complication, manifesting in up to 50% of recipients who were discharged from the hospital with normal cardiopulmonary function.[24] Hutter has reported a lower incidence of bronchiolitis obliterans and may imply improved incidences of this complication for the future.[20] The pathogenesis of bronchiolitis obliterans is unknown and at this time is not well understood. Unfortunately, this condition is irreversible and generally progressive. Potential causes may include mucociliary transport abnormalities, the inability to clear foreign antigens, chronic infection, pulmonary rejection, cyclosporine toxicity, long-term denervation, the lack of lymphatics, and the loss of bronchial blood supply. The emphasis in the late postoperative period is on possible prevention, early detection, and treatment of this condition.[18] These are achieved by close monitoring of the patient's pulmonary condition (PFTs, ABGs, auscultation of breath sounds, and chest x-ray evaluation) and noting development of dyspnea or coughing. Maintaining adequate levels of immunosuppression may help delay onset of bronchiolitis obliterans.[18]

SUMMARY

Treatment of chronic pulmonary parenchymal and vasculature disease leading to right ventricular failure remains an exceedingly difficult problem. One of the most promising developments in the treatment of these diseases has been the development of heart-lung transplantation. While currently heart-lung transplantation is limited by the lack of donors and by complication rates, which remain higher than desirable, heart-lung transplantation offers the best hope for returning to a near-normal life for patients with severe cardiopulmonary dysfunction. As transplantation techniques improve and management of complications advances, use of heart-lung transplantation may be extended to larger numbers of people.

Nurses must understand the pathophysiology of cardiopulmonary dysfunction and immune system suppression to identify development of complications and appropriate treatments. Nurses must also understand psychologic implications in transplantation to help patients and families adapt to the procedure and life changes after transplant surgery. Thus nurses have a major role in helping patients obtain optimal recovery and return to normal life.

REFERENCES

1. Reitz BA, Pennock JL and Shumway NE (1981). Simplified operative method of heart and lung transplantation. *Journal of Surgical Research, 31,* 1-5.
2. Robin ED (1987). The kingdom of the near dead: the shortened and unnatural life history of primary pulmonary hypertension. *Chest, 92,* 320-4.
3. Altman PL and Dittmer DS (1971). *Respiration and circulation.* Federation of American Societies for Experimental Biology. Bethesda, Md.
4. Wollschlager CM and Khan FA (1986). Secondary pulmonary hypertension: clinical features. *Heart and Lung, 15,* 4, 36-40.
5. Fishman A (1986). Pulmonary hypertension: preface. *Heart and Lung, 15,* 236-7.
6. Glanville AR, Burke CM, Thordore J and Robin ED (1987). Primary pulmonary hypertension: length of survival in patients referred for heart/lung transplantation. *Chest, 191,* 675-81.
7. Peil ML and Rubin LJ (1986). Therapy of secondary pulmonary hypertension. *Heart and Lung, 15,* 450-56.
8. Demikhov VP (1962). Some essential points of the techniques of transplantation of the heart, lungs and other organs. In Basi Haigh (trans): *Experimaental transplantation of vital organs.* Medgiz State Press for Medical Literature in Moscow, Moscow, 1960, New York Consultants Bureau.
9. Nakae S, Webb WR, Theordorides T et al (1967). Respiratory function following cardiopulmonary denervation in dog, cat and monkey. *Surgery Gynecology Obstetrics, 125,* 1285-1292.
10. Casteneda AR, Arnar O, Schmidt-Habelman P, Moller JH and Zamora R (1972). Cardiopulmonary autotransplantation in primates. *Journal of Cardiovascular Surgery,* 37:523-531.
11. Reitz BA, Burton NA, Jamieson SW, Bieber CP, Pennock JL, Stinson EB and Shumway NE (1980). Heart and lung transplantation: auto and allotransplantation in primates with extended survival. *Journal of Cardiovascular Surgery, 80,* 360-372.
12. Jamieson SW, Stinson EB, Oyer PE, Theodore J, Hunt S, Dawkins K, Billingham M and Shumway NE (1984). Heart and lung transplantation for pulmonary hypertension. *American Journal of Surgery, 147,* 740-742.
13. Fragomeni LS and Kaye MP (1988). The registry of the International Society for Heart Transplantation: fifth official report — 1988. *Journal of Heart Transplantation, 7,* 4, 249-253.
14. Heck CF, Shumway SJ and Kaye MP (1989). The registry of the International Society for Heart Transplantation: sixth official report — 1989. *Journal of Heart Transplantation, 8,* 271-276.
15. Hakim M, Higenbottam T, Dethune D, Cory-Pearce R, English TAH, Kneeshaw J, Wells FC and Wallwork J (1988). Selection and procurement of combined heart and lung grafts for transplantation. *Journal of Thoracic and Cardiovascular Surgery, 95,* 474-479.
16. Trento A, Griffith BP and Hardesty RL (1989). Heart-lung transplantation. In Shoemaker WC, Ayers S, Grenvik A, Holbrook PR and Thompson WL (eds). *Textbook of critical care medicine.* Philadelphia: WB Saunders Co.
17. Frist WH and Jamieson SW (1988). Heart/lung transplantation. In Cirelli GJ (ed). *Organ transplantation and replacement.* Philadelphia: JB Lippincott Co.
18. Chiles C, Guthauer DF and Jamieson SW (1985). Heart-lung transplantation: the postoperative chest radiograph. *Radiology, 154,* 299.
19. Jamieson SW (1985). Heart and lung: recent developments in heart and lung transplantation. *Transplantation Proceedings, 17*(1), 199-203.
20. Hutter JA, Despins P, Higenbottam T, Stewart S and Wallwork J (1988). Heart-lung transplantation: better use of resources. *American Journal of Medicine, 85,* 4-11.
21. Gao SZ, Schroeder JS, Hunt SA and Stinson EB (1988). Retransplantation for severe accelerated coronary artery disease in heart transplant recipients. *American Journal of Cardiology, 62,* 876-881.
22. Shinn JA (1984). Heart and lung transplantation for end stage pulmonary vascular hypertension. *Nursing Clinics of North America, 19*(3), 547-558.
23. Otulana BA, Higgenbottam TW, Clelland CA, Scott J, McGoldrick J and Wallwork J (1989). The detection of acute lung rejection in heart/lung transplantation patients by pulmonary function testing. *Journal of Heart Transplantation, 8,* 88.
24. Burke CMB, Glanville AR, Theodore J and Robin ED (1987). Lung immunogenicity, rejection, and obliterative bronchiolitis. *Chest, 92*(3), 547-549.

14

Lung Transplantation

Judy Elizabeth Boychuk and Jill Feldman Malen

HISTORICAL PERSPECTIVES ON LUNG TRANSPLANTATION

Largely as a result of the efforts of J. D. Cooper and the Toronto Lung Transplant Group, single- and double-lung transplantation has, within the past few years (1983 to present), become a viable clinical option for highly select patients with severe end-stage pulmonary disease. Before their efforts, 26 surgeons worldwide had attempted 40 human transplants between 1963 and 1978. Only two patients survived for more than 1 month.[1-4] In 1963 Hardy attempted the first human lung transplant in a patient with bronchogenic carcinoma.[5] The recipient survived for 18 days and died of renal failure. The major causes of death in the 40 transplanted patients were related to poor donor and recipient selection, respiratory failure, surgical technique, infection, rejection, and disruption of the airway anastomosis.

The next major development occurred in the late 1970s and early 1980s, when Cooper and the Toronto Transplant Group conducted a series of animal investigations, later applied to humans, to solve problems related to rejection and bronchial dehiscence. They were able to demonstrate successful bronchial healing with use of the following: (1) cyclosporine for initial immunosuppression, (2) avoidance of corticosteroids for 2 to 3 weeks postoperatively, and (3) use of an omental wrap to protect, vascularize, and nourish the bronchus.[6-9]

Single-lung transplantation

The Toronto Transplant Group published its initial successes with human single-lung transplantation in 1986 and 1988, reporting that since November 1983 they had performed 11 single-lung transplants.[4,10] Eight of these patients were alive up to 44 months after surgery, free of oxygen therapy and leading normal lives with good exercise tolerance. One patient celebrated the fifth anniversary of his single-lung transplant in November 1988. Causes of death in three patients were pneumonia at postoperative day 10 as a result of selection of an unsuitable donor, venous air embolism after removal of a large central venous catheter, and rejection at 7 months. A more recent report in January 1989 demonstrates that as of June 1988 they had performed 16 single-lung transplants[11]; no patient died as a result of bronchial complications. There were a total of four in-hospital deaths; three are described above. The fourth died of lymphoma, presumably as a result of immunosuppressive therapy. Of the 12 hospital survivors, two patients developed late bronchial stenosis that was successfully treated with bronchial dilation and introduction of a silicone stent.[11]

Physiologically, single-lung transplantation has been thought to have the best application in patients with pulmonary fibrosis. The native remaining lung has decreased compliance and increased pulmonary vascular resistance; therefore ventilation and blood flow are preferentially directed to the new lung. Lung perfusion scans have shown that blood flow to the transplanted lung significantly increases over time. Pulmonary function studies also show improvements in forced vital capacity (FVC), forced exhaled volume in 1 second (FEV_1), and diffusing capacity (DLCO).[4] Arterial blood gas levels improve also, and all surviving patients have been weaned from supplemental oxygen. Patients with emphysema and other forms of obstructive lung disease have been thought to be physiologically unsuited for single-lung transplantation. The increased lung compliance associated with these diseases could lead to problems with hyperinflation of the remaining native lung, mediastinal shift, and compression of the transplanted lung.[12] More recently, some lung transplant centers have performed successful single-lung transplantation for select patients with emphysema.

Double-lung transplantation

In 1988 and 1989 (after a series of successful experiments in the animal laboratory), the Toronto Lung Transplant Group was the first to report successes with en bloc double-lung transplantation in humans.[13] Bilateral lung transplantation is indicated in select patients with septic pulmonary disease or emphysema. A remaining septic lung would be a source of infection, and an emphysematous lung could result in functional impairments as described earlier.[14]

They performed en bloc double-lung transplants in seven patients, ages 16 to 47; four had emphysema, one had primary idiopathic bronchiolitis obliterans, one had eosinophilic granulomatosis, and one had pulmonary hypertension. Before transplant these patients had developed marked deterioration in condition as a result of their lung disease and severe exercise restriction, and most required continuous use of supplemental oxygen. All of these patients were severely ill, with a life expectancy of less than 12 to 18 months. They all underwent preoperative pulmonary rehabilitation. Right ventricular function was thought to be reasonably well preserved.[14,15] None of the patients were receiving corticosteroid therapy at the time of surgery. Intraoperative and postoperative results showed the following: (1) average length of surgery was 5 hours, (2) total bypass time ranged from 2.5 to 3.6 hours, (3) aortic cross-clamp time was 33 to 52 minutes, and (4) ischemic time ranged from 2 hours to 4 hours and 20 minutes.[12,15] All patients showed improvement in right ventricular function, pulmonary function studies, and gas exchange. Six of the seven patients were discharged from the hospital with a normal functional level. One patient with primary pulmonary hypertension developed tracheal stenosis after a prolonged period of postoperative hypotension. Despite recovery of right ventricular function, the patient required retransplantation on the eleventh postoperative day and died 2 days later. One patient developed an airway stricture that required dilation and placement of a silicone stent. Ischemia caused partial airway necrosis and dehiscence of the tracheal anastomosis in two patients; these healed spontaneously without clinically significant problems.[13,14]

These successes support single- and double-lung transplantation as a viable, although highly risky, option for select patients with severe end-stage pulmonary disease. As a result, many centers across North America have, in the past 1 to 2 years, initiated clinical lung transplantation programs.

This chapter identifies intensive preoperative and postoperative nursing and rehabilitative care needs of lung transplant recipients. By using a holistic rehabilitative approach, patients can return to their optimal level of function, and complications can be prevented or treated early.

PATIENT SELECTION

The patient selection process may vary from center to center. Described below are the components of the selection process that we feel are essential.

Patient referrals

Referrals for single- and double-lung transplantation usually originate from pulmonologists or primary care physicians. Referrals are initially screened according to selection and disqualifying criteria (see the box on p. 262). Well-defined guidelines facilitate the process and increase both the quantity and quality of referrals.

CRITERIA FOR SELECTING LUNG TRANSPLANT RECIPIENTS

Selection
Single Lung

Idiopathic interstitial pulmonary fibrosis
Sarcoidosis
Primary pulmonary hypertension
Emphysema*

Double Lung

Emphysema
Alpha-1 antitrypsin deficiency
Eosinophilic granuloma
Lymphangiolyomyomatosis
Cystic fibrosis

Disqualification
Absolute

Age†
Steroid dependency
Systemic illness
Cardiac insufficiency
Right ventricular ejection fraction <20%
Evidence of right ventricular failure
Left ventricular ejection fraction <40%
Mechanical ventilation dependent

Relative

Evidence of psychopathology
Profound malnutrition
Nonrehabilitative pulmonary disability

From Malen JF and Boychuk JE (1989). Nursing perspectives on lung transplantation. *Critical Care Clinics of North America, 1*, 707-722.
*Indicates candidate for single-lung transplantation if patient exceeds age limitation for double-lung transplantation.
† >60 for single lung, >50 for double lung.

Adequate initial screening of inappropriate referrals is essential, because on-site evaluation is financially demanding, logistically tedious, and highly stressful for the patient. Patients meeting initial screening criteria move on to evaluation. A mechanism must be instituted for team communication and consultative review of laboratory data, chest x-ray reports, and multisystem diagnostic studies before a final in-hospital evaluation. The goal of initial screening is to select appropriate patients for final inpatient evaluation.

A 5-day inpatient evaluation is the final stage of referral. In most cases it involves a complete multisystem assessment of the patient's medical and psychosocial status (see the box on p. 263). Patients with end-stage lung disease referred for lung transplantation usually require 24-hour oxygen therapy, have limited mobility, and their condition may be clinically tenuous. For these reasons, this evaluation has required an inpatient admission in our experience.

When this extensive evaluation is completed, a multidisciplinary conference is held to share information. A team decision is made to (1) accept the patient, (2) defer a final decision and reassess after addressing unresolved issues, or (3) refuse the patient. Communication with the patient and referring physician about the results of the evaluation and the basis for the decision are very important.

Preparation and rehabilitation

Accepted patients are expected to reside locally while on the active recipient waiting list. During the waiting period, the patient is engaged in a comprehensive program that includes education and aggressive pulmonary rehabilitation. Problems identified in nutrition, exercise tolerance, life-style management, and functional status are addressed with an appropriate plan of care.

Patients attend daily rehabilitation and are progressed to their optimal level of exercise. Psychosocial support is provided by a team psychologist and social worker. Weekly patient support groups are provided to assist patients and their families with emotional and social stresses inherent in the waiting period. Pagers are provided to patients to ensure accessibility without imposing too many limitations on their daily lives.

Pulmonary rehabilitation is the focus of the patient's therapeutic regimen before and after lung transplantation. A pulmonary rehabilitation team follows patients from the time of their preoperative assessment until 3 to 6 months after transplant. The goal of pulmonary rehabilitation is to achieve the best overall physical condition and functional level possible both before and after lung transplantation.

A preprogram assessment of cardiopulmo-

LUNG TRANSPLANT EVALUATION STUDIES PERFORMED

Organ system evaluation

Heart

Electrocardiography
Echocardiography/tricuspid Doppler studies
Radionuclide ventriculography
Thallium stress testing
Cardiac catheterization

Lungs

Chest x-ray examination
Ventilation perfusion scan
Pulmonary angiography
Pulmonary function studies

Kidney/liver

CBC
SMA 6/12 with fasting glucose
24-hour creatinine clearance
Lipids
Coagulation profile
Liver function studies

Exercise capacity

6-minute walk/stair climbing
Ear oximetry (rest and exercise)
Cardiopulmonary stress testing
Arterial blood gases (rest and exercise)

Nutritional status

Calorie count
Indirect calorimetry
Triceps' skinfolds
Weight/diet evaluation
Plasma proteins
Creatinine/height index

Histocompatability

Human lymphocytic antigen screen (HLA)
Cytotoxic lymphocytic antibody screen
Lymphocytic cytotoxic antibody cross-match

Psychopathology

Millon Clinical Multiaxial Inventory
Minnesota Multiphasic Personality Inventory
Profile interview
Weschler Adult Intelligence Scale (revised)
Rorschach Thematic Apperception Test
Bender Visual Motor Gestalt Test
Projective drawings

Socioeconomic

Assessment of coping and support structure
Financial assessment

From Malen JF and Boychuk JE (1989). Nursing perspectives on lung transplantation. *Critical Care Clinics of North America, 1,* 707-722.

nary and nutritional status in relation to the patient's exercise performance and functional level is weighed heavily in the decision to accept candidates for transplantation. Extensive exercise testing is completed. From a rehabilitation standpoint, the ideal candidate is someone who (1) has severe end-stage restrictive or obstructive lung disease, (2) has been able to maintain adequate nutrition, (3) has been ambulatory and capable of participating in an outpatient exercise program, (4) does not have clinical evidence of right-sided heart failure, (5) has normal left ventricular function and absence of significant atherosclerosis or coronary angiography, and (6) has adequate psychosocial support and coping abilities.[16]

Once the patient is formally accepted into the program, intensive pulmonary rehabilitation begins. The program should include (1) endurance training with a bicycle and/or treadmill, (2) strengthening and flexibility exercises, (3) close monitoring of oxygen saturation (Sao_2), heart rate, and blood pressure, (4) chest physiotherapy (CPT) and pulmonary hygiene, and (5) oxygen therapy to keep Sao_2 greater than 90%.

A 6-minute walk test should be repeated every 2 to 4 weeks and arterial blood gases checked as needed. Many of these patients have severe gas exchange abnormalities with hypoxemia, acidosis, and hypercarbia. Despite the severity of their lung disease, many patients have been able to achieve significant improvements in their exercise performance. Six-minute walk tests have been shown to improve an average of 30% during pretransplant rehabilitation.[15] Most have achieved 30 to 40 minutes of endurance exercise (3 to 5 times per week) at 70% to 80% of predicted maximal heart rate while maintaining oxygen saturations greater than 85% to 90%. Patient progress is reviewed weekly. Any decline in pulmonary function or change in performance is immediately reported to the program's medical director. Close monitoring identifies problems early and helps to prevent and quickly treat any exacerbations.

SURGICAL PROCEDURE
Donor selection

Appropriate donor and recipient selection is the key to successful lung transplantation. The principal problem is the critical shortage of suitable donors.[17] Patients may wait 4 to 6 months or longer for an appropriate donor. Of the available donors, only 1 in 20 has suitable lungs for use in transplantation.[18,19] Complications such as pulmonary edema, contusion, aspiration, or infection may preclude organ viability.[18,20] Guidelines for the identification and management of lung donors have been formulated by the United Network for Organ Sharing (UNOS).[21] Education of local organ procurement agencies and growing support from intensivists and emergency room staff will help meet the needs of lung transplant programs, but much progress is still needed to expand the pool of suitable lung donors.

Lung donors should be younger than 55 years of age and have no significant smoking history or other active pulmonary disease. A suitable lung donor has clear chest x-ray findings and a Pao_2 of greater than 300 mm Hg when measured on 100% oxygen and 5 cm of positive end expiratory pressure (PEEP) for 5 minutes. A bronchoscopy is performed by the donor retrieval team on the donor's arrival to ensure that the lungs are free of purulent airway secretions or aspirated material. Trauma patients with chest injuries apparent on clinical or chest x-ray examination are not suitable donors. Previous thoracic or cardiac surgery, the presence of a unilateral infiltrate, pneumothorax, or pulmonary contusion will preclude double-lung recovery but allows for the possibility of single-lung retrieval.[17]

Surgical considerations

Single-lung transplantation has traditionally been applied to restrictive lung disease. The poor compliance and increased pulmonary vascular resistance of the native lung result in preferential ventilation and perfusion to the transplanted lung.[5] Size matching between donor and recipient is less critical than with double-lung transplantation. An oversized single donor lung can be accommodated by descent of the diaphragm and shift of the mediastinum to the contralateral side (Fig. 14-1).

Double-lung transplantation has recently proved a therapeutic alternative in the treatment of emphysema and cystic fibrosis, where the increased pulmonary compliance of emphysema and infectious nature of cystic fibrosis preclude single-lung transplantation. In such patients, right-sided heart function is often well preserved. Replacement of both heart and lungs is therefore unnecessary and significantly increases the patient's risk of postoperative complications. Double-lung transplantation also eliminates the need to secure a suitable donor with a combination of suitable cardiac and pulmonary function.[15] Finally, double-lung

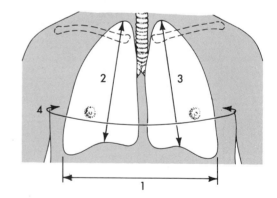

Fig. 14-1 Thoracic dimensions needed for lung donor–recipient matching. *1,* Horizontal measurement (costophrenic angle to costophrenic angle); *2,* right vertical (peak of diaphram to highest apical point on the x-ray view); *3,* left vertical; and *4,* circumference (outer chest circumference at nipple level). (From Brand P and Passaretti R (May 1988). Assessment of organ donors. *Diagnosis,* 168, STA Communications, Pointe-Claire, Quebec.)

transplantation permits the retrieval of both heart and lungs for use in more than one recipient.

Surgical techinque

The surgical technique involved in lung transplantation continues to be refined. All patients have radial and pulmonary arterial cannulation performed before induction of anesthesia. Final confirmation of organ suitability is received from the donor center on bronchoscopic and direct visualization of the donor lungs. The recipient is then anesthetized and a small upper midline laparotomy is performed, at which time the omentum is mobilized and tunneled beneath the sternum for subsequent retrieval. The abdomen is then closed. Single-lung transplantation can be performed on either side, but it is technically easier to perform a left lung transplant. Unlike double-lung transplantation, in which cardiopulmonary bypass is mandatory, the need for bypass in single-lung transplantation depends on the patient's tolerance of unilateral pulmonary support. If the patient undergoing single-lung transplantation does not tolerate contralateral single-lung ventilation, the ipsilateral side of the groin is prepared for subsequent femorofemoral bypass, should it be required. In single-lung transplantation, a standard posterolateral thoracotomy is performed through the bed of the excised fifth rib.[12] The main pulmonary artery is encircled and temporarily clamped to assess the impact on hemodynamic stability and gas exchange. If this procedure is not tolerated, the femoral artery and vein are cannulated so that at the time of extraction, femorofemoral venoarterial bypass can be instituted. Bypass has been required in a small percentage of patients. Mobilization and extraction of the single lung generally requires less time than that required of the double lung bloc; however, this will depend on the amount of adhesion present, tolerance of anesthesia, and intraoperative hemodynamic stability.

The recipient lung or lungs are removed, leaving a generous length of pulmonary artery and veins for reanastomosis to the transplant vessels. Technical problems have developed at the site of airway anastomosis because of precarious vascularity of the transplant bronchus/trachea, which must derive its blood supply from collaterals between the pulmonary and bronchial arteries. This has resulted in bronchial/tracheal leakage and stenosis as a result of varying degrees of ischemic necrosis of the transplanted airway. The use of the omental graft to aid in reestablishing blood flow to the airway was a landmark in the success of lung transplantation.[8,11,12] Improving tracheal/bronchial anastomotic reperfusion remains the focal point of ongoing research.

Implantation of the single-lung (Fig. 14-2, *A*) is achieved by placement of a left atrial clamp, which permits the opening and joining of the pulmonary vein orifices to create a generous left atrial cuff. The left atrial anastomosis is followed by pulmonary artery anastomosis and finally end-to-end anastomosis of donor and recipient bronchus approximately two rings proximal to the origin of the upper lobe. The atrial clamp is then removed to permit back bleeding and venting of the atria. The omentum is then retrieved from the anterior mediastinum and placed circumferentially around the bronchial anastomosis. Care is taken to avoid injury to the vagus, phrenic, and recurrent laryngeal nerves so as to ensure transmission of respiratory center impulses controlling diaphragmatic action as well as maintain speech, swallowing, and gastric emptying.

Implantation of the double lung bloc (Fig. 14-2, *B*) is preceded by the institution of cardiopulmonary bypass and insertion of a right ventricular vent subsequent to omental mobilization. The recipient lungs are excised, with the empty heart beating after the pulmonary veins have been stapled to prevent systemic air embolism.[23] The double-lung graft is inserted by passing each lung separately through the respective pleural-pericardial windows. The donor trachea is brought up into the posterior mediastinum and anastomosed to the recipient trachea immediately above the carina. Once the tracheal anastomosis is complete, the aorta is cross-clamped, aortic route cardioplegia initiated, and the heart arrested. Left atrial and main pulmonary arterial anastomoses are completed, followed by systemic reperfusion. The omental pedicle is then wrapped circumferentially around the tracheal anastomosis and tacked to the wall of the airway. Fiberoptic bronchoscopy is performed on completion of

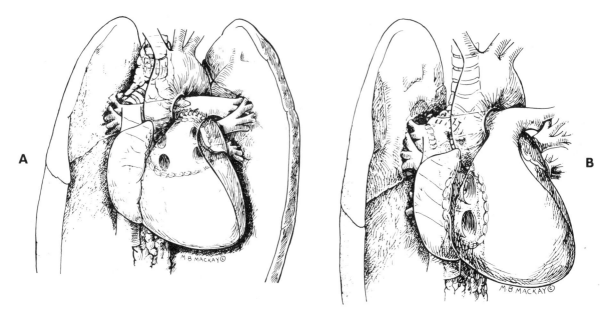

Fig. 14-2 Anastomoses for **A,** double-lung and **B,** single-lung transplantation.

single- and double-lung transplant procedures to evaluate the airway and document a satisfactory anastomotic lumen.[23]

This procedure has recently been modified as two single-lung transplants performed through an anterior thoracic incision. In most cases this minimizes and in some cases avoids the use of cardiopulmonary bypass.

POSTOPERATIVE CARE

This section describes the postoperative problems and intensive nursing care needs after lung transplantation. Patients usually require two nurses per shift for 24 to 48 hours, followed by 2 to 3 weeks of one-on-one nursing care. Their stay in the intensive care unit is usually 3 to 7 days.

Immunosuppression

It is well established that administration of corticosteroids immediately before, during, or up to 2 weeks after lung transplantation seriously jeopardizes the healing of the tracheal and bronchial anastomoses.[9] An immunosuppressive regimen of cyclosporine and azathioprine is standard in the immediate postoperative period. Corticosteroids are avoided for the first 7

to 14 days and replaced by OKT-3 or antilymphoblast globulin immediately after transplant surgery. At 2 to 3 weeks, oral prednisone is prescribed if the thoracotomy wound is healing well and the airway anastomosis appears satisfactory on bronchoscopy.[23] Thereafter, maintenance immunosuppression consists of cyclosporine, azathioprine, and prednisone.

Pulmonary complications

Ineffective airway clearance. Ineffective postoperative airway clearance and breathing pattern may occur and are related to denervation of the transplanted lung, impaired cough, infection, pain, surgery, analgesia, and/or altered chest wall musculoskeletal function.

Ineffective airway clearance usually remains a problem for the first 2 to 3 months after transplantation. In addition to the usual postoperative factors that contribute to stagnation of mucus, the transplanted lung has inherent problems because of denervation, loss of cough reflex, and slowing of mucociliary clearance. Mucociliary clearance, as assessed by removal of inhaled radiolabeled aerosol, is diminished in the graft compared to the native lung. The primary defect in the mucociliary apparatus has not yet been determined.[16] Complications that can further interfere with airway clearance include opportunistic infections in an immuno-compromised host and ischemic airway changes.[11] As described, hypotensive and hypoxemic episodes in the initial postoperative period can lead to ischemic insults to the airway followed by airway necrosis, dehiscence, and/or stenosis. With good pulmonary hygiene and adequate and prompt reperfusion, many of these necrotic airway changes can be prevented.[13,14] If stenosis occurs in the airway, silicone stents have been successfully placed to maintain airway patency. Necrosis and dehiscence can also progress to mediastinal abscess formation, mediastinitis and air leaks. Death can then ensue as a result of pulmonary and mediastinal sepsis, hemorrhage from erosion of a major vessel, and/or complete airway dehiscence.

Nursing and physiotherapy interventions can maintain adequate pulmonary clearance and prevent atelectasis and pneumonia. Bronchoscopy is performed frequently during the initial posttransplant period to assess airway secretions, healing of the anastomoses, and the condition of the bronchial mucous membrane. Sputum specimens and bronchiole alveolar lavage (BAL) fluid are obtained for culture and analysis of cell type to determine whether signs of infection and/or rejection are present.[25]

Aggressive chest physiotherapy should be implemented every 2 to 4 hours while the patient is awake. It should include postural drainage to all involved lobes, vibration, deep breathing, and coughing. Trendelenburg and high Fowler's or sitting positions can be used once the patient is hemodynamically stable. During the first few days, while the patient is intubated, sterile suctioning with saline lavage should be done after each drainage position and as needed. It is interesting to note that saline lavage, the presence of tracheobronchial secretions, and suctioning distal to the anastomosis do not stimulate cough. Patients need to be verbally coached to cough and expectorate their mucus. Incentive spirometry should be used after extubation to encourage deep breathing and coughing.

The importance of aggressive daily chest physiotherapy every 2 to 4 hours while awake cannot be overemphasized. Mucous plugging can lead to volume loss and consolidation in the transplanted lung. Daily assessments of chest x-ray changes, breath sounds, and sputum characteristics help to guide the chest physiotherapy regimen. Mucus is usually thick and blood tinged in quantities of 20 to 60 ml/day for several weeks.

Proper positioning of the patient is imperative in the postoperative period. In the single-lung transplant, the operative side should be kept up as much as possible by having the patient lie in the lateral decubitus position with the nonoperative side down. This position reduces postsurgical edema and aids in gravitational drainage of the airway. It also helps to minimize mediastinal shifting toward the operative side, thereby promoting optimal inflation of the new lung.

In some cases of acute rejection of a single-lung allograft, perfusion to the transplanted lung may be severely reduced. Placing the patient on the side of the transplanted lung may increase its perfusion.[18] Placing the patient prone for short periods aids in clearing secretions from posterior lower lobes.

In double-lung transplantation, the patient should be turned side-to-side, 90 degrees each way, every 1 to 2 hours. Prolonged periods in the supine position are avoided to minimize secretion retention. In the first 12 to 24 hours after surgery, turning is initiated gradually, beginning with 20- to 30-degree turns and assessing blood pressure, Sao_2, and heart rate, because these may drop rapidly in the initial postoperative period. Slowly the patient is progressed to full 90-degree turns and prone or semiprone postures. Increased fractions of inspired oxygen may be required during initial turning and when sitting the patient up or getting out of bed for the first time. Cardiovascular instability and ventilation/perfusion inequalities are probably responsible for these initial drops in Sao_2, heart rate, and blood pressure.

Pulmonary complications

Alteration in gas exchange. During the first 1 or 2 postoperative days, abnormalities in gas exchange usually occur as a result of reperfusion edema in the transplanted lung. This reimplantation response may lead to hypoxemia and the need for increased concentrations of supplemental oxygen and mechanical ventilation. The edematous lung is managed by keeping the patient as dry as possible without compromising blood pressure or renal function.[16] The nurse must closely assess cardiovascular, pulmonary, and renal function, reporting any changes immediately.

The next major causes of gas exchange abnormalities are infection and rejection. Since therapy is quite different for each of these causes, it is important to recognize the signs and symptoms that differentiate one from the other.[23] Both can result in a worsening of hypoxemia caused by ventilation and perfusion inequalities. In the initial postoperative period, lung transplant patients have some degree of hypoxemia requiring oxygen therapy. With infection and rejection, the hypoxemia worsens, particularly during exercise. Increased hypoxemia caused by rejection usually occurs twice before the end of the third postoperative week, at 5 to 9 days and after 11 days. Rejection is usually associated with a low-grade fever, general malaise, desaturation with minimal activity level, and a diffuse hilar infiltrate. Worsening hypoxemia resulting from infection may occur at any time. Infection is also associated with fever (usually spike in temperature), and is accompanied by an increased white blood cell count and positive findings on sputum cultures. Fatigue and decreased exercise tolerance can also occur with infection.

To further differentiate these two complications, several diagnostic tests are performed. Pulmonary function test results may worsen with infection or rejection. Chest x-ray changes with rejection may include perihilar infiltrates, ground-glass infiltrate with interstitial fluid, and/or rapid development of pleural effusion. These changes respond rapidly to bolus dose corticosteroid. In infection, localized infiltrates may be seen with signs of consolidation, although many of the opportunistic infections (e.g., pneumocystis and herpes simplex) can cause more diffuse interstitial infiltrates that may progress to consolidation. These do not clear after corticosteroid administration, and symptomatology may actually worsen.[22]

Bronchoscopy is usually done to obtain spu-

tum, transbronchial biopsy specimens, and BAL fluid. Rejection is associated with an increased lymphocyte count in BAL fluid. In infection, neutrophils are increased in the BAL fluid and infectious organisms are usually isolated.[25] Transbronchial biopsy specimens indicate rejection when perivascular lymphocytic infiltrates are seen in and around pulmonary arterioles and veins.

In single-lung transplantation, quantitative perfusion scans are helpful in following rejection and response to therapy. With acute rejection, perfusion decreases in the transplanted lung; this is reversed with steroid administration.

Open-lung biopsy is rarely indicated, but may be used as a final step in differentiating lung rejection from infection when all other studies have not confirmed the diagnosis. In rejection, alveolar exudates are seen that are fibrous or contain desquamated pneumocytes, and inflammatory cells or perivascular exudates with round cells or lymphocytes.[16] In infection, organisms are usually isolated; pneumocystis, herpes simplex, gram-negative infections, aspergillus fumigatus, and cytomegalovirus (CMV) have been reported.

It is very important for nurses to be aware of the differences between rejection and infection so that detection of any slight changes or trends in body temperature, hemodynamics, chest x-ray findings, blood gases, pulmonary function studies (especially forced expiratory volume in 1 second [FEV_1]), fatigue, and exercise tolerance can be immediately reported and more closely investigated. Early detection and prompt treatment of infection and rejection are key to the successful long-term viability of the transplanted lung.

Nursing staff should report signs of hypoxemia immediately, especially a widening of the alveolar-arterial oxygen difference, desaturation with activity or exercise, and increasing fatigue or decreasing exercise tolerance. Oxygen is administered to keep SaO_2 over 90% and PaO_2 above 60 mm Hg. In the initial post operative period, the PaO_2 is kept closer to 100 mm Hg in anticipation of cardiovascular instability. Rejection, infection and/or reperfusion edema should be promptly treated to reduce the length of intubation and/or prevent the need for reintubation.

Cardiovascular complications

Hemodynamic instability secondary to hypovolemia, myocardial irritability, and depressed myocardial contractility may occur in the immediate postoperative period. A delicate balance is needed to maintain adequate circulatory volume and cardiac filling pressures while preventing fluid overload and the propensity for pulmonary edema. Initial alterations in pulmonary capillary permeability, resulting from cardiopulmonary bypass and graft ischemia coupled with lymphatic interruption, lead to extravasation of fluid to interstitial and intraalveolar spaces.[26] Liberal use of diuretics is balanced with maintaining adequate renal function by replacing fluid volume.

After cardiopulmonary bypass, supraventricular dysrhythmias are common. These are thought to occur as a result of poor atrial protection during aortic cross-clamp and prolonged atrial ischemia. In the face of altered hemodynamics, supraventricular dysrhythmias are treated in much the same fashion as in other postcardiothoracic procedures, by digitalization, administration of calcium channel blockers, and cardioversion.[26] Ventricular dysrhythmias indicate underlying electrolyte abnormalities or myocardial ischemia and should be treated promptly.[26]

Cardiac output may decrease transiently as a result of the effects of anesthesia and cold hypokalemic arrest during cardiopulmonary bypass. Perivascular and interstitial edema resulting from lung ischemia, cardiopulmonary bypass, and increased levels of circulating catecholamines may be reflected in an elevated pulmonary vascular resistance. The use of pulmonary vasodilators such as prostaglandin E_1 are effective in reducing right ventricular afterload during this period.[26]

Inotropic support in the face of adequate filling pressures can facilitate renal perfusion and maintain urine output while eliminating the need for administration of copious intravenous fluids.[26] Alpha-adrenergic agents may serve to temporarily elevate systemic vascular resistance and thereby increase perfusion pressure. It is important to remember that prolonged or excessive use of peripheral vasoconstricting agents may ultimately impair blood flow, causing further hypoperfusion irrespective of systemic pressures.[26]

Hematologic complications

Coagulopathy may occur after lung transplantation as a result of the use of cardiopulmonary bypass, heparinization, and perioperative blood loss requiring excessive blood product replacement.[26] Patients with pleural adhesions or previous thoracic surgery are particularly susceptible to postoperative bleeding. Mediastinal bleeding in excess of 200 ml/hr for several hours, despite attempts to restore hemostasis, justifies reexploration. Measuring the platelet count, fibrinogen level, fibrin degradation products, and prothrombin and activated partial thromboplastin times will facilitate early identification of coagulopathy. Administration of cryoprecipitate, platelets, and fresh frozen plasma will aid in the restoration of hemostasis.

Nutritional complications

Prevention of malnutrition is of primary importance during the pretransplant and posttransplant periods. Malnutrition in the pulmonary patient can lead to weight loss, muscle wasting, depletion of visceral (serum) proteins, negative nitrogen balance, impaired wound healing, and decreased resistance to infection. To avoid these problems, a detailed nutritional assessment is performed preoperatively and nutritional status optimized before transplantation. The cause of weight loss in severe lung disease is not entirely understood but is believed to result largely from the increased caloric expenditure by increased work of breathing. The caloric requirements for breathing may be 10 times the normal level.[27]

After surgery the goals of nutritional care are to maintain positive nitrogen balance and ideal body weight. The basal energy expenditure should be calculated to determine energy needs. Additional stress factors after surgery further increase the patient's caloric needs. These may include fever, secondary surgical procedures, infection, sepsis, and mechanical ventilation. If oral intake is inadequate, nutritional supplements by the enteral or parenteral route are implemented. Vitamins A and D will aid in wound healing and are given before and after surgery.

Because the peritoneum is entered during surgery, paralytic gastric ileus is frequently seen and results in delayed gastric emptying, distended stomach with a normal-sized bowel, and large amounts of gastric drainage. Since it is a gastric ileus, bowel sounds are usually present and audible. To initiate nutritional support immediately after surgery, the parenteral route may have to be taken until enteral or oral feedings are tolerated. The nurse should take all necessary precautions to avoid complications related to enteral and parenteral nutrition. As described, malnutrition has far-reaching implications in the postoperative period. Nurses should work closely with the dietitian to assess the needs of the patient, ensure delivery of adequate calories daily, monitor serum electrolytes including sodium, potassium, chloride, magnesium, calcium, glucose, and phosphate, and weigh the patient daily. Cholesterol and triglyceride levels are monitored closely because they can be elevated as a result of cyclosporine therapy.

Pain

Altered comfort may be related to pain, dyspnea, fatigue, and sleep deprivation. During the initial rehabilitation phase, it is important to allow the patient adequate rest and pain control. Before each physiotherapy treatment is initiated, pain control measures should be implemented and assessed. Initial postoperative pain usually results from intubation and the surgical incision. Use of morphine by epidural or intravenous route is usually the most effective pain control measure during the immediate postoperative period. As incisional pain subsides, more diffuse chest wall pain may develop. This pain may be related to changes in thoracic musculoskeletal configuration. Fig. 14-3 compares the before and after double-lung transplant chest x-ray films of a patient with severe emphysema. Postoperatively, the diaphragms descend and the intercostal spaces decrease.

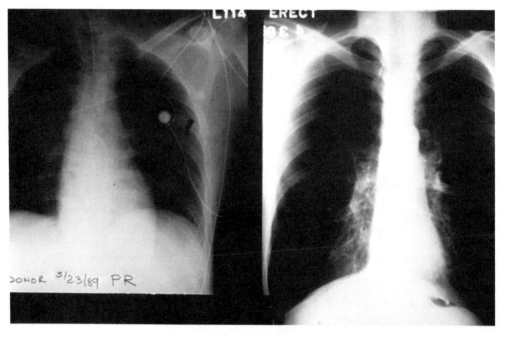

Fig. 14-3 Chest x-ray film before *(right)* and after *(left)* double lung transplantation in a patient with severe emphysema secondary to alpha-1 antitrypsin deficiency.

Excessive coughing can also add to muscle pain. Use of oral analgesic agents before chest physiotherapy, flexibility exercises, and such modalities as massage and TENS units aids in relieving these discomforts.

Suboptimal exercise performance

Decreased exercise tolerance also occurs and is related to surgery, pain, fever, preoperative musculoskeletal deconditioning, and cardiopulmonary instability.

Rehabilitation resumes within 12 to 24 hours after lung transplantation. It begins with aggressive CPT, proper positioning of the patient, and active and passive range of motion exercises. Usually within the first 3 to 5 days, the patient sits up in a chair and begins resistance exercises. Ambulation for short distances is initiated as soon as possible. Assessment of patient tolerance, blood pressure, heart rate, and Sao_2 change with CPT and exercise help to guide progression of therapy. Supplemental oxygen is increased during therapy to keep the Sao_2 greater than 90%. A daily schedule is developed that should include rest periods, physiotherapy, personal care, assessment, and diagnostic procedures. Exercise is progressed as rapidly as tolerated toward the goal of having the patient walk a mile during the course of the day (usually within 2 to 4 weeks). At that time the patient is advanced to the treadmill room where long-term rehabilitation is begun. The patient's preoperative level of function can be used as a baseline for setting initial goals postoperatively.

For the first 3 months the patient is seen 5 days per week for endurance exercising, which usually consists of a combination of walking, treadmilling, and bicycling. Oxygen saturation, heart rate, performance, and perceived exertion are closely monitored. As oxygenation improves, the patient is weaned off oxygen therapy.

Exertional dyspnea is usually more pronounced in single-lung transplant patients with pulmonary fibrosis, because native lung juxtacapillary (J) receptors are still activated and can presumably send messages to the respiratory center via the vagus nerve, which can result in rapid, shallow breathing.[28] Use of the oximeter for reinforcement along with support and encouragement by staff will facilitate gradual weaning from oxygen therapy and resumption of a more normal breathing pattern. Many emphysema patients still purse-lip breathe for some time after their transplant.

Strengthening, flexibility, and CPT exercises are also carried out under the close supervision of the physical therapy staff. Significant amounts of retained pulmonary secretions usually persist for several weeks in the denervated transplanted lung. The mucus can be adequately controlled and mobilized with hydration, CPT, and exercise, thereby preventing bronchial infections and pneumonia. Between 3 and 6 months, the patient and family are usually discharged with a rigorous home exercise program, including all of the components mentioned. After discharge from rehabilitation, patients are followed indefinitely every 3 to 6 months, with 6-minute walk tests and follow-up teaching and evaluation as needed.

SUMMARY

Lung transplantation has become a viable — although highly risky — therapeutic option for select patients with end-stage lung disease. Lack of donor suitability is a major obstacle to a more widespread application of the procedure. Many patients wait months and sometimes a year or more for an appropriate donor; some die waiting.

Careful evaluation and selection of patients, rigorous pretransplant and posttransplant pulmonary rehabilitation and intensive nursing and medical care significantly improve posttransplant recovery. Improved preoperative exercise tolerance and muscle strength prepare patients for the surgery and ensuing postoperative course. Likewise, long-term posttransplant rehabilitation is essential to the patient's ultimate recovery and return to a normal, healthy life.

REFERENCES

1. Nelems JMB, Rebuck AS and Cooper JD (1980). Human lung transplantation. *Chest, 78*, 569-573.
2. Kamholz SL, Veith FL, Mollenkopf FP et al (1983). Single lung transplantation with cyclosporin immunosuppression. *Journal of Thoracic and Cardiovascular Surgery, 86*, 537-542.
3. Derom F, Barbier F, Ringoir S et al (1971). Ten-month

survival after lung transplantation in man. *Journal of Thoracic and Cardiovascular Surgery, 61,* 835-846.

4. Toronto Lung Transplant Group (1988). Experience with single-lung transplantation for pulmonary fibrosis. *Journal of the American Medical Association, 259,* 2258-2262.

5. Hardy JD, Webb WR, Dalton ML et al (1963). Lung homotransplantation in man. *Journal of the American Medical Association, 186,* 1065.

6. Dubois P, Chiniere L and Cooper JD (1984). Bronchial omentopexy in canine lung allotransplantation. *Annals of Thoracic Surgery, 38,* 11-14.

7. Lima O, Cooper JD, Peters WJ et al (1981). Effects of methylprednisolone and azathioprine on bronchial healing following lung autotransplantation. *Journal of Thoracic and Cardiovascular Surgery, 82,* 211-215.

8. Morgan WE, Lima O, Goldberg M et al (1983). Improved bronchial healing in canine left lung reimplantation using omental pedicle wrap. *Journal of Thoracic and Cardiovascular Surgery, 85,* 134-139.

9. Goldberg M, Lima O, Morgan E et al (1983). A comparison between cyclosporine A and methylprednisolone plus azathioprine on bronchial healing following canine lung autotransplantation. *Journal of Thoracic and Cardiovascular Surgery, 85,* 821-826.

10. Todd T, Goldberg M, Koshal A et al (1988). Separate extraction of cardiac and pulmonary grafts from a single organ donor. *Annals of Thoracic Surgery, 46,* 356-359.

11. Cooper JD (1989). Lung transplantation. *Annals of Thoracic Surgery, 47,* 1-17.

12. Patterson A and Cooper JD (1988). Status of lung transplantation. *Surgery Clinics of North America, 68,* 545-558.

13. Dark JH, Patterson GA, Al-Jilaihauri AN et al (1986). Experimental en bloc double lung transplantation. *Annals of Thoracic Surgery, 42,* 394-398.

14. Patterson GA, Cooper JD, Dark JH et al (1988). Experimental and clinical double lung transplantation. *Journal of Thoracic and Cardiovascular Surgery, 95,* 70-74.

15. Cooper JD, Patterson GA, Grossman R and Maurer J et al (1989). Double lung transplant for advanced chronic obstructive lung disease. *AARD, 139,* 303-307.

16. Maurer JR (1987). Unilateral lung transplant. *Pulmonary Perspective, 4,* 1-3.

17. Boychuk JE and Patterson GA (1988). Assessing heart and lung donors. *Diagnosis, 5,* 165-173.

18. Krull K and Hatswell E (1989). Single-lung allograft: a nursing perspective. *Critical Care Nurse, 8,* 35-57.

19. Cooper JD (1984). Experience with lung transplantation at the Toronto General Hospital. *Transplantation Today, 1,* 26-27.

20. Toronto Lung Transplant Group: Sequential bilateral lung transplantation for paraquat poisoning. *Journal of Thoracic and Cardiovascular Surgery, 89,* 734-742.

21. Toronto Lung Transplant Group. Unilateral lung transplantation for pulmonary fibrosis. *New England Journal of Medicine, 314,* 1140-1145.

22. Cooper JD (1987). Lung transplantation: a new era. *Annals of Thoracic Surgery, 44,* 447-448.

23. Grossman R and Cooper JD. *Lung transplantation.* Book chapter (In press).

24. Kamholz SL (1988). Current perspectives on clinical and experimental single lung transplantation. *Chest, 94,* 390-396.

25. Higenbottam T, Stewart S, Penketh A, and Wallock J (1987). The diagnosis of lung rejection and opportunistic infection by transbronchial lung biopsy. *Transplantation Proceedings, XIC,* 3777-3778.

26. Ream AK and Fogdall RP (1982). *Acute cardiovascular management: anesthesia and intensive care.* Philadelphia: JB Lippincott Co.

27. Burtis G, Davis J and Martin S (1988). *Applied nutrition and diet therapy.* Philadelphia: WB Saunders Co.

28. West JB (1979). *Respiratory physiology—the essentials.* Baltimore: Williams & Wilkens Co.

15

Liver Transplantation

Susan L. Smith and Maria Ciferni

HISTORICAL PERSPECTIVE

According to Van Thiel et al, "The ultimate therapeutic step in the treatment of hepatic disease is the provision of a new liver with or without removal of the affected native organ."[1] The road to successful liver grafting in humans, however, has been a long one, fraught with many obstacles. Experimental attempts at liver transplantation began in the 1950s. In 1955 Welch[2] unsuccessfully attempted heterotopic liver transplantation in dogs; in 1956 Cannon[3] was also unsuccessful at orthotopic liver transplantation in dogs. The first successful heterotopic liver transplant in a dog was performed by Moore[4] in 1960, and in that same year Starzl[5] and Moore[6] performed successful orthotopic liver transplants in dogs.

Human liver transplantation did not become a reality until 1963.[7] Although unsuccessful, Dr. T.E. Starzl's accomplishment was a milestone in surgery. It was not until 1967, however, that a human liver transplant was finally successful, again performed by Dr. Starzl.[8] Starzl attributed the success to the addition of antilymphocyte globulin (ALG) in the immunosuppressive regimen. This early success, however, was just the beginning.

For 20 years, from 1963 to 1983, liver transplantation was considered experimental, but it was during this time that major advances were made in clinical and immunologic aspects of liver transplantation.[9,10] By 1983 most of the technologic challenges had been conquered, but the challenge of the immune system still re-

mained to be overcome. In 1983 the National Institutes of Health (NIH) held a Consensus Development Conference on Liver Transplantation. The most important outcome of this conference was that liver transplantation was considered an accepted therapeutic modality for some patients with end-stage liver disease.[11] At the time of this conference there was only one liver transplant center (University of Pittsburgh) in the United States with a sizable patient experience. Currently 82 liver transplant centers are registered with the United Network of Organ Sharing (UNOS).[12] The growth of liver transplantation, in numbers alone, is staggering: In 1981 just 26 liver transplants were performed in the United States[13]; by 1988 it was estimated that 2000 had been performed in the United States, and another 1000 throughout the rest of the world.[1]

The development in the late 1970s of cyclosporine as a powerful immunosuppressant dramatically changed the world of organ transplantation. In the pioneering days of liver transplantation, triple-drug therapy (corticosteroids, azathioprine, and ALG) was used to prevent and treat rejection. By 1984 all transplant centers in the United States were primarily using double therapy consisting of corticosteroids and cyclosporine.[14]

Before the advent of cyclosporine, 5-year survival after liver transplantation was less than 20%.[15] Currently the 63% 5-year survival across the entire spectrum of patients transplanted is three times higher than with conventional azathioprine-steroid immunosuppression.[16] The longest-surviving recipient is a young woman transplanted in 1970 for biliary atresia.[17]

Other factors are responsible for the increased success of liver transplantation. They include advances in surgical techniques, particularly the standardization of biliary tract reconstruction and advances in retransplantation; advances in medical and surgical technology, such as pump-driven venovenous bypass that does not require recipient heparinization[18] and rapid infusion and autologous autotransfusion devices[19]; improved procurement and preservation techniques for the donor liver[20]; and increased knowledge about management of potentially fatal complications. Now that liver transplantation is considered a therapeutic option for many patients with end-stage liver disease, social and ethical issues related to equal access, availability, and affordability of liver transplantation are preeminent. It is estimated that 5000 individuals in the United States alone can benefit from liver transplantation.

PATIENT SELECTION
Indications

Liver disease is a major problem in the United States. Alcohol is one of the most abused drugs in our society,[21] affecting more than 9 million Americans.[22] Cirrhosis is the fourth leading cause of death in adults over age 40 in the United States, and the third leading cause of death, after heart disease and cancer, in men between the ages of 40 and 55.[23]

To be considered a candidate for orthotopic liver transplantation the patient must have irreversible end-stage liver disease, either acute or chronic, that is refractory to other forms of conventional medical or surgical therapy. In addition, the patient must also have no absolute contraindications to liver transplantation.

Indications for orthotopic liver transplant in adults include (1) advanced cirrhosis resulting from cholestatic syndromes or posthepatitic disease, (2) hepatocellular disease, (3) metabolic liver disease, (4) unresectable hepatic malignancies, and (5) fulminant hepatic failure. For a complete list of current indications see the box on p. 275. In adults the most frequent indications include cirrhosis, primarily from chronic

active hepatitis, cryptogenic cirrhosis, primary biliary cirrhosis, and primary sclerosing cholangitis, and in children, biliary atresia (extrahepatic and intrahepatic type, biliary hypoplasia, and Alagille's syndrome), inborn errors of liver metabolism (alpha-1 antitrypsin deficiency, Wilson's disease, and tyrosinemia), and posthepatitic cirrhosis.[16] The clinical syndromes of primary biliary cirrhosis, primary sclerosing cholangitis, chronic active hepatitis, and Budd-Chiari as indications for liver transplantation are described next. Variceal bleeding as an indication for liver transplantation versus shunt surgery is also discussed.

Primary biliary cirrhosis. The patient with primary biliary cirrhosis (PBC) is generally considered a good candidate for liver transplantation.[24,25] This disease, which occurs primarily in middle-aged women, involves a progressive destruction of the small intralobular bile ducts that leads to cholestasis and to eventual liver failure. The cause is unknown.[26] Hepatocyte function is preserved, because it is the bile ducts that are damaged from the disease, not the hepatocytes. Although there may be no clinical manifestations of the disease for many years, once signs and symptoms present, deterioration is progressive. Timing of transplantation in the patient with PBC will ideally precede progressive jaundice, variceal bleeding, uncontrollable ascites, osteodystrophy, malnutrition, hepatic encephalopathy, and spontaneous bacterial peritonitis. In general, when the serum bilirubin exceeds 5.0 mg/dl, the albumin is less than 3.0 g/dl, and there is evidence of portal hypertension, the patient with primary biliary cirrhosis is a candidate for liver transplantation.[26]

Primary sclerosing cholangitis. Primary sclerosing cholangitis is a progressive cholestatic hepatobiliary disorder that leads to stricturing of the extrahepatic and intrahepatic biliary ducts, cholestasis, and ultimately cirrhosis. In most cases no discernible cause can be found.[28] This disease occurs most commonly in young men with a history of chronic inflammatory bowel disease.[29,30] Recurrent sepsis and the potential for the development of cholangiocarcinoma in the preoperative period are major concerns in the patient with primary sclerosing

INDICATIONS FOR ORTHOTOPIC LIVER TRANSPLANTATION

Advanced chronic liver disease

Predominantly cholestatic diseases
  Primary biliary cirrhosis
  Primary sclerosing cholangitis
  Biliary atresia
  Familial cholestatic syndromes
Predominantly hepatocellular disease
  Chronic viral-induced liver disease
  Chronic drug-induced liver disease
  Alcoholic liver disease
  Idiopathic autoimmune liver disease
Predominantly vascular disease
  Budd-Chiari syndrome
  Venoocclusive disease

Hepatic malignancies that are not resectable

Hepatocellular carcinoma
Cholangiocarcinoma
Rare nonhepatocellular or bile ductular tumors
  that arise within the hepatic parenchyma
Isolated hepatic metastatic disease
  Carcinoid
  Pancreatic islet cell tumor
  Others

Fulminant hepatic failure

Viral hepatitis
  A, B, D, non-A, non-B, EBV, other
Drug-induced liver disease
  Halothane
  Gold
  Disulfiram
  Acetaminophen
  Others
Metabolic liver disease
  Wilson's disease
  Reye's syndrome
  Organic acidurias

Metabolic liver disease

Alpha-1 antitrypsin deficiency
Wilson's disease
Homozygous type II hyperlipoproteinemia
Crigler-Najjar syndrome type I
Erythropoietic protoporphyria
Urea cycle deficiencies
Glycogen storage diseases type I and IV
Tyrosinemia
Hemochromatosis

From Van Thiel DH, Makowka L and Starzl TE (1988). Liver transplantation: where it's been and where it's going, *Gastroenterology Clinics of North America, 17*(1), 1-18.

cholangitis. These factors obviously place a premium on the optimal timing of transplantation.

Chronic active hepatitis. Acute hepatitis is followed by complete resolution in most patients. However, there are three forms of chronic sequelae of acute hepatitis: the asymptomatic carrier state, chronic persistent hepatitis, and chronic active hepatitis. A carrier state occurs when the infected individual's system is unable to clear the antigen from the serum. Immunosuppressed individuals such as organ transplant recipients, oncology patients, and those with chronic renal failure are at high risk of becoming chronic carriers. The common etiologic factor in this group of patients is an ineffective cellular immune response.[31] When

the virus is hepatitis B virus (HBV), the hepatitis B surface antigen (HBsAg) and the antibody to surface antigen (anti-HBsAg) are found in the serum. The chronic carrier suffers no liver damage but can transmit the virus to others. There are approximately 200 million carriers in the world.[32] In the United States about 5% to 10% of the population and 1% of health care workers are carriers.[33] Carrier states develop after HBV and non-A, non-B hepatitis (NANB) infections, but not after hepatitis A virus (HAV) infections.

A chronic persistent state develops in about 5% to 10% of those that contract acute hepatitis B or NANB. With chronic persistent hepatitis there are usually no signs or symptoms and liver damage is limited.

In chronic active hepatitis (CAH), liver damage is progressive. A weak cellular immune response is ineffective in clearing the virus. Continued viral replication in the liver leads to progressive hepatocellular necrosis. Chronic active hepatitis is more likely to occur in a person who had a mild or asymptomatic case of acute HBV or NANB infection.[32-34] The most worrisome sequela of CAH is primary hepatocellular carcinoma,[34] whereas the most common complication, cirrhosis, can develop after a severe case of acute hepatitis. In this case it is called posthepatitic cirrhosis, and it can develop as the end stage of CAH.[31]

Budd-Chiari syndrome. Budd-Chiari syndrome or hepatic vein thrombosis is a form of liver disease that can result from a variety of conditions, including retrohepatic tumors resulting in vena caval obstruction, liver tumors, hypercoagulable states secondary to paroxysmal nocturnal hemoglobinuria, and oral contraceptives, myeloproliferative disorders such as polycythemia vera, and venoocclusive disease. In this syndrome, a noncirrhotic outflow block from the sinusoidal bed of the liver leads to centrilobular necrosis and the clinical syndrome of refractory ascites.[35] A causal relationship between Budd-Chiari and use of oral contraceptives has been assumed, but may be coincidental, since very few cases are actually documented.[36] Budd-Chiari represents a spectrum of pathologic changes and clinical symptoms, from the patient with acute Budd-Chiari who does not have cirrhosis but does have ascites with severe congestive hepatomegaly, to the patient with chronic Budd-Chiari who has a fibrotic liver, signs of portal hypertension, and liver failure. A goal of preoperative and postoperative management of the patient with Budd-Chiari syndrome is to treat the underlying cause to decrease the risk of recurrence of the disease.

Variceal bleeding. Iwatsuki[16] has added yet another condition to the list of indications for liver transplantation: variceal bleeding. The survival rates of 302 variceal bleeders who received transplants were compared to 698 patients with other indications for liver transplant. The survival rates of variceal bleeders after transplantation were significantly higher than those with other indications (5-year survival 71% versus 59%). Iwatsuki suggests that liver transplantation is a treatment option for patients with variceal bleeding for whom sclerotherapy has not been successful.

Acute hepatic necrosis. Acute hepatic necrosis is defined as the clinical and biochemical presence of liver disease in someone whose liver function was normal before the development of signs and symptoms, and the development of hepatic encephalopathy within 8 weeks of the onset of signs and symptoms.[37,38] A subacute form of hepatic necrosis can also occur, in which encephalopathy can occur as long as 20 weeks after the initial manifestation of clinical signs and symptoms. Both of these conditions are characterized by a sudden onset of altered mental status, progressive jaundice, and encephalopathy.

The prognosis associated with this condition is very poor. With the exception of acute hepatic necrosis resulting from acetaminophen toxicity, the condition is nearly always fatal. Overall mortality, regardless of cause, is 75% to 95%.[37] The depth of encephalopathy and the age of the patient play a role in survival.

The most common causes of acute hepatic necrosis are viral hepatitis, drug toxicity, and fulminant Wilson's disease.[38] Viral hepatitis (primarily hepatitis B), however, accounts for the majority of cases (80%), whereas drug toxicity (halothane and acetaminophen) accounts for 15%.[37] Other causes include industrial toxins (e.g., carbon tetrachloride, pesticides, and herbicides), toxic mushroom poisoning, infection, acute fatty liver of pregnancy, Reye's syndrome, and acute hepatic artery thrombosis.[39-41]

Although the efficacy of liver transplantation for acute hepatic necrosis has not been clearly shown, it is the only option for the patient with an acutely, irreversibly necrotic liver. Limited experience at a few transplant centers has shown, however, that some patients can be saved with liver transplantation.[42-44] At the University of Pittsburgh survival rates have increased from less than 20% without transplantation to 55% with transplantation.[44]

Contraindications

As the status of liver transplantation has changed and long-term success rates rival all other types of solid organ transplantation, the absolute and relative contraindications have also changed. At the time of the NIH Consensus Development Conference, contraindications included alcoholism, tumors other than primary hepatic tumors, and psychosocial and economic factors such as inability to understand the procedure and inability to pay. However, patients with all of these conditions and situations have been and continue to be transplanted as the treatment becomes more successful. The combination of preexisting local or systemic infections outside the hepatobiliary system such as peritonitis, pneumonia, or bacteremia and the necessity of postoperative immunosuppressive therapy place the patient at great risk for a fatal infection and therefore preclude successful liver transplantation. Likewise, because the operative procedure is so rigorous, significant cardiovascular or pulmonary disease decreases the likelihood of surviving the perioperative or postoperative period.[45]

Hepatic malignancy. Ironically, the initial indications for human liver transplantation mandated that the patient have a hepatic malignancy. The rationale for this criterion was that because of the highly experimental nature of the procedure and the low survival rates, it was not justifiable to subject a patient with nonneoplastic disease to the procedure. Today, hepatic malignancy is, in most cases, considered a contraindication to liver transplantation.

The clinical picture for a patient with a malignant tumor of the liver is much different than that for the typical patient who is evaluated for liver transplantation. Unlike a patient with chronic liver disease, a patient with a primary hepatic malignancy who is in relatively good physical condition does not manifest cutaneous stigmata of advanced liver disease and rarely has cirrhosis or portal hypertension. For most types of liver tumors there is no effective chemotherapy, and the resectability rate is quite low. Conceptually, then, total hepatectomy and orthotopic liver transplantation represent the only possible therapy for most patients with a primary malignancy of the liver.

It is ironic that the first survivor of an orthotopic liver transplant was transplanted for hepatoma; she died 13 months after the transplant as a result of tumor recurrence.[8] The fact that the surgical procedure for this group of patients is generally simpler than other organ transplant procedures from a technical perspective added to the initial enthusiasm for the treatment of hepatic tumors with orthotopic liver transplantation. This enthusiasm, however, has dampened over the years as it has been realized that the results are not as good as initially expected. In the era before cyclosporine was introduced, for example, 13.5% of Starzl's patients (Denver/Pittsburgh) were transplanted for malignancy, whereas in the cyclosporine era only 5.6% of patients have been transplanted for hepatic malignancy.[46] Although liver transplantation has provided long-term cure for a few patients with hepatic tumors, the overall actuarial survival at 3 years is 20% to 40%.[47]

The most common cause of death after 3 months is tumor recurrence.[47] Immunosuppressive regimens necessary for prevention and treatment of rejection are thought to accelerate tumor growth. Of those patients whose primary indication for transplantation is hepatocellular carcinoma and who live long enough for occult tumor recurrence to be evident, 85% develop overt recurrent disease.[1] However, if hepatocellular carcinoma is found incidentally at the time of transplant, the recurrence rate is very low.

Calne et al,[48] at the Kings College program in Cambridge, reported the results of 93 patients with primary or secondary malignant disease of the liver who underwent orthotopic liver transplantation. In patients with primary hepatocellular carcinoma who survived for longer than 3 months, the recurrence rate was 64.9%. Starzl[49] reported the results of 54 patients with malignant disease treated with orthotopic liver transplantation. The recurrence rate for primary hepatocellular carcinoma was 77.8%. The only patients without early recurrence were those with small hepatomas found incidentally at the time of transplant and those with the fibrolamellar variant of hepatocellular carcinoma. Fibrolamellar carcinoma, which is slow growing and nonaggressive, usually occurs in adolescents or young adults, is more common in females by a ratio of 2 to 1, and has a high resectability rate. More recently Koneru et al[46] reported the results of 34 patients treated for hepatocellular carcinoma with liver transplantation. In 14 patients the tumor was found incidentally, and in 20 hepatocellular carcinoma was the primary indication for transplantation. In the first group, tumor recurrence occurred in only one patient. In the second group, of the 15 patients who survived for longer than 2 months, eight developed tumor recurrence within 12 months.

Cholangiocarcinoma is frequently associated with sclerosing cholangitis. The prognosis for long-term survival after liver transplantation in a patient with cholangiocarcinoma is worse than for a patient with primary hepatocellular carcinoma. Van Thiel et al report a 100% recurrence rate and death in this group of patients. O'Grady et al transplanted seven patients with central cholangiocarcinoma and seven with peripheral cholangiocarcinoma. In each group, of those who lived for 3 months, six had documented tumor recurrence. Koneru et al[46] reported on nine patients transplanted for cholangiocarcinoma; seven developed early tumor recurrence. Because of the dismal results obtained from transplanting patients with cholangiocarcinoma, a percutaneous transhepatic or endoscopic brush biopsy of the biliary tree should be obtained in all patients with sclerosing cholangitis who are being evaluated for liver transplantation. At present, once cholangiocarcinoma develops, liver transplantation is contraindicated.[50]

The liver is the organ most frequently involved with metastatic tumors. Therefore, before any patient undergoes transplant surgery for malignant hepatic disease, every attempt is made to rule out metastatic disease. Computed tomography (CT) of the abdomen, lungs, and head, chest x-ray evaluation, nuclear magnetic resonance imaging (MRI), bone scanning, and other tests are commonly performed. Unfortunately, micrometastases are frequently undetectable and may not be discovered until abdominal exploration at the time of transplant. For patients with a high index of suspicion for metastatic disease, despite workup findings that do not confirm the diagnosis, it is explained to the patient before surgery that the transplant may not be able to be done, and a backup patient is prepared so that the organ does not go unused. Survival after transplant for metastatic disease is rare. In a series reported by O'Grady,[48] only three patients survived for 6 months and all died of recurrent disease.

In spite of the unfavorable prognosis for long-term survival after liver transplantation for malignant hepatic disease, controversy continues as to whether the results justify continued efforts in this field of liver transplantation. Pilchmayer et al[51] consider orthotopic liver transplantation acceptable palliative treatment despite short-term survival, whereas Iwatsuki et al stated, "Transplantation for malignant disease is conceptually unsound."[52] Makowka et al[53] reported transplanting five patients with unresectable hepatic metastases originating from endothelial tumors of the gastrointestinal tract. At the time of their report, three patients were still living at 7, 16, and 34 months after transplant. This is an area that is certain to attract more research in the future.

Alcoholic cirrhosis. The most common cause of cirrhosis in the United States and the western hemisphere is alcoholic liver disease. At least 50% of cases of cirrhosis in the United States are attributable to alcohol abuse.[54] Therefore patients with alcoholic cirrhosis represent the largest number of potential adult liver transplant recipients.[55]

Alcoholic cirrhosis, however, has been considered a relative contraindication to liver transplantation for several reasons: (1) the high risk of patient noncompliance associated with the alcoholic life-style, (2) other medical disorders associated with alcoholism, such as cardiomyopathy, chronic pancreatitis, cerebral atrophy, and protein-calorie malnutrition, and (3) based on early reports, the outcome in alcoholics is generally worse than in nonalcoholics.[56] However, in the Pittsburgh experience since 1980, the results with alcoholic patients have been as good as in adult patients transplanted for nonalcoholic liver disease.[57]

The criteria used to decide whether to transplant the alcoholic cirrhotic patient vary among transplant centers. Clearly, the patient who is an active alcoholic is at very high risk for psychologic morbidity and an unsuccessful outcome and is not usually considered a candidate. On the other hand, the patient who has demonstrated some period of sobriety is considered by most transplant teams to be a potential candidate. Although the establishment of arbitrary waiting periods is not yet supported by the medical literature, the minimal length of time that a patient must have been sober before being considered for transplantation ranges from 6 months to 2 years.[54,58] A further step taken by many transplant centers to ensure the best chance for successful outcome is the requirement that patients also have completed an established alcohol treatment program.

Active hepatitis. Recurrence of hepatitis B is common in the patient who is actively replicating virus at the time of transplant.[58,59] In the past the presence of active disease from hepatitis B, as manifested by positive serologic test results for HBsAg or HBeAg, was considered an absolute contraindication to transplantation because of the very high incidence of recurrence of hepatitis.[60-64] In addition, the presence of Delta virus represents a high risk of recurrence of disease.[65] Recurrence of hepatitis B is initially manifested by elevated liver enzyme levels accompanied by malaise, nausea, and jaundice; a biopsy reveals changes that are different from rejection and consistent with acute hepatitis. These changes typically occur at least 2 months after transplantation.[66] One of the clinical problems associated with these findings is the differential diagnosis between rejection and hepatitis. The treatment for these two conditions is very different — in fact, opposite — immunosuppressive therapy is increased for rejection and decreased for hepatitis. Making the incorrect diagnosis and subsequently the wrong treatment choice can have disastrous results in the patient. The eventual outcome of recurrent hepatitis spans the spectrum from a self-limiting process without sequelae to acute fulminant hepatitis requiring retransplantation.[66] All patients with active hepatitis at the time of transplant have recurrence. The severity of the recurrence, though, is unpredictable. Recently, because of preliminary results obtained with the use of long-term immunoprophylaxis against hepatitis B virus begun in the anhepatic phase, active hepatitis at the time of transplant is now considered to be a relative contraindication.[59,65,67]

Patient evaluation

Evaluation of the appropriateness of a candidate for liver transplantation is a complex process and involves a multidisciplinary approach. These patients are usually chronically ill with end-stage liver disease. The goals of the evaluation are to (1) determine the medical necessity for and proper timing of transplantation, (2) determine the technical feasibility of the procedure, (3) identify any precluding extrahepatic disease, (4) determine physiologic and psychologic suitability, and (5) identify organ systems that may require being brought to optimal conditions before transplantation.

Medical necessity. The medical necessity for liver transplantation is usually straightforward as determined by the patient's specific disease (or diseases). Optimal timing for transplantation is much less clear. The NIH Consensus Conference report states that liver transplant should be performed before the patient is too debilitated to tolerate the rigors of the surgical procedure.[11] At present there are no definitive guidelines to define optimal timing for surgery. Reliance on traditional methods of evaluating liver function can be misleading. Liver "function" tests such as liver and biliary enzymes, bilirubin, coagulation factors, and albumin do not really assess liver function; instead they assess liver dysfunction. There is no way to estimate functional hepatocyte mass using these laboratory tests. This becomes evident when comparing patients with liver disease according to their "numbers." Patients with the worst numbers will often "look" better than those whose numbers may be within normal range or slightly abnormal according to textbook parameters. Reliance on a traditional method of evaluation of liver function can result in unnecessary delays of referral for liver transplantation and can adversely affect the patient's prognosis for a successful transplant. Assessment of quantitative liver function has been used, however, by some centers (see the box on p. 280) to better define hepatic reserve and therefore provide a rational basis as to optimal timing for transplantation.[27,68]

Liver function can be quantified by assessing metabolic and clearance functions of the liver that are dependent on functional liver cell mass and blood flow. Some of the more useful quantitative tests are the galactose elimination capacity (GEC), antipyrine metabolism and clearance, galactose clearance, and protein load.

EMORY HEPATIC DATABASE

Child score
Liver biopsy
Quantitative liver function
   Galactose elimination capacity
   Amino acid tolerance score
   Antipyrine clearance
Liver volume
Hemodynamics
   Cardiac output
   Liver blood flow
   Portal flow
EEG
Liver package angiography

From Millikan WG et al (1988). Orthotopic liver transplantation, *Emory University Journal of Medicine, 2*(3), 192-198, JB Lippincott, Philadelphia.

The GEC measures the functional hepatocyte mass by calculating the maximal removal rate of galactose, which is exclusively and rapidly converted to glucose in the liver. In this test a known quantity (500 mg/kg) of galactose is administered intravenously and blood samples are drawn at intervals over 20 to 60 minutes. Plasma galactose concentrations are plotted against time. The maximal rate of galactose removal is calculated from the slope of this curve and the volume of distribution of galactose. Normal GEC is 500 mg/min or 33 mg/kg/min.[69]

The antipyrine clearance test measures mixed-function oxidase reactions in the liver.[69] Antipyrine is a drug similar to aspirin that is completely absorbed in the GI tract, metabolized by the liver, and excreted in the saliva. In this test a known quantity of antipyrine is administered orally and saliva samples are analyzed over the following 24 to 48 hours.

Low-dose galactose clearance is used as an index of "nutritive" liver blood flow. In this test a 5% solution of galactose is given by continuous infusion at 65 mg/min and blood samples are taken at intervals over 60 to 100 minutes when the plasma steady state has been reached. Galactose clearance is calculated in milliliters per minute, with normal galactose clearance being between 1100 and 1600 ml/min.[69]

The protein load test measures amino acid and ammonia tolerance. Six ounces of oral protein solution is administered. Baseline fasting levels of serum and urine amino acids and ammonia are subtracted from levels after administration of the protein load. A plasma response curve similar to a glucose tolerance test is plotted to evaluate the liver's ability to metabolize protein, and the patient's clinical tolerance is assessed.

Although some quantitative studies of liver function are more invasive than qualitative assessment techniques, the precision of the studies is beneficial when determining optimal treatment for the patient with liver disease. Increasing use of quantitative evaluation to determine the optimal timing for transplantation should assume increasing importance in patient assessment.

Technical feasibility. Technical advancements have made it possible to transplant most patients, but some factors will increase the operative risks. For example, portal vein thrombosis, prior biliary bypass operations, multiple intraabdominal procedures, and major arterial anomalies increase technical difficulty. Evaluation of technical problems involves radiologic evaluation to detect conditions that would complicate transplantation or require modification of standard surgical procedures.[69]

Until recently, patency of the portal vein was considered a prerequisite for liver transplantation. However, if the surgeons have considerable experience with surgery of the portal vein, liver transplantation is considered feasible even if the recipient portal vein is abnormally small or thrombosed.[70]

Physiologic and psychologic suitability. This component of the evaluation begins with a thorough patient history and physical examination, including a psychiatric and psychosocial evaluation.[71] Because chronic liver disease can affect all major organ systems, various laboratory and other diagnostic tests are performed to evaluate the major organ systems and identify any contraindications to transplantation. In addition, various specialists are often consulted to give their impressions and recommendations regarding suitability for transplantation. It should be noted that this process is complex and time consuming. From the patient and family perspective, it is often physically and psychologically stressful. Although the evaluation may be done on an outpatient basis, it commonly requires hospitalization.

Once considered an acceptable candidate for transplantation, the patient may require considerable treatment for sequelae of end-stage liver disease. Paracenteses and thoracenteses may be required for the control of ascites and pleural effusions, and antibiotics may be needed for the treatment or prevention of infection. Sclerotherapy may be necessary to control variceal bleeding, and frequent transfusions with blood products may be necessary to optimize the preoperative coagulation status.

Optimal timing for transplantation is highly individualized, depending primarily on the hepatic and systemic sequelae of liver disease. In general, a rapid elevation in serum bilirubin, ascites that is refractory to diuretics, the onset of spontaneous encephalopathy, recurrent variceal hemorrhage, and recurrent sepsis are signs of deterioration that warrant expedient transplantation.

LIVER RECOVERY

According to Millikan et al, "The donor harvest is the most difficult part of liver transplantation because of the logistics involved."[68] Harvest or recovery of the donor liver is most often performed in conjunction with removal of the heart and kidneys for donation and now, occasionally, with the pancreas. Therefore three surgical donor teams are coordinating efforts to remove organs from one cadaver donor as quickly and effectively as possible. The goals of liver procurement are to (1) recognize an organ unacceptable for transplantation, (2) perform a technically perfect operation, (3) avoid warm ischemia, and (4) minimize cold ischemia of the donor organ.

Suitability of the donor liver cannot be determined until the liver is visually inspected in the donor's abdomen by an experienced liver transplant surgeon. Even then the ultimate outcome of graft function will not be known for up to 48 hours or longer after transplantation. Peters et al at the University of Tennessee reported that 20% of livers recovered could not be transplanted because of congenital arterial anomalies, contamination of the abdominal cavity, an abnormal liver, hepatic malignancy, or cardiac arrest in the donor.[72]

Matching the size of the potential recipient with the donor is a critical consideration in liver transplantation. Though criteria vary, in general, the donor weight should be 10 kg less than the recipient,[73] or the variance in weights should not exceed 20%.[55]

Surgical procedure for recovery of the donor liver

Recovery of the donor liver involves two essential steps—incision of the restraining ligaments that secure the liver to the diaphragm and the anterior abdominal wall, and dissection of the vessels and bile duct that will be anastomosed to the native companion structures. Removal of the donor liver is done through a long midline incision from the sternal notch to the pubis and begins with dissection of the major vessels around the liver. The aorta is isolated at its bifurcation and at the diaphragm to allow cross-clamping of the aorta for an in situ flush. The common bile duct is transected proximal to the ampulla, and the gallbladder is flushed with cool saline solution to remove stagnant bile. The liver is flushed in situ, first with cold heparinized lactated Ringer's solution to remove stagnant blood and then with cold heparinized Euro-Collins solution or University of Wisconsin (UW) solution for preservation during transport. The suprahepatic vena cava is transected at the level of the right atrium, and the infrahepatic vena cava just above the renal veins, thereby preserving them for renal transplantation. The portal vein is divided at the confluence of the splenic vein and the superior mesenteric vein, and the abdominal aorta with the hepatic arterial blood supply is excised. The distal aorta, iliac arteries, vena cavae, and iliac veins are also recovered and preserved for potential use as vascular grafts. The liver is packed in Euro-Collins or UW solution in ice and transported to the recipient's transplant center.

THE SURGICAL PROCEDURE

The surgical procedure for orthotopic liver transplantation involves three separate procedures: the donor hepatectomy, the recipient hepatectomy, and graft insertion. The procedure is a long one, typically taking from 8 to 10 hours to complete. For the operative care of the liver transplant recipient alone, participation of more than 40 team members is necessary, including surgeons, anesthesiologists, nurses, perfusionists, hematologists, and blood bank and laboratory personnel. Strong leadership in the operating room is critical to ensure effective communication and cooperation among all those involved.

Two very different surgical approaches to liver transplantation exist: the orthotopic and the heterotopic approach. In *orthotopic* liver transplantation the patient's diseased liver is removed and replaced with a donor liver with normal or near-normal anatomic reconstruction. In *heterotopic* liver transplantation the patient's diseased liver is left in place and an auxiliary liver is grafted into an ectopic site.[74] The first attempts at liver transplantation were heterotopic to avoid sacrifice of functional hepatic reserve should the graft fail or reject. Currently experimental indications for heterotopic liver transplantation are for treatment of the patient with acute hepatic failure or the patient who has had surgery in the right upper quadrant that prohibits orthotopic liver transplantation.[73] Other indications are currently under study.

The donor hepatectomy has been described. In this section the procedures for recipient hepatectomy and graft insertion will be described and discussed. Before the actual beginning of the procedure, multiple invasive monitoring devices and large-bore intravenous cannulas are placed in the patient, and baseline laboratory data are obtained.

Because the surgery is long, proper positioning of the patient on the operating room table is crucial to allow prevention of peripheral nerve injuries and pressure-related ischemia. The patient's knees are slightly flexed, with the toes pointing upward to prevent hyperextension of the knees. The legs are taped together below the knees to prevent external rotation of the hips.

Recipient hepatectomy

The recipient hepatectomy can be the most difficult phase of the surgery because of the underlying effects of chronic liver disease on the vasculature and hepatic system. However, in patients with no prior surgery and/or minimal portal hypertension, this phase may be relatively straightforward. Usually the average patient requiring transplant does have a significant degree of portal hypertension and coagulopathy; therefore hemorrhage is the major potential risk during this phase. Another reason for hemorrhage during this stage of the surgery is often the presence of adhesions vascularized with fragile collaterals that formed as a result of prior surgery. Patients with chronic liver disease frequently have a hyperdynamic cardiovascular state (cardiac output often exceeds 10 L/min). This state must be maintained during surgery and often requires use of a specially equipped rapid infusion device that prevents the coagulation factor depletion and hyperkalemia commonly associated with massive transfusion. Another advance in the intraoperative management of liver transplant patients is the autologous cell-saver device that allows the patient's own red blood cells lost to the operative field to be washed out and autotransfused. This decreases the amount of banked packed red blood cells required and limits exposure of the patient to non-A, non-B hepatitis and cytomegalovirus. However, with this device the plasma is not returned, so there is still a need for fresh frozen plasma and platelets.

The recipient hepatectomy begins with opening the abdomen with a bilateral subcostal incision and a midline incision extending up to the xiphoid and identifying all pertinent portal structures. At this time, the donor liver has usually not arrived, so nothing irreversible is done at this stage. However, since the maximum cold ischemic time for the donor liver is 12 hours using Euro-Collins preservation solution (or up to 24 hours using UW solution), this is considered a time-saving step in the procedure. It is important that before consenting for surgery the patient and family be made aware that the procedure may have to be aborted during this stage if the condition of the donor or the donor liver deteriorates before completion of recovery.

Once the donor liver arrives, some time is required for its final preparation, which involves removal of diaphragmatic remnants, and dissection of the vena cavae, hepatic artery, and portal vein. The native liver is removed intact, leaving behind the inferior vena cava (IVC) from just below the diaphragm to just above the renal veins. Removal of the diseased liver requires clamping of the infrahepatic and suprahepatic IVC and division of the portal vein. Venous return from the IVC is interrupted and the infrahepatic IVC and portal vein outflow is occluded. In adults this traditionally led to engorgement of all subdiaphragmatic vessels, resulting in increased portal hypertension and congestion of the bowel. Congestion of the bowel can lead to significant interstitial (third-space) fluid loss and contamination of the peritoneum with bowel flora. In addition, clamping of the infrahepatic IVC is often associated with damage to the kidneys and hemodynamic instability as a result of an interruption of venous return to the heart.

However, with the advent of venovenous bypass without the need for heparin in 1982, venous return to the heart can be maintained and venous engorgement avoided by shunting systemic venous return and portal flow to the superior vena cava (SVC). In other words, normal hemodynamics can be maintained during the anhepatic phase. Heparinless venovenous bypass is accomplished by use of a centrifugal blood pump (Bio-Medicus, Inc.) equipped with large-bore drainage and return cannulas (Fig. 15-1). Blood is drained from the infrahepatic IVC and the portal vein to a centrifugal pump that returns blood to the ipsilateral axillary or internal jugular vein. Usually a flow rate of 1.5 to 6.0 L/min can be maintained.[75]

Orthotopic liver transplantation has been greatly enhanced by the use of venovenous

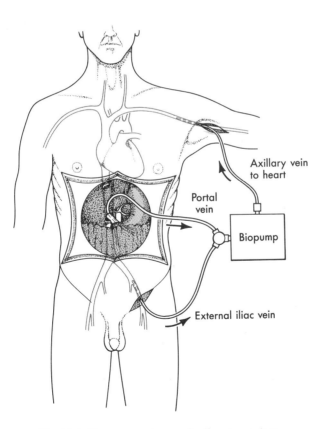

Axillary vein
to heart

Portal
vein

Biopump

External iliac vein

Fig. 15-1 Venovenous bypass for liver transplant.

bypass. Before this technology was available, timing of the anhepatic phase was critical and hemostasis was difficult to control. Venovenous bypass allows for a longer anhepatic phase, better hemostatic control, increased hemodynamic stability, and decreases risks to the kidneys and GI tract. McSteen et al[76] compared the intraoperative events of patients transplanted with heparinless venovenous bypass to those of patients transplanted with bypass requiring systemic anticoagulation. Blood and blood product replacement was significantly higher (associated with greater hemodynamic instability) in the second group, and the mean bypass time was significantly less in the first group (99 versus 160 minutes). However, Khoury et al[77] reported one case of severe air embolism with the use of venovenous bypass, which they attributed to air gaining entrance into the system at tubing connection sites. Present systems have an alarm device that activates with the presence of air bubbles in the tubing.

Graft insertion

Once venovenous bypass is established the liver can be removed, and graft insertion can begin. This phase involves four vascular anastomoses (Fig. 15-2) and the biliary anastomosis. The vascular anastomoses are usually performed in the following order: suprahepatic IVC, infrahepatic IVC, portal vein, and hepatic artery. After the suprahepatic and infrahepatic IVC anastomoses are completed, portal venovenous bypass is interrupted and an end-to-end anastomosis between the donor and recipient portal veins is performed. On completion of this anastomosis, venovenous bypass is discontinued and the liver is reperfused. Major bleeding is controlled and the hepatic arterial anastomosis is done by anastomosing the donor hepatic artery to the recipient hepatic artery.

Once the vascular anastomoses are completed, the surgeon must wait to see if the new liver will function. During this time the patient is rewarmed, which facilitates the production of clotting factors by the transplanted liver. There are several factors that contribute to hypothermia in the liver transplant patient: low ambient temperature of the operating room, wet prepa-

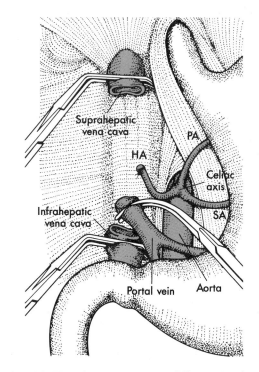

Fig. 15-2 Vascular anastomoses of liver transplant.

ration procedures, exposure of the abdominal viscera, long operative time, extracorporeal circulation, and cold preservation of the graft. Several important measures are routinely taken to prevent or counteract hypothermia. These include raising the ambient room temperature, use of plastic abdominal drapes, heating inspired gases, wrapping the patient's head and legs, intermittent packing and closing of the abdomen, and acute peritoneal dialysis with warmed saline.[68]

After rewarming and achieving hemostasis, the biliary anastomosis can be completed. Two types of biliary anastomoses are routinely performed: choledochocholedochostomy (common duct to common duct) and a Roux-en-Y choledochojejunostomy (common duct to jejunum) (Fig. 15-3). A choledochocholedochostomy with a T-tube stent is preferable unless there is concomitant disease of the common bile duct (as with sclerosing cholangitis). On completion of the biliary anastomosis a cholangio-

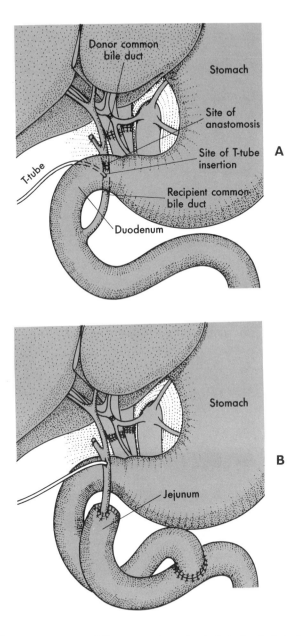

Fig. 15-3 Biliary anastomoses of liver transplant. **A**, choledochocholedochostomy.
B, choledochojejunostomy.

gram is performed, and the abdomen is closed after placement of (typically) three drains.

POSTOPERATIVE CARE

In the acute setting there are two distinct phases of care: the immediate postoperative or stabilization phase, and the transitional phase, after the need for intensive care but before discharge from the hospital. Because of the nature of end-stage liver disease, patients in need of a liver transplant are frequently hospitalized, often for prolonged periods, before transplantation. The goal then becomes stabilizing and optimizing the patient's condition, or in some cases simply keeping the patient alive until a compatible donor liver becomes available. Likewise, because of the complex nature of liver transplantation (the majority of patients suffer a major postoperative complication),[78] patients who have received a transplanted liver are likely to be readmitted for treatment of complications, usually related to the infectious problems of long-term immunosuppression or rejection. The following discussion, however, will focus on the acute care of liver transplant patients after surgery. Optimal outcomes for the patient and family are dependent on a coordinated interdisciplinary approach and a collaborative relationship among nurses, physicians, and ancillary personnel.

The critical phase: immediate postoperative care

Basic to care of the liver transplant patient is a thorough understanding of normal liver function, the pathophysiology of acute and chronic liver failure, and the clinical sequelae of liver disease — specifically portal hypertension and its major physiologic consequences of collateral vessel formation, ascites, splenomegaly, and encephalopathy. Critical to nursing assessment of the liver transplant patient is recognition of normal versus abnormal liver (graft) function and patient responses to a vast and complex array of nursing and medical interventions. The following discussion of nursing care centers around prevention and treatment of complications that commonly occur after liver transplantation.

The following, although somewhat oversimplified, is a description of the experience of a typical liver transplant patient admitted to the intensive care unit (ICU). The patient has been told sometime in the past year that he or she has a terminal liver disease and that the only hope for a cure is a liver transplant. After dealing with the initial disbelief and shock, the patient and family are given technical and practical information about liver transplantation and are supported through what is often a difficult decision-making process about whether to accept the option of transplantation. Next comes the wait, sometimes prolonged, for a compatible donor, and then "the telephone call" comes beckoning them to the transplant center now that a compatible donor has become available. The attendant preoperative psychologic stresses endured by the liver transplant patient are transferred to the nursing staff, who must support the family during the surgical procedure, and this stress carries over additively into the postoperative period.

The surgery averages about 8 to 10 hours (although some centers are reporting shorter operative times), during which time the patient is put to the ultimate test of physiologic stress: prolonged general anesthesia, the most complex surgical procedure performed to date, venovenous bypass, hypothermia, hemorrhage, and immunosuppression. After surgery, on admission to the ICU, the patient may be barely recognizable to those who know him or her. Edema from massive fluid resuscitation and third-spacing of fluids may disfigure the patient; the patient's head is wrapped to prevent heat loss; and a multiplicity of tubes, catheters, and drains are entering and exiting the various orifices, veins, and arteries. The patient's eyes may be taped shut. In short, underneath the equipment and blankets, there may be but a vague resemblance of the person who went off to surgery the day before. It is imperative that the family be prepared to see the patient for the first time after surgery. They will usually require several reassurances that what they will see is normal, and not unusual resulting from early complications. This perspective is an important starting point for care of the liver transplant patient.

Hypothermia. Many liver transplant patients will be hypothermic to some degree. And although it is a temporary problem, it deserves considerable attention from the nurse. Contributing factors to hypothermia in the liver transplant patient are numerous: the ambient temperature in the operating room, wet surgical preparation procedures, preoperative and postoperative narcotics and muscle relaxants, prolonged general anesthesia, prolonged exposure of the peritoneum and bowel to the atmosphere, unwarmed intravenous fluids and surgical field irrigants, and the cold preservation technique used in the donor liver. The recognition and modification of these factors as is appropriate can prevent or limit the unwanted physiologic consequences of severe hypothermia.

The physiologic consequences of hypothermia can contribute to an unstable course in the immediate postoperative period. Severe hypothermia is associated with cardiac dysrhythmias, which can add to the usual state of cardiovascular instability during this time. Although severe hypothermia is no longer the norm, moderate hypothermia is common and can prolong anesthetic recovery, alter platelet function and clotting ability, shift the oxyhemoglobin dissociation curve to the left causing metabolic alkalosis and hypokalemia, and increase systemic vascular resistance (SVR).

Since the majority of adult liver transplant patients have an indwelling pulmonary artery catheter, monitoring of the core temperature is easily accomplished. The patient's thorax, hands, and feet should remain covered until rewarming is complete, and the head should be wrapped in some fashion to prevent heat loss. This is difficult to accomplish when operating room equipment is being removed from the patient, ICU equipment is being attached to the patient, and when the anesthesiologist and nurse are assessing the patient's condition after transport. The tendency is to leave the patient's upper body exposed to accomplish these tasks at a time when the body most needs to be covered. For this reason, and because frequent assessments will be necessary during the first few hours after admission of the patient, the use of radiant warming devices and an overlying thin blanket layer are preferred over piling thick layers of blankets on the patient that must be removed to perform the simplest task. Intravenous fluids may also need to be warmed before infusion.

The patient's hemodynamic status is monitored continuously during the rewarming phase. The cardiovascular instability discussed below will be exacerbated near the end of the rewarming phase as the SVR decreases, resulting in vasodilation and relative hypovolemia. At this time the amount of intravenous fluids required will increase, and the flow rate of any continuous infusions of antihypertensive agents will need to be decreased. Anticipating this problem of hypothermia and being prepared to intervene when the patient arrives from the operating room is an important nursing priority.

Primary nonfunctioning graft. One of the less well understood dilemmas of liver transplantation is the phenomenon of the primary nonfunctioning graft (PNFG). This refers to the graft that despite all efforts by the organ recovery and transplant teams to ensure its viability fails to function. In most cases a PNFG will be clinically evident almost immediately. On vascularization of the graft in the operating room, the functional liver should produce bile. If it does not, this is an early clue that there may be a problem.

Assessment of graft function is an immediate and ongoing responsibility of the critical care nurse. Several factors can be analyzed in assessment of graft function and for recognition of PNFG. As stated, bile production is one such factor. A primary function of the liver is to produce and secrete bile. In the patient with a T-tube, assessment of bile for quality and quantity is done on admission and on a regular basis thereafter. The bile should be thick or viscous and range in color from dark gold to brown. If the patient does not have a T-tube—common in patients with sclerosing cholangitis, for example—then this "window" of liver function is not available.

The most sensitive laboratory indices of liver function are the coagulation factors, prothrombin time (PT), and partial thromboplastin time (PTT). Alteration in liver function is reflected very early by prolonged coagulation times. The PT and PTT in the immediate postoperative period will vary, depending on the preoperative levels and intraoperative events. What should occur, though, is a steady downward trend toward normalcy in both the PT and PTT.

Hypokalemia is another sign in the immediate postoperative period that the liver is functional.

Before grafting, the liver was flushed of all preservation solution, which is rich in potassium. The liver cells thus give up potassium, and when the graft is vascularized functional hepatocytes extract potassium from the blood. Therefore for a variable period slight to moderate hypokalemia is seen. Although this may require potassium supplementation, it is a favorable sign. On the other hand, hyperkalemia, which may signify cell death, in this early period would indicate that the hepatocytes are not functional and is therefore an unfavorable sign.

Hyperglycemia is another favorable sign in the immediate postoperative period. This indicates that the liver is able to store glycogen and convert it to glucose and respond to the metabolic effects of corticosteroids. This often requires a short-term continuous insulin infusion and frequent monitoring of serum glucose. Hypoglycemia, like hyperkalemia, would indicate nonfunctional hepatocytes and is also an unfavorable sign.

The serum transaminases (SGOT, SGPT) and phosphatases (alkaline phosphatase and gamma GT) and the serum bilirubin should show a progressive downward trend after transplantation. The exact values after transplantation vary widely from patient to patient and depend on the degree of recovery ischemia of the liver and intraoperative events. For instance, if the patient required massive blood transfusion, the initial levels may be very low as a result of hemodilution. More accurate levels will be manifested at approximately 6 to 12 hours after surgery. With PNFG the enzyme and bilirubin levels increase as the liver begins to necrose.

Finally, the clinical status of the patient provides an early clue to liver function. The importance of liver function on other vital systems becomes evident in the setting of PNFG and acute liver failure. Evaluation of mental status for development of encephalopathy is difficult because the patient is intubated and still partially anesthetized. Failure of the patient to gradually wake up may be the only neurologic manifestation of PNFG. Acute hepatorenal syndrome will accompany PNFG, which will lead to hypervolemia and pulmonary edema, manifested by elevated filling pressures of the right and left sides of the heart, hypoxemia, failure to wean from mechanical ventilation, and peripheral edema.

The differential diagnoses for PNFG include reversible recovery ischemia, hyperacute rejection, and unknown causes. PNFG is a life-threatening situation: the only treatment is immediate retransplantation, usually within 48 hours. From a psychologic perspective, this is devastating to the family (and patient if he or she is aware of the situation), who have anticipated the safe return of their loved one to the ICU. Temporary support measures until retransplantation include continued mechanical ventilation, ultrafiltration for management of fluid and electrolyte imbalances and supplementation of coagulation factors with fresh frozen plasma (FFP), cryoprecipitate, and platelets if necessary.

Cardiovascular instability. There are two major causes of cardiovascular instability in the immediate postoperative period: hypovolemia and systemic arterial hypertension. Intensive cardiovascular monitoring and assessment are often the major and most important focus of nursing care for the first 24 to 48 hours after surgery. Most adults will have a pulmonary artery catheter for monitoring filling pressures of the right and left sides of the heart, cardiac output, and systemic and pulmonary vascular resistance (SVR and PVR), which facilitates the necessary titration of fluids and cardioactive and vasoactive drugs.

Patients with end-stage liver disease are usually hyperdynamic (high cardiac output and low SVR) before surgery. With progressive liver disease portal venous flow decreases and hepatic arterial flow increases compensatorily to maintain a constant liver blood flow. This is reflected in an increased cardiac output. Another result of decreased portal blood flow is the widespread development of splanchnic collateral vessels, which causes decreased resistance in the splanchnic vasculature. Decreased splanchnic resistance is manifested clinically as a decreased SVR. This altered hemodynamic profile generally persists into at least the early postoperative period; therefore it is important to use the patient as his or her own control when assessing these hemodynamic parameters. Left-side heart filling pressures are the most useful guide to monitoring cardiovascular pharmacologic interventions.

Hypovolemia can result from the massive shift of intravascular fluid to the interstitial spaces (third-space loss), the reaccumulation of ascites, and hemorrhage. The major factors contributing to third-space loss are the abdominal surgical procedure, the physiologic stress of surgery, the massive fluid resuscitation that occurs intraoperatively, and hypoalbuminemia. Hypovolemia will frequently be exacerbated during rewarming of the hypothermic patient.

There is a confluence of lymphatic vessels in the area of the porta hepatis that is severed during the recipient hepatectomy. Damage to these lymphatics can result in a significant accumulation of ascitic fluid in some patients. Large volumes of ascites may be removed by abdominal surgical drains, particularly if the drains are connected to suction. Abdominal drainage must be considered in the calculation of fluid balance as one mechanism for the prevention of hypovolemia. Resolution of postoperative ascites may take several weeks.

The most frequent technical complication requiring early reoperation is hemorrhage.[78,79] Causes of early postoperative hemorrhage include dilutional coagulopathy secondary to massive intraoperative blood transfusion, potential bleeding from numerous raw peritoneal surfaces, and surgical technical errors such as bleeding from vascular anastomoses, or from small untied vessels of the donor organ or the recipient. Late postoperative hemorrhage can most frequently be attributed to complications from percutaneous liver biopsy and percutaneous biliary tract procedures. The abdominal drains, commonly Jackson Pratt drains (Fig. 15-4), require frequent stripping to maintain their patency for the assessment of the extent of abdominal ascites or the presence of blood or bile in the abdomen. These drains are also a potential source of infection and as such must be handled in a manner to prevent the entry of potentially pathogenic organisms into the abdomen.

Hypertension is an almost expected phenomenon after liver transplantation. The patient

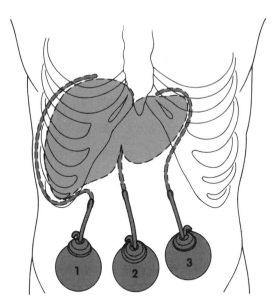

Fig. 15-4 Abdominal drainage with Jackson-Pratt (JP) drains after orthotopic liver transplant. JP1 is placed in the right subphrenic space, JP2 in the area of the porta hepatis, and JP3 in the left subphrenic space.

normally has severe hypertension; mean arterial pressures frequently exceed 120 mm Hg. It may be present for only a few days or weeks or may persist for months after transplant. The exact cause of hypertension in this setting is not well understood. However, proposed etiologic factors include increased SVR resulting from catecholamine release during the stress response, manipulation of the right adrenal gland during surgery, hypothermia, hypervolemia, renal insufficiency, and administration of cyclosporine. To determine the cause and institute the appropriate treatment, a total hemodynamic profile—blood pressure, cardiac output, SVR, CVP, and urine output—is necessary. Various vasoactive agents have been employed for control of hypertension, including nitroprusside, labetalol, hydralazine, captopril, nifedipine, and diltiazem.

Unfortunately, hypertension does not exist as a solitary problem. Complicating matters in these patients with chronic liver disease are the coexisting problems of thrombocytopenia and fragile cerebral vessels (particularly in the older patient). Failure to control hypertension in this patient population can thus result in intracerebral hemorrhage.

Electrolyte, chemical, and acid-base imbalances. Virtually any imbalance can occur after liver transplantation. This is not surprising, considering the magnitude of the physiologic stress of surgery, fluid shifts that occur, the multitude of pharmacologic agents administered, and the multisystem complications that frequently occur. The most common imbalances, however, are hypokalemia, hyperglycemia, hypomagnesemia and metabolic alkalosis.

Hypokalemia, as previously discussed, is a temporary problem in the early postoperative period resulting from flushing of the preserved liver and hypothermia that is easily corrected with IV potassium supplementation. Hypokalemia will also occur as a side effect of potassium-wasting diuretic therapy, intracellular shifts secondary to metabolic alkalosis, hypothermia, insulin therapy, and steroid therapy. In the late postoperative period hypokalemia can result from excessive GI fluid loss (e.g., from diarrhea). Rarely, if serum potassium is monitored regularly and supplementation given when indicated, is hypokalemia from any cause significant enough to produce physical signs. Hyperkalemia in the early postoperative period, as previously discussed, can indicate a nonfunctional graft and can also herald acute vascular thrombosis with subsequent cell death and release of potassium.

The main causes of hyperglycemia have also been previously discussed. Other causes include corticosteroid therapy, stress-induced diabetes mellitus, and sepsis. Some patients will develop diabetes mellitus as a permanent condition as a result of liver transplantation and steroid therapy. This results in increased morbidity and represents added physiologic and psychologic burdens to the patient. This is also an example of how liver transplantation is not a panacea, but often amounts to trading one set of problems for another. In the euglycemic patient, hyperglycemia may be one of the earliest signs of sepsis, particularly in the immunosuppressed patient, who may not manifest the normal inflammatory response.

Hypomagnesemia is another almost expected phenomenon after liver transplantation. Although many patients are hypomagnesemic from malnutrition before transplantation, the condition is exacerbated in the postoperative period. The exact nature of this problem is not completely understood. However, contributing postoperative factors are thought to include diuretic therapy, administration of cyclosporine, and hypocalcemia that occurs as a result of the massive transfusion of stored blood. Unlike hypokalemia, the clinical manifestations of hypomagnesemia are frequently evident and include neuromuscular irritability and sleeplessness. In extreme cases, seizures can occur. Routine monitoring of the serum magnesium and supplementation with intravenous or oral magnesium sulfate as indicated will prevent these problems.

Metabolic alkalosis is the most common acid-base disturbance in the immediate postoperative period and is most prominent during the first 24 to 48 hours after surgery. Precipitating factors include the large citrate load (from stored blood) that is metabolized to bicarbonate; hypokalemia; diuretic therapy; and the administration of large volumes of fresh frozen plasma (fresh frozen plasma is deficient in chloride). Metabolic alkalosis can present a problem with weaning the patient from mechanical ventilation. The patient will hypoventilate in response to the alkalosis and become hypercarbic. Generally this problem resolves spontaneously as the other factors are diminished. Intravenous hydrochloric acid by continuous infusion or acetazolamide (Diamox), a carbonic anhydrase inhibitor, can be administered to correct the metabolic alkalosis.

Pulmonary compromise. The liver transplant patient is at great risk for the development of pulmonary complications. First, the patient is subjected to a very long surgical procedure in the supine position and a prolonged course of general anesthesia, both of which contribute to atelectasis. Second, endotracheal intubation and mechanical ventilation are necessary for a variable length of time to support ventilation and oxygenation during and after surgery. This predisposes the extremely immunosuppressed patient to the development of pulmonary infections. Third, immobility for extended periods of time can be a problem after the long and complex operation or in the unstable patient. A primary goal even in the immediate postoperative period is to wean the patient from mechanical ventilation so that the endotracheal tube can be removed and normal ventilation can be resumed. Efforts to wean the patient from mechanical ventilation can be thwarted by paresis or paralysis of the right hemidiaphragm (secondary to phrenic nerve damage as a result of retraction and dissection during surgery), decreased vital capacity resulting from upper abdominal wall incisions, atelectasis, pleural effusion, and metabolic alkalosis. Wood et al[66] reported a 50% mortality in patients requiring prolonged mechanical ventilation and tracheostomy.

Pulmonary compromise in the liver transplant patient can be classified as either ineffective ventilation or ineffective oxygenation. The various factors and conditions that contribute to these forms of pulmonary compromise, along with their nursing and medical interventions, will be discussed.

Ineffective ventilation. The two major factors that contribute to ineffective ventilation are damage to the right hemidiaphragm and ascites. During the recipient hepatectomy phase of the surgical procedure the right hemidiaphragm may be damaged due to difficulties in dissection. There are no specific interventions for this problem, but fortunately, over time, this problem will resolve spontaneously. Ineffective ventilation is manifested by a decreased ventilation/perfusion ratio and an increased $paco_2$.

Ineffective oxygenation. Ineffective oxygenation is a more common problem with multiple causes: preexisting pulmonary shunting, atelectasis and intrapulmonary shunting, pneumonia, pleural effusions, hypervolemia, immobility, and adult respiratory distress syndrome (ARDS) related to intraoperative events and sepsis. Ineffective oxygenation is manifested by an increased intrapulmonary shunt fraction, decreased pao_2, and decreased Sao_2. Frequent

pulmonary assessment, evaluation of arterial blood gases, and chest physical therapy are the mainstays of pulmonary care for the liver transplant patient with ineffective oxygenation.

Pleural effusions are extremely common. They are commonly confined to the right side and result from the nature of the surgical procedure and the presence of ascites. As previously stated, the diaphragm is easily injured during the recipient hepatectomy. Inflammation from the injury and the translocation of intraabdominal fluid into the pleural space contribute to the development of effusions. Frequent assessment of the lungs for diminished sounds at the right base caused by a pleural effusion is necessary. It is not uncommon, during the recovery phase, for a liver transplant patient to accumulate effusions requiring several thoracenteses or placement of a chest tube for drainage. Although these are common and frequent procedures, they are not to be taken lightly in the posttransplant patient.

The most common pulmonary complications are infectious in nature.[78] Bacterial, viral, fungal, and protozoal pulmonary infections are common problems in this group of patients. A variety of bacterial infections can occur, and usually occur earlier than infections from other types of organisms. Viral infections predominantly originate from cytomegalovirus (CMV). Rubin stated, "CMV is the single most important infection affecting the liver transplant patient."[80] CMV pneumonia is diagnosed by bronchiole alveolar lavage (BAL) and frequently occurs simultaneously with CMV hepatitis in the highly immunosuppressed patient.

Renal insufficiency. The potential is great for postoperative renal insufficiency in the liver transplant patient. A number of patients have varying degrees of renal insufficiency before transplant surgery and are thus at greater risk for morbidity and mortality than the patient with normal renal function. The preoperative serum creatinine level is an accurate predictor of poor survival in this group of patients.[81]

Intraoperative and postoperative factors that contribute to renal insufficiency include intraoperative events such as massive hemorrhage and hypotension, postoperative hypovolemia, infection, graft failure, broad-spectrum antibacterial and antifungal therapy, and cyclosporine. Frequently there are several simultaneous contributing factors. In the majority of patients these factors cause a short-term acute tubular necrosis that usually resolves within 3 to 4 weeks. During this time supportive measures such as hemofiltration or hemodialysis may be necessary. In one series acute renal failure requiring hemodialysis was the only statistically significant predictor of decreased patient survival.[82]

Daily assessment of the serum creatinine level and creatinine clearance in response to the above-mentioned factors is prudent. Regular monitoring of serum drug levels and manipulation of antibiotic and immunosuppressant regimens is frequently necessitated.

Coagulopathy. Coagulopathy, to one degree or another, is a preexisting condition in all liver transplant patients. Primary liver dysfunction and splenomegaly with pancytopenia are the major preexisting contributing factors. Intraoperative hemostasis is complicated by coagulopathy, frequently necessitating the transfusion of large volumes of blood, which can create further coagulopathy via dilutional mechanisms. Thus a vicious intraoperative cycle is established that can persist into the postoperative period. Additional postoperative factors that can contribute to the development of coagulopathy include hypothermia, disseminated intravascular coagulation, drug-related bone marrow toxicity, and graft failure.

Coagulopathy in the early postoperative period can be disastrous when one considers the major vascular anastomoses that have just been created and the invasive monitoring required for optimal assessment and treatment of the patient. Coagulopathy can also interfere with postoperative care by contraindicating necessary procedures such as a liver biopsy.

Frequent assessment of coagulation times, clotting factor assays, serum fibrinogen, and degradation products of fibrinolysis in the early postoperative period is imperative. Fresh frozen plasma is routinely administered to replenish coagulation factors. Platelets and cryoprecipitate are less frequently required. As is true for any patient with a coagulopathy, care must be taken to prevent trauma to the skin and mucous membranes.

Vascular complications. The two major vascular complications that can occur after liver transplantation are hepatic artery thrombosis and portal vein thrombosis. Both events are associated with increased morbidity and mortality.

The diameter of the hepatic artery in the adult is approximately 4 to 6 mm, and the intima of the hepatic artery is very fragile. These factors, along with the presence of atherosclerosis in the older ault, predispose the artery to intraoperative and postoperative thrombosis. Acute hepatic artery thrombosis usually occurs within the first few days after transplantation. Rejection also plays a role in hepatic artery thrombosis.[83]

Acute hepatic artery thrombosis is a catastrophic event that occurs in up to 12% of adults.[83] Acute occlusion of the hepatic artery denies the liver of its chief source of oxygen and results in acute massive hepatic necrosis. The sudden onset of hepatic gangrene is manifested by acute liver failure and sepsis with fever, hypotension, and acute renal and respiratory failure. On abdominal x-ray examination, gas can often be seen in the liver. When hepatic artery thrombosis is suspected, it should be confirmed by Doppler ultrasound[84] and/or arteriogram. Interventions for the patient with acute hepatic artery thrombosis include multisystem supportive measures until retransplantation can be performed. Late onset hepatic artery thrombosis is insidious and may be seen as a delayed biliary leak (the donor bile duct depends on the right hepatic artery for its blood supply) or intermittent sepsis.[83,85] Late onset hepatic artery thrombosis is usually a less emergent situation than acute hepatic artery thrombosis because of the formation of collateral vessels.

Portal vein thrombosis can occur in the immediate postoperative period or can be delayed. Associated factors include a hypoplastic portal vein, previous surgery of the portal vein, and surgical technical error. Portal vein thrombosis is also diagnosed by Doppler ultrasound and/or a venous phase superior mesenteric artery arteriogram. Acute portal vein thrombosis is a dramatic event manifested by severe liver dysfunction and variceal bleeding in the patient with preoperative varices. Delayed portal vein thrombosis manifests as portal hypertension with its attendant physiologic consequences: varices, ascites, splenomegaly, and encephalopathy. Portal vein thrombosis may be treated with a distal splenorenal shunt procedure, reanastomosis of the portal vein anastomosis, and declotting; the bleeding varices are managed with sclerotherapy until a shunt can be performed.

Gastrointestinal complications. A variety of gastrointestinal (GI) complications can occur after liver transplantation. Expected complications that resolve spontaneously include ileus, mild to moderate gastric outlet obstruction, and loss of appetite. Stress ulceration is anticipated and prevented by administration of prophylactic H2 receptor blockers and antacids.

Malnutrition is both a preoperative problem associated with chronic liver disease and a postoperative complication. The stress of surgery, the healing requirements of the body and other postoperative complications, mainly infection, contribute to increased metabolic needs at a time when appetite and patient motivation may be poor. Laboratory nutritional assessment parameters include serum albumin, serum transferrin, serum cholesterol, and urine urea nitrogen, which reflects the patient's metabolic response to stress. Enteral and peripheral or central hyperalimentation are frequently necessary to provide adequate calories and protein to maintain the patient in positive nitrogen balance. Central hyperalimentation is avoided if possible because of the increased incidence of fungal sepsis associated with this therapy in the immunosuppressed patient.

An acute condition of the abdomen, in a variety of presentations, is an unexpected complication of liver transplantation. The causes include small bowel obstruction, bowel infarction, bowel perforation, peritonitis, pancreatitis, hemorrhage secondary to anastomotic leaks, and abdominal abscess. Assessment for peritoneal signs of an acute condition of the abdomen — sudden onset of ileus, nausea and/or vomiting, abdominal tenderness, abdominal rigidity, and rebound tenderness — is an important component of the abdominal assessment of

the liver transplant patient. It is also important to note that recognition of this process may be delayed, primarily because of the effects of the corticosteroids, and thus heightened awareness is necessary. With the possible exception of pancreatitis, an acute abdominal condition is a surgical emergency. Nursing care then includes preparation of the patient for diagnostic procedures, surgery, and postoperative wound care, often involving complex management of surgical tubes and drains.

In patients with a choledochojejunostomy (common bile duct anastomosed to the jejunum), bowel perforations can occur at the jejunostomy site secondary to an anastomotic leak. Bowel perforation can also occur in other areas of the small bowel, cecum, or colon as a result of denuded areas of serosa.[78] Long-term steroid therapy, which inhibits normal tissue healing, is also a contributing factor to breakdown of anastomoses. Clinical manifestations of bowel perforation in the liver transplant patient include cloudy abdominal drainage, the presence of enteric organisms in the abdominal drainage, and wound or systemic candidal infection.[78,85] Surgical intervention is necessary whenever a bowel perforation occurs at any site.

Biliary complications. As discussed previously, there are two preferred techniques for the biliary anastomosis: choledochocholedochostomy (common bile duct to common bile duct) and choledochojejunostomy. A choledochocholedochostomy is performed unless the recipient common bile duct is damaged, infected, or abnormal in some respect. In the adult, this is the case with sclerosing cholangitis. When a choledochocholedochostomy is performed, it is routinely stented with a T-tube that exits percutaneously and drains externally. A choledochojejunostomy can also be internally stented, but this is a matter of individual physician preference.

Care of the T-tube is part of the complex tube and drain management of the postoperative liver transplant patient. It is critical that the tube be kept clean, because it is a potential source of ascending cholangitis. T-tube cholangiograms are routinely performed at regular intervals to assess the status of the biliary tree. Since this procedure is associated with sepsis, it is critical that antibiotics be administered before the cholangiogram is performed. A cephalosporin is usually the antibiotic of choice, because gram-negative organisms colonize the common bile duct. An important nursing intervention is teaching the patient how to care for his or her T-tube and assessment of the T-tube exit site, because the tube will remain in place for as long as 6 months.

Biliary complications include biliary anastomotic leaks leading to cholangitis, peritonitis, and abdominal sepsis; biliary strictures; and dislodgement of the T-tube requiring surgical replacement. Biliary leaks can be detected by laboratory analysis of abdominal drainage for bilirubin and by a dye study through the T-tube, or in the absence of the T-tube, by a transhepatic study in the radiology suite. Biliary complications always require surgical intervention.[86]

Neurologic complications. Occasionally neurologic complications occur in liver transplant patients. Most often they are related to idiosyncratic central nervous system (CNS) effects of cyclosporine therapy or the metabolic abnormalities caused by this drug. These temporary, dose-related side effects include confusion, cortical blindness, quadriplegia, encephalopathy, seizures, and coma. Seizures may be aggravated by high-dose corticosteroids, hypomagnesemia, and hypertension. The differential diagnosis for confusion includes meningitis, graft dysfunction, cyclosporine toxicity, psychosis, sleep deprivation, cerebrovascular accident, and intracerebral bleeding.

Hypocholesterolemia is a common problem among liver transplant patients. This presents a special problem when the patient is given cyclosporine because it is a highly lipophilic drug. DeGroen et al[87] reported an inverse relationship between toxic CNS effects and total serum cholesterol. When cholesterol levels are less than 120 mg/dl, the cyclosporine drug level increases dramatically and CNS effects are more likely to occur.[87] This can be especially distressing to the family of the patient, and thus family members need to be assured that the effects are temporary.

Infection. Infection is the major cause of morbidity and mortality in the liver transplant patient,[79] with an overall infection rate of 80%.[88]

Early infections are primarily bacterial in origin and late infections are primarily fungal in origin. However, viral infections may occur at any time, and as previously noted, are the most important infections in this patient population. The associated mortality for severe bacterial and fungal infections is approximately 70%.[89] The potential infections are too numerous to list. However, the most common ones are pneumonias; subphrenic, subhepatic, and other abdominal abscesses; and peritonitis and generalized sepsis.[78,80] Most systemic infections are secondary to an abdominal abscess.[88]

General factors that predispose the liver transplant patient to infection are long-term immunosuppressive therapy, the abdominal surgery itself, prolonged operative time, a debilitated preoperative state, preoperative derangement of the hepatic reticuloendothelial system, hemodialysis, GI and vascular complications, and a prolonged ICU stay. The most significant preoperative prognostic indicator for infection is the serum albumin, i.e., the hypoalbuminemic patient is likely to acquire a postoperative infection.[90] The major postoperative risk factor is an increased serum creatinine level.[91] Additional factors predispose the patient to the development of fungal infections. They include the use of broad-spectrum antibiotics in both the preoperative and postoperative periods and the use of steroids for the prevention and treatment of rejection. The most common fungal infections are caused by *Candida* spp.[89] *Aspergillus* spp. infections, although uncommon, are associated with 100% mortality.[89] Failure to correctly differentiate between rejection and infection or other conditions that cause elevations in serum bilirubin, transaminases, and phosphatases results in overtreatment with steroids, thereby increasing the risk of serious infection. Timely liver biopsy can be extremely helpful in this dilemma.

Assessment of the liver transplant patient for signs of infection is, unfortunately, not straightforward. As with any immunosuppressed patient, the signs may be diminished or masked altogether. Furthermore, there are so many potential sites of infection that diagnosis is both difficult and often time consuming.

Prevention of infection in the liver transplant

patient is, also unfortunately, not something that the health care team can completely control. Some centers advocate routine preoperative bowel decontamination regimens. Colonna et al[90] recommended a combination of erythromycin base, neomycin sulfate, and nystatin. Krom[92] recommends a regimen of polymyxin B sulfate, gentamycin sulfate, and nystatin. This topic deserves additional research efforts, particularly using a controlled, randomized approach.

There are several sites that routinely become colonized with bacteria and fungi: abdominal drains, T-tube, NG tube, oral cavity (and sputum), and wounds. Differentiating between colonization and true infection is important (and often difficult) to ensure accurate treatment with antimicrobials. In addition to culture reports, the patient's clinical status must be taken into consideration when making the diagnosis of infection.

Treatment of infection in the liver transplant patient often includes surgical exploration and drainage of the abdomen combined with the aggressive use of broad-spectrum antibiotics. Immunosuppressant doses are often decreased as well, to balance their toxic and therapeutic effects.

Care of the liver transplant patient is extremely labor intensive. Because of the need for extensive invasive monitoring equipment and procedures for assessment and treatment, the patient comes in contact with numerous members of the health care team, all of whom are potential vectors of pathogenic organisms. Adherence to infection control standards is of paramount importance in preventing infection in this patient population. Unfortunately, this may place the nurse in the position of "traffic controller" and watchdog for those who dismiss the importance of handwashing as the most important infection control measure. For specific nursing implications, refer to Chapter 3, Immunologic Aspects of Transplantation.

Rejection. The most important consideration of graft survival is the ability to control rejection. The relatively short maximum cold ischemic time of the liver precludes HLA typing and leukocyte cross-matching (although clinically these factors do not seem as important in liver

ABO type	Identical ABO type	Compatible but non-identical ABO type	Incompatible ABO type
(A)	A	O	B,AB
(B)	B	O	A,AB
(AB)	AB	O,A,B	
(O)	O		A,B,AB

Fig. 15-5 ABO matching for liver transplant.

transplantation). ABO matching between donor and recipient is the only prospective histocompatibility testing done for liver transplantation.

ABO matching for liver transplantation is shown in Fig. 15-5. The ideal situation is an ABO identical match; however, in emergent situations such as PNFG or acute vascular thrombosis, ABO nonidentical but compatible matches are acceptable. Survival of ABO identical grafts is better than that of compatible, nonidentical grafts.[93] A major complication associated with ABO nonidentical liver transplantation is hemolysis. Hemolysis results from a form of graft-versus-host response in which B lymphocytes in donor lymphoid tissue produce antibodies to recipient ABO antigens. Hemolysis in this setting typically occurs between the fifth and eighth postoperative day.[94] The patient will usually develop a spiking fever initially. The reticulocyte count and serum bilirubin level will be elevated, and the serum hemoglobin level will decrease. A direct Coomb's test will also yield positive results. Interventions for severe hemolysis may include aggressive intravenous hydration, diuretics, packed red blood cell transfusion, plasmaphoresis, and, rarely, splenectomy.

Although the liver is not as antigenic as other solid organs, assessment of rejection of the transplanted liver is a major focus of patient care. Acute allograft rejection occurs in approximately 80% of liver transplants.[95] The liver has immune characteristics that logically should promote graft rejection. The liver contains Kupffer cells, vascular and sinusoidal endothelial cells, and portal dendritic and inflammatory cells, all of which should make the liver highly antigenic. On the contrary, there is minimal expression of class I HLA antigens on the hepatocytes, which favors decreased antigenicity. It is also thought that donor Kupffer cells may be replaced with host macrophages, which would promote graft acceptance.[95]

Acute, accelerated, and chronic rejection are known to occur after liver transplantation, but there is debate as to whether hyperacute rejection occurs, even when there is a positive antidonor (anti–T lymphocyte) cross-match between the donor and recipient. Iwatsuki et al from Pittsburgh, in two separate reports,[96,97] noted that the liver is resistant to hyperacute rejection and that a positive anti–T lymphocyte cross-match is not an absolute contraindication to liver transplantation. There are two possible explanations as to why hyperacute rejection does not occur.[95] First, the large liver mass, via the reticuloendothelial function of the Kupffer cells, is thought to be capable of sequestering cytotoxic antibodies formed against the graft. The presence of a sinusoidal rather than a capillary system in the liver may allow for removal of antigen by the Kupffer cells lining the sinusoids. Second, the cytotoxic antibody titer may be diluted sufficiently as a result of intraoperative blood loss and volume exchange to inhibit the humoral immune response. However, Rego et al[93] report a case of hyperacute rejection after an ABO incompatible liver transplant.

The focus of this discussion will be on acute liver rejection because it occurs so frequently and because it can be both prevented (presumably) and treated. It is therefore a primary consideration to the nurse caring for the liver transplant patient. Chronic liver rejection cannot be prevented or successfully treated: when chronic rejection occurs, retransplantation is indicated.

The basic mechanism of acute liver rejection is that described as the cellular immune response in Chapter 3, Immunologic Aspects of Transplantation. Sensitization of host T lymphocytes occurs when antigen-presenting cells carry the antigenic markers to the peripheral lymphoid tissue. Circulating lymphocytes are also exposed to foreign antigen within the graft, where Kupffer cells act as antigen-presenting cells.

Acute liver rejection occurs as early as 7 to 10 days after transplantation. Clinical signs and symptoms include tachycardia, fever, malaise, right upper quadrant and right flank tenderness or pain, hepatomegaly, and increased ascites accumulation. The patient's mental status may also change and disorientation may be noted. Bile flow decreases and the characteristics of the bile change, with the bile becoming lighter in color and less viscous. The serum transaminase and phosphatase and serum bilirubin levels will elevate, but these are not sensitive indicators of rejection. Cyclosporine toxicity, hepatitis B reinfection, CMV hepatitis, and ischemia may cause similar elevations.

Diagnosis of acute rejection is done most expeditiously by serial liver biopsies. Early histologic changes of acute rejection are lymphocytic infiltration in the portal tracts beneath the endothelial lining of the sinusoids and the walls of the central veins and bile ducts. The diagnosis in the early postoperative period is often clouded by bile duct damage, which can occur as a result of recovery-related ischemic injury or damage caused by preservation solutions. For this reason an intraoperative biopsy is done for later comparison. Interestingly, it is not until rejection is moderately advanced that the hepatocytes are involved, because although central vein and bile duct epithelia are rich in class I and II major histocompatibility complex (MHC) antigens, hepatocytes are relatively lacking in these antigens.

Although the definitive method for diagnosing rejection is the liver biopsy, this practice is not without complications. The technique usually involves percutaneous insertion of a needle into the liver parenchyma via a midaxillary intercostal approach while the patient is in a sustained exhalation phase of respiration. Because of the vascularity of the liver and the relative position of the right lung to the liver, potential complications of liver biopsy include intraperitoneal bleeding, intrahepatic and subcapsular hematoma, pseudoaneurysm of the hepatic artery, and hemothorax and pneumothorax. The patient must be carefully assessed for at least 8 hours after a liver biopsy for signs and symptoms of these complications. A new technique, successfully used in other areas—fine needle biopsy—may be applicable here, and may have a lower complication rate.

Care of the patient experiencing acute liver rejection is highly individualized and depends on the degree of rejection, patient responses to and complications of immunosuppression, and the effect of resultant liver dysfunction on other organ systems. The immunosuppressant agents used to treat acute rejection and nursing implications are discussed in detail in Chapter 4, Immunosuppressive Agents Used in Transplantation. The focus of care is often on the side effects of these agents rather than on any actual physical problems resulting from the rejection. However, emotional responses to the diagnosis of acute rejection need to be addressed as well as the physical responses. For nursing implications related to this problem, see Chapter 7, Psychiatric Aspects of Transplantation.

The survival and well-being of the liver transplant recipient in the postoperative period depends to a great extent on the nurse's having a sufficient knowledge base and commitment to quality nursing care. The liver transplant recipient can present a challenge—intellectual, physical and emotional—to the most experienced nurse. The outcome, however, is sufficient reward when the majority of patients receiving a liver transplant, whose life expectancies were less than a year, leave the hospital planning what to do with their second chance at life.

REFERENCES

1. Van Thiel DH, Makowka L and Starzl TE (1988). Liver transplantation: where it's been and where it'g going. *Gastroenterology Clinics of North America, 17*(1), 1-18.
2. Welch CS (1955). A note on transplantation of the whole liver of dogs. *Transplant Bulletin, 2,* 54-55.
3. Cannon JA (1956). Organs (communication). *Transplant Bulletin, 3,* 7.
4. Moore FD, Smith LL, Burnap TK, Dallenbach FD, Dammin GJ, Gruber VF, Shoemaker WC, Steenberg RW, Ball MR and Belko JS (1959). One stage homotransplantation of the liver following total hepatectomy in dogs. *Transplant Bulletin, 6,* 103-107.
5. Starzl TE, Kaupp HA, Brock DR, Lazarus RE and Johnson RV (1960). Reconstructive problems in canine liver homotransplantation with special reference to the postoperative role of the hepatic venous flow. *Surgery, Gynecology and Obstetrics, 111,* 733-743.
6. Moore FD, Wheeler HB, Demissianos HV, Smith LL, Balankura O, Abel K, Greenburgh JB and Dammin GJ (1960). Experimental whole-organ transplantation of the liver and the spleen. *Annals of Surgery, 152,* 374-387.
7. Starzl TE, Marchiaro TL, Von Kulla KN, Hermann G, Brittain RS and Waddell WR (1963). Homotransplantation of the liver in humans. *Surgery, Gynecology and Obstetrics, 117,* 659-676.
8. Starzl TE, Groth CG, Brettschneider L, Penn I, Fulginiti VA, Moon JB, Blanchard H, Martin AJ and Porter KA (1968). Orthotopic homotransplantation of the human liver. *Annals of Surgery, 168,* 392-415.
9. Starzl TE, Iwatsuki S, Van Thiel DH, Gartner JC, Zitelli BJ, Malata KJ, Schade RR, Shaw BW, Hakala TR, Rosenthal JT and Porter KA (1982). Evolution of liver transplantation. *Hepatology, 2,* 614-636.
10. Calne RY, Rolles K, White DJG, Thiru S, Evans DB, McMater P, Dunn DC, Craddock GN, Henderson RG, Aziz S and Lewis P (1979). Cyclosporin A initially as the only immunosuppressant in 34 recipients of cadaveric organs: 32 kidneys, 2 pancreases, and 2 livers. *Lancet, 2,* 1033-1036.
11. National Institutes of Health (1983). National Institutes of Health Consensus Development Conference Statement: Liver transplantation. *Hepatology, 4*(1S), 107S-110S.
12. Maddrey WC (1990). *Conference on liver transplantation.* The National Digestive Diseases Advisory Board. February 11. Arlington, Va.
13. Medical Technology and Practice Patterns Institute, Inc., Washington D.C., Nov. 21, 1988.
14. Starzl TE, Iwatsuki S, Shaw BW and Gordon RD (1984). Orthotopic liver transplantation in 1984. *Transplantation Proceedings, 27,* 250-258.
15. Iwatsuki S, Starzl TE, Todd S, Gordon RD, Tzakis AG, Marsh JW, Koneru B, Stieber A, Klintmalm G and Husberg B (1988). Experience in 1000 liver transplants under cyclosporine-steroid therapy: a survival report. *Transplantation Proceedings, 20,* 498-504.
16. Iwatsuki S, Starzl TE, Todo S, Gordon RD, Tzakis AG, Marsh JW, Makowka L, Koneru B, Stieber A, Klintmalm G, Husberg B and Van Thiel D (1988). Liver transplantation for treatment of bleeding esophageal varices. *Surgery, 104,* 697-705.
17. Starzl TE, Iwatsuki S, Shaw BW, Gordon RD, Esquivel C, Todo S, Kam I and Lynch S (1985). Factors in the development of liver transplantation. *Transplantation Proceedings, 27*(2S), 107-119.
18. Shaw BW, Martin DJ, Marquez JM, Kang YG, Bugbee AC, Iwatsuki S, Griffith BP, Hardesty RL, Bahnson HT and Starzl TE (1985). Advantages of venous bypass during orthotopic transplantation of the liver. *Seminars in Liver Disease, 5,* 344-348.
19. Dzik WH (1985). Use of intraoperative blood salvage during orthotopic liver transplantation. *Archives of Surgery, 120,* 946-948.

20. Todo S, Nery J, Yanaga K, Podesta L, Gordon RD and Starzl TE (1989). Extended preservation of human liver grafts with UW solution. *Journal of the American Medical Association, 261,* 711-714.

21. Malin H (1981). *An epidemiologic perspective on alcohol use and abuse in the United States.* Rockville, Md: National Institute of Alcohol Abuse and Alcoholism.

22. Hubmayer RD and Pratter MR (1985). Alcohol overdose and withdrawal. In Rippe JM, Irwin RS, Alpert JS and Dalen JE (eds). *Intensive care medicine* (pp 920-925). Boston: Little, Brown & Co.

23. Swerdlow JL (1989). *Matching needs, saving lives.* Washington, DC: The Annenberg Washington Program.

24. Grambsch PM, Dickson ER, Wiesner RH and Langworthy A (1989). Application of the Mayo primary biliary cirrhosis survival model to Mayo liver transplant patients. *Mayo Clinic Proceedings, 64,* 699-704.

25. Markus BH, Dickson ER, Grambsch PM, Fleming TR, Mazzaferro V, Klintmalm GBG, Wiesner RH, Van Thiel D and Starzl TE (1989). Efficacy of liver transplantation in patients with primary biliary cirrhosis. *New England Journal of Medicine, 320,* 1709-1713.

26. Sherlock S (1987). Primary biliary cirrhosis. In Schiff L and Schiff ER (eds). *Diseases of the liver.* 6th Ed (979-1000). Philadelphia: JB Lippincott Co.

27. Millikan WJ, Henderson JM, Stewart MT, Marsh JW, Galloway JR, Jennings RH, Olson R and Warren WD (1988). Orthotopic liver transplantation: another surgical tool for complications of the portal hypertensive syndrome. *Emory University Journal of Medicine, 2,* 192-198.

28. Warren KW, Williams CI and Tan EGC (1987). Sclerosing cholangitis. In Schiff L and Schiff ER (eds). *Diseases of the liver.* 6th Ed (pp 1289-1335). Philadelphia: JB Lippincott Co.

29. Dickson RE, LaRusso NF and Weisner RH (1984). Primary sclerosing cholangitis. *Hepatology, 4,* 335-355.

30. Weisner RH and LaRusso NF (1980). Clinicopathologic features of the syndrome of primary sclerosing cholangitis. *Gastroenterology, 79,* 200-206.

31. Galambos JT (ed). (1979). *Cirrhosis. Major problems in internal medicine* (vol 17). Philadelphia: WB Saunders Co.

32. Sherlock S (1985). *Diseases of the liver and biliary system.* (7th ed) London: Blackwell Scientific Publications.

33. Gurevich I (April 1983). Viral hepatitis. *American Journal of Nursing,* 571-586.

34. Seef LB and Koff RS (1986). Evolving concepts of the clinical and serologic consequences of hepatitis B virus infection. *Seminars in Liver Disease, 6,* 11-22.

35. McDermott WV, Stone MD, Bothe A and Trey C (1984). Budd-Chiari syndrome. *American Journal of Surgery, 147,* 463-467.

36. Reynolds TB (1987). Budd-Chiari. In Schiff L and Schiff ER (eds). *Diseases of the liver.* 6th Ed (pp 1446-1473). Philadelphia: JB Lippincott Co.

37. Bonnice CA (1985). Fulminant hepatic failure. In Rippe JM, Irwin RS, Alpert JS and Dalen JE (eds). *Intensive care medicine.* (pp. 747-754). Boston: Little, Brown & Co.

38. Willson RA (October 1977). Acute hepatic failure. *Hospital Medicine,* 8-23.

39. Gould BE and Pratter MR (1985). In Rippe JM, Irwin RS, Alpert JS and Dalen JE (eds). *Intensive care medicine.* (pp 962-965). Boston: Little, Brown & Co.

40. Mar DD (January 1982). Drug-induced hepatotoxicity. *American Journal of Nursing,* 124-126.

41. Frank IC and Cummins L (1987). Amanita poisoning treated with endoscopic biliary diversion. *Journal of Emergency Nursing, 13,* 132-136.

42. Iwatsuki S, Esquivel CO, Gordon RD, Shaw BW, Starzl TE, Shade RR and VanThiel DH (1985). Liver transplantation for fulminant hepatic failure. *Seminars in Liver Disease, 5,* 325-328.

43. Buckels JAC (1987). Liver transplantation in acute fulminant hepatic failure. *Transplantation Proceedings, 19,* 4365-4366.

44. Stieber AC, Ambrosino G, Van Thiel D, Iwatsuki S and Starzl TE (1988). Orthotopic liver transplantation for fulminant and subacute hepatic failure. *Gastroenterology Clinics of North America, 17,* 157-165.

45. Shaw BW, Wood RP, Stratta RJ, Pillen TJ and Langnas NA (1989). *Archives of Survery, 124,* 895-900.

46. Koneru B, Cassavilla A, Bowman J, Iwatsuki S and Starzl TE (1988). Liver transplantation for malignant tumors. *Gastroenterology Clinics of North America, 17*(1), 177-193.

47. Busuttil R (1990). Neoplastic liver disease. *Conference on liver transplantation.* The National Digestive Diseases Advisory Board. February 12. Arlington, Va.

48. O'Grady JG, Polson RJ, Rolles K, Calne RY and Williams R (1988). Liver transplantation for malignant disease: results in 93 consecutive cases. *Annals of Surgery, 207,* 373-379.

49. Starzl TE, Iwatsuki S, Shaw BW, Nalesnik MA, Farhi DC, and Van Thiel DH (1986). Treatment of fibrolamellar hepatoma with partial or total hepatectomy and transplantation of the liver. *Surgery, Gynecology and Obstetrics, 162,* 145-148.

50. Vierling JM (1984). Epidemiology and clinical course of liver diseases: identification of candidates for hepatic transplantation. *Hepatology, 4,* 84S-94S.

51. Pichlmayr R, Brolsch C and Wonigeit K (1984). Experience with liver transplantation in Hannover. *Hepatology, 4,*(1S), 56S-60S.

52. Iwatsuki S, Gordon RD, Shaw BW and Starzl TE (1985). Role of liver transplantation in cancer therapy. *Annals of Surgery, 202,* 401-407.

53. Makowka L, Tzakis AG, Mazzaferro V, Teperman L, Demetris J, Iwatsuki S and Starzl TE (1989). Transplantation of the liver for metastatic endocrine tumors of the intestine and pancreas. *Surgery, Gynecology and Obstetrics, 168,* 107-111.

54. Flavin DK, Niven RG and Kelsey JE (1988). Alcoholism and orthotopic liver transplantation. *Journal of American Medical Association, 259,* 1546-1547.

55. Maddrey WC, Friedman LS, Munoz SJ and Hahn EG (1988). Selection of the patient for liver transplantation and timing for surgery. In Maddrey WC (ed). *Transplantation of the liver.* (pp 23-58). New York: Elsevier.

56. Scharschmidt BF (1984). Human liver transplantation: analysis of data on 540 patients from our four centers. *Hepatology, 4*, 95S-101S.

57. Starzl TE, Van Thiel D, Tzakis A, Iwatsuki S, Todo S, Marsh JW, Koneru B, Staschak S, Stieber A and Gordon RD (1988). Orthotopic liver transplantation for alcoholic cirrhosis. *Journal of the American Medical Association, 260*, 2542-2544.

58. Stock PG, Najarian JS and Ascher NL (1988). Liver transplantation. In Gallagher TJ and Shoemaker WC (eds). *Critical care: state of the art*. vol 9 (pp 21-40). The Society of Critical Care Medicine.

59. Lauchert W, Muller R and Pichlmayr R (1987). Long-term immunoprophylaxis of hepatitis B virus reinfection in recipients of human liver allografts. *Transplantation Proceedings, 5*, 4051-4053.

60. Johnson PJ, Wansbrough-Jones M, Portman B, Eddleston AL and Williams R (1978). Familial HBsAg-positive hepatoma: treatment with orthotopic liver transplantation and specific immunoglobulin. *British Medical Journal, 1*, 216.

61. Calne RY, Williams R and Rolles K (1986). Liver transplantation in the adult. *World Journal of Surgery, 10*, 422-431.

62. Rolles K, Williams R, Neuberger J and Calne RY (1984). The Cambridge and King's College Hospital experience of liver transplantation, 1968-1983. *Hepatology, 4*, 50S-55S.

63. Starzl TE, Iwatsuki S, Shaw BW, Van Thiel DH, Gartner JC, Zitelli BJ, Malatak JJ and Schade RR (1984). Analysis of liver transplantation. *Hepatology, 4*, 47S-49S.

64. Van Thiel DH, Schade RR, Gavaler SJ, Shaw BW, Iwatsuki S and Starzl TE (1984). Medical aspects of liver transplantation. *Hepatology, 4*, 79S-83S.

65. Colledan M, Gilson M, Doglia LR, Fassati LR, Ferla G, Gridelli B, Rossi G and Galmarini D (1987). Liver transplantation in patients with B viral hepatitis and delta infection. *Transplantation Proceedings, 19*, 4073-4076.

66. Demetris AJ, Jaffe R, Sheahan DG, Burnham J, Spero J, Iwatsuki S, Van Thiel DH and Starzl TE (1986). Recurrent hepatitis B in liver allograft recipients. *American Journal of Pathology, 125*, 161-172.

67. Lanchert W, Muller R, Pichlmayr R (1987). Immunoprophylaxis of hepatitis B virus reinfection of human liver allografts. *Transplantation Proceedings, 19*, 2387-2389.

68. Henderson JM and Warren WD (1986). A method of measuring quantitative hepatic function and hemodynamics in cirrhosis: the changes following distal splenorenal shunt. *Japanese Journal of Surgery, 16*, 158-168.

69. Zajko AB, Campbell WL, Bron KM, Schade RR, Koneru B and Van Thiel DH (1988). Diagnostic and interventional radiology in liver transplantation. *Gastroenterology Clinics of North America, 17*(1), 105-141.

70. Zajko AB, Bron KM, Starzl TE, Van Thiel DH, Gartner JC, Iwatsuki S, Shaw BW, Zitelli BJ, Malatack JJ and Urbach AH (1985). Angiography of liver transplantation patients. *Radiology, 157*, 305-311.

71. House RM and Thompson TL (1988). Psychiatric aspects of organ transplantation. *Journal of the American Medical Association, 260*, 535-539.

72. Peters TG, Williams JW, Vera SR, Van Voorst SJ, Hall G and Britt LG (1986). Liver procurement: lessons from the first sixty liver transplants at the University of Tennessee. *Transplantation Proceedings, 18*, 602-604.

73. Van Thiel DH, Gavaler JS, Tarter RE and Starzl TE (1988). Past, present, and future of liver transplantation. In Maddrey WC (ed). *Transplantation of the liver* (pp 1-22). New York: Elsevier.

74. Terpstra OT, Schalm SW, Weimar W, Willemse PJA, Baumgartner D, Groenland THN, Ten Kate FWJ, Porte RJ, de Rave S, Reuvers CB, Stibbe J and Terpstra JL (1988). Auxiliary partial liver transplantation for end-stage chronic liver disease. *New England Journal of Medicine, 319*, 1507-1511.

75. Griffith BP, Shaw BW, Hardesty RC, Iwatsuki S and Bahnson HT (1985). Veno-venous bypass without systemic anticoagulation for transplantation of the human liver. *Surgery, Gynecology and Obstetrics, 160*, 271-273.

76. McSteen F, Hackett J, Rhodes W and Merritt P (1984). Heparinless bypass for liver transplantation. *Proceedings of the American Academy of Cardiovascular Perfusionists, 5*, 28-29.

77. Khoury GF, Mann ME, Porot MJ, Abdul-Rasool IH and Busuttil RW (1987). Air embolism associated with veno-venous bypass during orthotopic liver transplantation. *Anesthesiology, 67*, 848-851.

78. Wood RP, Shaw BW and Starzl TE (1985). Extrahepatic complications of liver transplantation. *Seminars in Liver Disease, 5*, 377-384.

79. Koneru B, Tsakis AG, Bowman J, Cassavilla A, Zajko AB and Starzl TE (1988). Postoperative surgical complications. *Gastroenterology Clinics of North America, 17*(1), 71-90.

80. Rubin RH (1988). Infectious disease problems. In Maddrey WC (ed). *Current topics in gastroenterology. Transplantation of the liver.* (pp 279-308). New York: Elsevier.

81. Cuervas-Mons V, Starzl TE, Van Thiel DH, Millan I and Gavaler JS (1986). Prognostic value of preoperatively obtained clinical and laboratory data in predicting survival following orthotopic liver transplantation. *Hepatology, 6*, 922-927.

82. Brems JJ, Hiatt JR, Colonna JO, El-Khoury G, Quinones WJ, Ramming KP, Ziomek S and Busuttil RW (1986). Variables influencing the outcome following orthotopic liver transplantation. *Archives of Surgery, 122*, 1109-1111.

83. Wozney P, Zajko AB, Bron KM, Point S and Starzl TE (1986). Vascular complications after liver transplantation: a 5-year experience. *American Journal of Radiology, 147*, 657-663.

84. Segel MC, Zajko AB, Bowen A, Skolnick ML, Bron KM, Penkrot RJ, Slasky RS and Starzl TE (1986). Doppler ultrasound as a screen for hepatic artery thrombosis. *Transplantation, 41*, 539-541.

85. Carithers RL, Fairman RP, Mendez-Picon G, Posner MP, Mills AS and Friedenberg KT (1988). Postoperative care. In Maddrey WC (ed). *Current topics in gastroenterology. Transplantation of the liver.* (pp 111-142). New York: Elsevier.

86. Wilson BJ, Marsh JW, Makowka L, Steiber AC, Koneru B, Todo S, Tzakis A, Gordon RD and Starzl TE (1988). Biliary tract complications in orthotopic adult liver transplantation. *American Journal of Surgery, 158,* 68-70.

87. DeGroen PC, Allen JA, Rakela J, Forbes GS and Krom RAF (1987). Central nervous system toxicity after liver transplantation. *New England Journal of Medicine, 317,* 861-866.

88. Ho M, Wajszczuk CP, Hardy A, Drummer JS, Starzl TE, Hakala TR and Bahnson HT (1983). Infections in kidney, heart and liver transplant recipients on cyclosporine. *Transplantation Proceedings, 15,* 2768-2772.

89. Wajszczuk CP, Dummer SJ, Ho M, Van Thiel DH, Starzl TE, Iwatsuki S and Shaw BW (1985). Fungal infections in liver transplant recipients. *Transplantation, 40,* 347-353.

90. Colonna JO, Winston DJ, Brill JE, Goldstein LL, Hoff MP, Hiatt JR, Quinones-Baldrich W, Ramming KP and Busuttil RW (1988). Infectious complications in liver transplantation. *Archives of Surgery, 123,* 360-364.

91. Dindzans VJ, Schade RR and Van Thiel DH (1988). Medical problems before and after liver transplantation. *Gastroenterology Clinics of North America, 17*(1), 19-31.

92. Krom RAF (1986). Liver transplantation at the Mayo Clinic. *Mayo Clinic Proceedings, 61,* 278-282.

93. Rego J, Prevost J-L, Rumeau A, Modesto G, Foutanier G, Durand D, Suc J-M, Ohayon E and Ducos J (1987). Hyperacute rejection after ABO-incompatible orthotopic liver transplantation. *Transplantation Proceedings, 19,* 4589-4950.

94. Angstadt J, Jarrell B, Maddrey W, Munoz S, Yang S-L, Moritz M and Carabasi A (1987). Hemolysis in ABO-incompatible liver transplantation. *Transplantation Proceedings, 19,* 4595-4597.

95. Ascher NL, Freese DL, Paradis K, Snorer DC and Bloomer JR (1988). Rejection of the liver. In Maddrey WC (ed). *Current topics in gastroenterology. Transplantation of the liver.* (pp 167-190). New York: Elsevier.

96. Iwatsuki S, Iwaki Y, Kano T, Klintmalm L, Koep J, Weil R and Starzl TE (1981). Successful liver transplantation from crossmatch-positive donors. *Transplantation Proceedings, 13,* 286-288.

97. Iwatsuki S, Rabin BS, Shaw BW and Starzl TE (1984). Liver transplantation against T cell–positive warm crossmatches. *Transplantation Proceedings, 16,* 1427-1429.

16

Pancreas Transplantation

Becky G. Wills and Luana C. Post

It is estimated that every year more than 12,000 persons are diagnosed as having insulin-dependent diabetes mellitus (IDDM) in the United States.[1] As the fourth leading cause of death in this country, diabetes affects morbidity and mortality not only as a primary disease, but also through secondary complications associated with the disease. For example, retinopathy resulting from diabetes is the second leading cause of new blindness in all persons and is the leading cause of blindness in persons between the ages of 20 and 60.[2,3] Nephropathy resulting from diabetes accounts for 25% of end-stage renal failure patients who require dialysis.[1] Ten percent of diabetic patients will require a major amputation during their lifetime as a result of microvascular abnormalities.[4] Diabetes also accelerates the atherosclerotic process, which results in cardiovascular disease — the leading cause of death in the diabetic population.[5,6] Because the diabetic population accounts for 12% of hospitalized persons, these and other complications of this disease have a great impact on the cost of health care in the United States.

Exogenous insulin administration is an inadequate mechanism for consistently maintaining normal blood glucose levels in many patients.[7] Newer administration techniques, such as the insulin pump, have been shown to provide inconsistent glucose control and may also produce life-threatening hypoglycemia.[8] Persistent fluctuations in glucose levels create metabolic derangements that promote the development of secondary complications.[7,9] Because diabetes may decrease life expectancy by one fourth,[2] a more consistent method for maintaining euglycemia is desired.

Pancreas transplantation is a viable therapeutic option for insulin-dependent diabetics. Grafting a functioning endocrine pancreas into the insulin-dependent patient provides the optimal physiologic means of correcting altered metabolism. The goal of pancreas transplantation is twofold: to promote an insulin-independent life-style for the individual, and to prevent, arrest, or reverse the secondary complications associated with diabetes. Pancreas transplantation is not an immediate lifesaving measure, but successful transplantation may greatly improve the quality of life among diabetic patients and reduce the millions of dollars spent yearly on management of the disease and its sequelae.

HISTORICAL PERSPECTIVE

Although the characteristic symptoms of diabetes have been documented since the time of the ancient Egyptians, the disease had not been linked to the pancreas until 1788, when Thomas Cawley noticed pancreatic changes in a diabetic patient on autopsy.[10] In 1889 Minkowski and Von Mering substantiated the link between the pancreas and diabetes when they observed diuresis and glucosuria in a dog following total pancreatectomy. The first attempt to graft pancreas tissue was performed on a dog by Hedon in 1892. The transplant prevented the development of diabetes, and this outcome further strengthened theories of the link between the pancreas and diabetes.[1]

As more knowledge was gained regarding the identification of pancreatic hormonal influence on diabetes, scientists focused efforts on identifying the hormone responsible for euglycemia. In 1921 Frederick Banting and Charles Best discovered insulin and proved its success in lowering blood glucose levels in dogs.[1,10,11] The discovery of insulin was considered a cure for diabetes, and research efforts toward developing the field of pancreatic transplantation diminished.

The introduction of insulin marked a medical breakthrough in the management of the diabetic patient. The prognosis for survival for a newly diagnosed diabetic before the availability of insulin was approximately 1 year, with patients usually succumbing to ketoacidosis.[10,11] Insulin therapy greatly reduced the number of deaths and prolonged diabetic patients' life spans considerably.

Although insulin was a relatively safe and natural mode of lowering blood glucose levels, it was ineffective in maintaining consistent euglycemia over extended periods of time. Patients receiving insulin still experienced wide fluctuations in blood glucose levels. Attempts to develop better insulin compounds were also unsuccessful. As diabetics began to live longer, secondary complications associated with the disease became apparent. Scientists in the 1930s, 1940s, and 1950s noticed pathologic lesions in the glomeruli, on the retina, and in the blood vessels of insulin-dependent diabetics.[10] Although patients were surviving ketoacidosis, they were dying years later from renal and cardiac disease. Medical advances such as the development of hemodialysis were significant in reducing mortality, but impacted only the secondary effects of diabetes rather than the underlying cause of the disease. Control of metabolic dysfunction was necessary.

During the early insulin era, the first successful pancreas transplants were performed on dogs by Gayet and Guillaumie in 1927, and Houssay in 1929.[1] Trials in animal models continued into the 1950s and 1960s. These pioneering efforts provided the basis for the first human pancreas transplant, which was performed at the University of Minnesota in 1966.[12] The patient was a uremic diabetic woman who underwent a simultaneous kidney-pancreas transplant. The patient survived surgery but succumbed 2 months after transplant to sepsis and rejection. Thirteen additional pancreas transplants were performed by the Minnesota group between 1969 and 1973, but only one pancreas graft functioned longer than 1 year.[1]

The technique of performing a simultaneous kidney-pancreas transplant in the diabetic patient was employed by the Minnesota group, based on the philosophy that transplant of the kidney alone in the uremic diabetic patient was treatment of a secondary rather than the primary problem.[12] Other transplant centers, however, reported no outcome differences postoperatively in uremic diabetics who received both organs rather than a single kidney.[13] Because of difficulties in recovering suitable pancreas grafts and poor success rates associated with pancreas transplantation, most centers transplanted only kidneys into uremic diabetics.

Other efforts in pancreas transplantation during the 1960s and 1970s were also unsuccessful. According to the final report of the American College of Surgeons/National Institute of Health Organ Transplant Registry (ACS/NIHOTR) in 1977, the 1-year graft and patient survival rates were 3% and 40%, respectively.[14] Poor success resulted from (1) difficulties in maintaining adequate immunosuppression without subjecting the patient to overwhelming infection and (2) complications in surgical technique with respect to organ grafting and exocrine management of the donor organ.[15]

Research focused on developing an alternative to tissue grafting to decrease both technical difficulty and the amount of immunosuppression required to prevent rejection. The concept of transplanting only the islet cells by injection decreased the risks associated with surgical technique, but poor results were reported in both animal and human trials. Problems related to islet cell transplantation included imperfect methods of procuring the islets from the donor pancreas and severe rejection of the highly antigenic beta cells within the transplanted islets.[15,16] None of the patients undergoing this type of procedure at the University of Minnesota remained insulin independent.[16] Although it was recognized that islet cell transplantation might eventually be the optimal method of glucose control, practical application of the technique depended on further research. Attention again turned toward organ grafting.

Over the last decade, interest in pursuing pancreas transplantation as a cure for diabetes has increased. This interest has been reflected by the exponential increase of transplants performed since 1978. The International Pancreas Transplant Registry (IPTR), which succeeded the ACS/NIHOTR in 1977, published a report in 1989 that summarized all known cases of pancreas transplantation performed between December 17, 1966, and October 17, 1988. The number of transplants performed from 1983 to 1988 increased (n = 1129), compared with the years 1978 to 1982 (n = 201) and 1966 to 1977 (n = 64). Success rates increased during each era as well. Based on the 1129 reported cases since 1982, the overall graft and patient survival rates for 1 year were 46% and 82%, respectively, compared with the 1966 through 1977 statistics of 3% and 40%, respectively.[17] Factors that influenced the improved success of pancreas transplantation are those which influenced other transplant populations—namely, refinement of surgical technique, greater understanding of immunobiology, and wider availability of specific immunosuppressive therapy. It is worthy of mention that by 1986 graft survival rates had doubled to 42%, compared with 21% before 1982. This reflects the impact of cyclosporine, which became widely available in 1983, on controlling rejection in the transplanted patient.

There are several technical considerations in pancreas transplant surgery: (1) how much of the donor pancreas to transplant, (2) how to manage exocrine drainage of the donor organ once transplanted, and (3) whether to simultaneously transplant a kidney from the same donor into the uremic diabetic. Various methods have been developed and used among transplant centers. These techniques and associated survival rates will be discussed.

INDICATIONS

Criteria for pancreas transplantation vary among centers. Pancreas transplant generally is indicated in the patient with insulin-dependent diabetes whose secondary complications are more serious than are the risks of major surgery and immunosuppression. At present the procedure is most commonly performed in diabetic patients who, because of end-stage renal disease, have received or will receive a kidney transplant. This population would already require surgery and immunosuppression.

Ideally, pancreas transplant should be performed in the diabetic patient who has not yet developed, but is likely to develop, secondary lesions. Transplanting patients at this time would theoretically prevent the progression of microvascular complications. Unfortunately, it is difficult to predict which individuals will follow this course, since no definitive clinical indicators exist. Because overaggressive transplantation may unnecessarily subject patients to hazards of surgery and immunosuppression, most centers transplant diabetics who have demonstrated such complications as nephropathy, neuropathy, and retinopathy but are not so advanced in the disease course to place them at increased risk for complications of transplantation.

CONTRAINDICATIONS FOR PANCREAS TRANSPLANTATION

Contraindications to pancreas transplantation are similar to those for other solid organ transplants, such as the presence of metastatic cancer, infection, or overwhelming immunosuppressive disease. Specific disabilities caused by diabetes, such as persistent peripheral gangrene, severe coronary artery disease with angina, and incapacitating peripheral and autonomic neuropathies, may contraindicate transplantation. Since pancreas transplant is not an immediate lifesaving intervention, the patient's condition should be evaluated carefully to determine whether the benefits outweigh the risks of the procedure. The patient's willingness to accept the uncertainty of potential benefits and risks is also necessary.

CANDIDATE SELECTION

Candidate selection involves multidisciplinary evaluation of all major body systems. Data collected are used to evaluate eligibility of the patient and to provide baseline information with which to evaluate posttransplant cessation or reversal of complications of IDDM.

Because of the angiopathy associated with diabetes, the cardiovascular assessment is an important portion of the evaluation. Workup includes a 12-lead ECG and a thallium scan to detect coronary artery perfusion abnormalities. If cardiovascular abnormalities are identified, cardiac catheterization is indicated. Some centers have incorporated mandatory cardiac catheterization into the evaluation protocol because of the high incidence of posttransplant myocardial infarction among their population.[18] Severe vessel occlusion not correctable by angioplasty or bypass grafting contraindicates simultaneous kidney-pancreas transplantation, although renal transplantation may be performed.

Neurologic tests, such as nerve conduction studies, provide information regarding the extent of neuropathy. Urologic testing is done to determine the degree of bladder dysfunction and assists in determining the feasibility of specific operative techniques, which will be discussed in subsequent sections of this chapter. An ophthalmologic examination to detect the degree of retinopathy is performed. Metabolic studies include glucose tolerance tests, urine and serum C-peptide levels, and glycosylated hemoglobin levels. A thorough psychosocial evaluation is also included during this phase. A complete educational evaluation should be completed and appropriate learning measures instituted.

SURGICAL TECHNIQUES

Pancreas transplantation may involve grafting the entire organ, a segment of the organ, or the islet cells. The pancreas may be transplanted alone, or if the patient is uremic, a kidney from the same donor may be transplanted simultaneously. It is also possible to transplant a pancreas into a patient who has previously received a kidney graft. This allows pancreas transplant as an option for diabetic patients who underwent transplant for end-stage renal disease (ESRD) before pancreas transplant was an option.

The pancreas in the insulin-dependent diabetic has no endocrine function. Exocrine function, however, is generally not affected by the disease. Therefore, during transplant, the native pancreas is left in situ for continued exocrine function. The donor pancreas is transplanted to correct altered glucose metabolism.

Islet cell transplantation

Transplantation of islet cells, which contain the insulin-secreting beta cells, is the least perfected of pancreas transplant techniques and has been successful only in animal trials. The cells are isolated and extracted from a donor pancreas and then inoculated into the recipient. Care is taken to provide adequate separation of exocrine cells, because these cells tend to digest the viable transplant tissue. Ideal inoculation sites are those which have sufficient vascularity, accessibility for biopsy, durability to avoid damage from exocrine cells, portal venous drainage, and a decreased propensity for rejection. Sites for transplanting islet cells include the peritoneal cavity, liver, spleen, capsule of the kidney, testes, omentum, and cerebral ventricles. Greater success rates have been reported when sites with portal venous drainage have been used, because insulin from the transplanted islets flows directly into the liver.[11,19]

Unfortunately, islet cell transplantation has achieved limited success in human trials. Complications associated with this procedure include inadequate yield of islet cell mass, imperfect separation of islet tissue from exocrine tissue, unsuccessful preservation techniques, damage of cells during procurement and inoculation, failure of cells to implant, and rejection. If pancreatic islet cell transplantation is perfected, it will probably become the treatment of choice for the insulin-dependent diabetic. The relative technical ease of this method poses little discomfort or risk to the patient. Research is underway to develop techniques that reduce the antigenicity of islet allografts so that the amount of immunosuppression required after transplant may be reduced.[20,21] New isolation techniques make possible the procurement of 250,000 to 500,000 islet cells from one organ, enabling donation from one donor to several recipients. As research continues, islet cell transplantation may emerge as the future cure for diabetes.

Segmental transplantation

Segmental transplantation generally includes grafting the body and tail of the pancreas, which composes approximately 60% of the organ. Segmental pancreas transplantation allows for simultaneous recovery of the donor liver, because the splenic artery, which is the blood supply for the pancreas graft, may be divided from the celiac axis without damage to the hepatic artery.[1] Venous drainage is accomplished by retaining, when possible, the splenic vein and a short segment of portal vein during organ recovery.

The success of segmental transplantation is comparable to whole organ grafting with respect to graft survival, incidence of infection, and vessel thrombosis.[22] Because 70% to 80% of the islet mass is located in the middle to distal portion of the pancreas, metabolic control can be readily achieved. Segmental transplant also allows for living-related donation, a technique that remains controversial.

Whole-organ transplantation

The donor organ is recovered with the superior mesenteric and splenic arteries. The hepatic and celiac arteries may be salvaged for donor liver recovery. The pancreas is resected along with a cuff of donor duodenum, which nestles the head of the pancreas, and the spleen is used as a "handle" to remove the organ from the donor. Depending on the technique used, the

duodenal cuff may be resected or retained once the organ is recovered. Advantages to whole-organ grafting are that a larger mass of islet cells are transplanted, the duodenal cuff is a secure conduit for pancreatic enzymes, and better perfusion occurs over the vessel anastomoses, which reduces the risk of thrombosis.

Placement of the pancreas graft

Early attempts at pancreas transplantation involved placement of the graft extraperitoneally to decrease the risk of fistula development and peritonitis. More recently, grafts are being placed intraperitoneally because the peritoneum is abundantly vascular and can absorb the exocrine drainage that exudes from the surface of the organ.[23]

The pancreas graft is placed into the right iliac fossa, and the donor arterial supply is anastomosed to the recipient common iliac artery. The donor venous drainage is anastomosed to the common iliac vein (Fig. 16-1). If a simultaneous pancreas-kidney transplant is performed, the kidney is grafted into the left iliac fossa (Fig. 16-2). The right iliac fossa is pre-

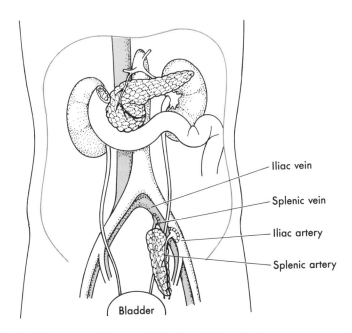

Iliac vein

Splenic vein

Iliac artery

Splenic artery

Bladder

Fig. 16-1 Graft placement and revascularization during single-organ segmental pancreas transplantation.

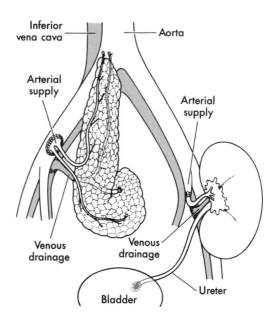

Fig. 16-2 Placement of organs during simultaneous kidney-pancreas transplant.

ferred for pancreas placement, because the relationship among donor and recipient veins makes obstruction of venous outflow less likely.[24]

EXOCRINE MANAGEMENT

Normally, the acinar cells secrete digestive enzymes via the pancreatic ductal system into the duodenum to aid in digestion of proteins, starches, and fat. Although the recipient's native pancreas is left in situ and performs exocrine function, enzymal secretion occurs in the grafted pancreas as well. It is therefore necessary to provide for exocrine drainage of the donor pancreas. Exocrine drainage management has proved to be the greatest technical challenge of pancreas tranplantation. Several methods for handling exocrine drainage have been developed; these techniques are ductal occlusion, enteric drainage, and urinary diversion.

Ductal occlusion

Ductal occlusion may be used in segmental and whole-organ transplantation and is accomplished by injecting a polymer substance into the main pancreatic duct, which hardens and occludes the duct (Fig. 16-3). In the early 1980s this method was the most common method of exocrine management and represents the majority of ductal management techniques used in all reported clinical cases to date.[1] Early postoperative complications such as leakage, wound infection, and fistula formation are usually transient, but they have influenced the preference for other methods.[25] A long-term complication of ductal injection is progressive fibrosis of the organ associated with graft failure.[26] Despite these complications, graft survival rates are comparable to those associated with other methods of exocrine drainage in the early postoperative phase.[11] Long-term follow-up, however, has revealed complications such as fibrosis and failure.

Enteric drainage (pancreaticojejunostomy)

Enteric drainage involves anastomosing the graft to a Roux-en-Y loop of recipient jejunum (Fig. 16-4). This method provides the most physiologic means for exocrine management, mimicking the normal enteric drainage of pancreatic enzymes. Patients with enteric drainage

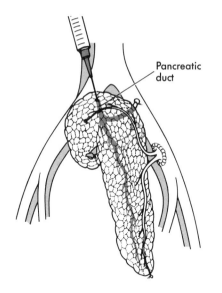

Fig. 16-3 Exocrine management by ductal injection.

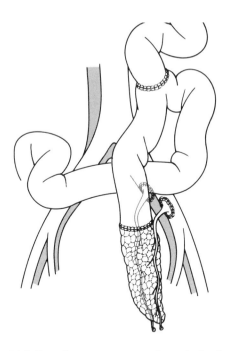

Fig. 16-4 Exocrine management by enteric drainage (Roux-en-Y jejunum).

suffer fewer metabolic imbalances, because pancreatic secretions are reabsorbed into the system. This method is required for pancreatic transplantation in patients who have undergone total pancreatectomy and in whom both endocrine and exocrine function are needed.[27]

Initial attempts at enteric drainage were associated with a high incidence of delayed wound healing, anastomotic leaks, and fistula formation. Refined surgical techniques and the availability of nonsteroidal immunosuppressive drugs such as cyclosporine have led to better results. Sepsis, however, remains a major complication of this technique.[11] Another disadvantage of this method is that diagnosis of rejection is difficult because secretion of enzymes, one parameter of assessing graft function, cannot be directly monitored.[28] Graft and patient survival rates, however, are comparable to those associated with other methods of exocrine drainage.[22]

Urinary diversion (pancreaticoduodencystostomy)

Urinary diversion offers an alternative to enteric drainage and ductal injection. Urinary drainage is established by anastomosing the pancreas to the recipient's bladder. The anastomosis is best accomplished by retaining an

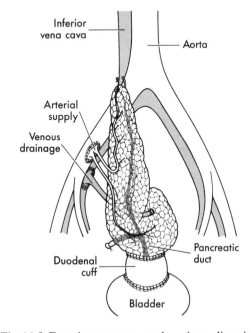

Fig. 16-5 Exocrine management by urinary diversion.

attached segment of donor duodenum during recovery and using this cuff to provide a suturing point between the donor pancreas and recipient bladder (Fig. 16-5). Recipients who receive this method of exocrine management must not have advanced bladder dysfunction.

One complication associated with urinary diversion is the potential for metabolic acidosis resulting from bicarbonate loss into the urine. Normal renal buffering can partially compensate for this loss, but patients usually require supplemental bicarbonate. Other complications with urinary diversion are ulceration and bleeding of the duodenal segment and the development of cystitis related to irritation by pancreatic drainage.[29]

There are several advantages associated with this method. For example, the urinary tract is bacteria free, thereby reducing the risk of infection. Pancreatic enzymes do not become activated in urine, so the incidence of fistula formation is also reduced. The greatest advantage of this drainage procedure is that it offers a direct method for assessing graft exocrine function. Urine amylase levels have been shown to be an earlier indicator of pancreas rejection than serum glucose levels.[30]

Success rates among techniques

According to the IPTR, 1-year graft survival rates for whole-organ and segmental grafts transplanted during the 1983 to 1986 era were similar at 42% and 46%, respectively. The 1-year survival rate for duct management, including polymer injection, enteric drainage, and urinary drainage, were 46%, 44%, and 43%, respectively. Within each category of ductal management, there were no significant differences in survival rates between whole and segmental pancreas transplants.[31]

POSTOPERATIVE CARE

Postoperative care of the pancreas transplant recipient involves promoting resumption of homeostasis and the prevention and early identification of complications. Although the surgical procedure is not usually as complex as other transplant procedures (e.g., heart and liver), postoperative care of the pancreas transplant recipient requires meticulous nursing assessment, planning, intervention, and evaluation.

Procedure varies among institutions regarding patient placement in the immediate postoperative period. Some centers admit patients to the postanesthesia care unit (PACU) for recovery and extubation, and then place the patient in either a general care area or an intensive care unit (ICU). Other centers may bypass the PACU and admit the patient directly to an ICU. Such factors as hosptial policy and patient condition influence postoperative patient placement.

Most often the patient is recovered from anesthesia, extubated, and awake on arrival in the patient care area. Oxygen deliverd by face mask or nasal cannula is usually required for a variable length of time after surgery. Invasive lines generally include a central venous catheter, peripheral intravenous line, urinary drainage catheter, and several surgical drains. If the patient is admitted to an ICU, an arterial line may be available for invasive blood pressure monitoring and blood specimen collection. The presence of a nasogastric tube depends on the length of the operation, type of anesthesia, and presence of preoperative ileus.

All elements of standard postoperative care provide the foundation for care for the pancreas transplant patient. These elements include invasive and/or noninvasive hemodynamic monitoring, assessment of oxygenation and tissue perfusion, and fluid and electrolyte management. Frequent measuring of vital signs is necessary to detect hypotension and tachycardia, which might indicate hemorrhage. Assessment of respiratory effort, aggressive pulmonary toilet, and evaluation of arterial blood gasses will assist the nurse in weaning the patient from oxygen therapy. Intake and output is measured frequently and is evaluated in accordance with the central venous pressure to determine adequacy of circulating plasma volume and tissue perfusion. If the patient has received a simultaneous kidney graft, urinary output is measured as often as every half-hour, and replacement fluids are infused to keep pace with the spontaneous diuresis that occurs with a functioning kidney graft.

Other general interventions include prophylactic antibiotic and antacid therapy. The patient remains NPO until bowel sounds are auscultated and the nasogastric tube, if present, is removed. Liquids are usually begun 24 to 48 hours postoperatively, and the diet is advanced as tolerated. The patient who receives a pancreas transplant also requires specific care aimed at preventing and detecting graft injury and rejection, and monitoring and management of metabolic status. These aspects of care are discussed below.

Prevention of thrombosis

Transplanting the pancreas graft into the right iliac fossa versus the left iliac fossa decreases the high risk of vessel thrombosis because of better graft vessel relationship to the recipient iliac artery and vein. However, thrombosis of graft vessels continues to be a postoperative complication leading to graft dysfunction in the immediate postoperative period. Many of the early postoperative interventions are directed at preventing vessel occlusion and injury. Activity is restricted to protect the vascular anastomoses and prevent shifting of the organ, which might cause thrombosis. Bed rest is continued for 3 to 5 days, and there should be no hip flexion on the side of the pancreas graft. Skin care can be accomplished by gently log-rolling the patient 20 degrees every 2 hours and by having the patient pull up off the bed using an overhead trapeze while back care is provided. An air mattress provides extra skin protection and patient comfort. When bed rest is discontinued, it is still necessary to prevent hip flexion for several more days. At that time the patient may stand to walk, but sitting is generally restricted until the seventh postoperative day.

Other measures used to reduce the risk of thrombosis in the immediate postoperative period are hemodilution and anticoagulation therapy. Low-molecular-weight dextran is infused intravenously for 5 to 7 days to decrease blood viscosity. Anticoagulation is achieved by subcutaneous heparin injection, or aspirin therapy when oral intake has resumed. Doppler flow studies are obtained periodically in the postoperative period to assess vessel patency.

Prevention of rejection

Immunosuppression is accomplished with corticosteroids, azathioprine, cyclosporine, and antilymphocyte globulin. These agents may be used in any combination, and standard immunosuppression regimens differ among institutions. According to a report issued by the IPTR,[17] higher graft and patient survival rates are associated with immunosuppressive regimens that consist of both cyclosporine and azathioprine, versus a regimen that does not include both of these agents. If the patient is a recipient of a kidney-pancreas graft, the regimen is likely to consist of antilymphocyte globulin, corticosteroids, and azathioprine until kidney graft function is documented. By that time the patient has usually resumed oral intake and oral cyclosporine can be administered; the oral form is considered less nephrotoxic than the intravenous form.

Monitoring rejection

Monitoring rejection in the patient who has received a pancreas transplant continues to be a challenge. Blood glucose levels are monitored closely in the immediate postoperative period, but upward trends are more helpful in detecting thrombosis than rejection. Rising glucose levels are a late sign of rejection, and by the time this occurs, the rejection is usually too advanced to respond to treatment.[30]

Some parameters that reflect exocrine function of the pancreas graft are unreliable indicators of rejection. Serum amylase levels are typically elevated in the immediate postoperative period but quickly return to normal. Causes of elevated serum amylase are preservation injury, abscess, pancreatitis, and rejection. Inconsistent trending patterns have been associated with rejection and are therefore not useful in most cases.

Urine amylase, bicarbonate, and pH levels have been shown to be good predictors of rejection in cases in which exocrine drainage has been accomplished by urinary diversion. Timed urine specimens are collected and analyzed for trends. Decreasing urine amylase and bicarbonate and a decline in urine pH have been shown to precede rejection.[30,32] The Registry report indicates that patients who receive a single pancreas graft with urinary diversion have higher graft survival rates than those who receive a single pancreas graft with other exocrine management techniques[17] because of the ability to directly monitor graft exocrine function and therefore rejection. Despite more favorable survival rates, some centers report inconsistency in reliability of urinary exocrine levels as early indicators of rejection.[20,33]

Patients who receive simultaneous kidney-pancreas grafts from the same donor have higher success rates than those who receive a pancreas graft alone or a pancreas graft years after a kidney.[17] This is because an additional parameter, the serum creatinine level, can be used to monitor rejection of both organs. Serum creatinine is a reliable indicator of rejection of the kidney graft, and it is frequently true that when the kidney is being rejected, the pancreas is also being rejected. Detection of kidney graft rejection most often precedes detection of pancreas graft rejection, and antirejection therapy can be instituted early, thereby possibly avoiding overwhelming rejection of the pancreas graft.

Assessment of endocrine function

Blood glucose levels are monitored frequently in the immediate postoperative period as an indicator of graft perfusion. Increasing levels during this time may indicate graft dysfunction as a result of vessel thrombosis, which would become evident as a tender graft. The significance of mildly elevated levels is difficult to interpret in light of concurrent corticosteroid use, which causes hyperglycemia by decreasing uptake of glucose by cells.

Assessment of acid-base status

Metabolic acidosis is frequently seen when urinary diversion is used for exocrine drainage of the pancreas graft. Causes stem from urinary loss of pancreatic electrolytes. There is a fixed loss of bicarbonate from the pancreas graft in the urine, which can be compensated for by the kidney. In cases in which renal function is compromised, however, the acidosis may be severe, because obligatory retention of chloride exacerbates this condition. Sodium bicarbonate may be added to intravenous infusions, and the patient may require supplemental oral bicarbonate after fluid therapy has been discontinued.

Hemorrhage

Postoperative hemorrhage is a risk associated with any type of surgery. Besides anastomotic leakage, other conditions predispose the patient to hemorrhage. Erosion of the bladder and persistent ulceration of the duodenal cuff often used in the urinary diversion technique have been reported.[29] Mild hematuria in the early postoperative period is not uncommon in patients who receive simultaneous kidney-pancreas transplants or who have urinary diversion for exocrine management, but gross hematuria is indicative of anastomotic leak of the duodenocystostomy site or ulceration of the duodenal cuff or bladder. Anticoagulant therapy can exacerbate the condition and may need to be discontinued until hemostasis is achieved. It is important to avoid overaggressive urinary catheter irrigation, because this can disrupt sutures. Irrigation and recatheterization are therefore most often physician responsibilities.

Graft pancreatitis

Graft pancreatitis, which is demonstrated by hyperamylasemia, and pain and tenderness over the graft site, may occur both early and late in the postoperative period. Early pancreatitis and hyperamylasemia are most likely to result from technical factors that occur during organ recovery and transplantation. Such factors include cold ischemia time greater than 6 hours, manipulation of the organ during recovery and transplant, and technique of exocrine management. For example, serum amylase levels remain elevated longer in grafts treated by ductal occlusion. Late graft pancreatitis has been correlated to several factors. Some centers report a relationship between enteric exocrine drainage and the development of late pancreatitis. Other causative factors include rejection and trauma.

Treatment for graft pancreatitis is similar to that of ordinary pancreatitis. The patient must remain on NPO status, and intravenous therapy is administered. Anticoagulant therapy should be instituted to prevent thrombosis, which is associated with pancreatitis. In extreme cases the graft must be removed. Patients who experience graft pancreatitis are at risk for developing other complications, such as ascites, pseudocyst, fistula, and abscess formation.

REFERENCES

1. Sutherland DER, Moudry K and Najarian J (1988). Pancreas transplantation. In Cerilli GJ (ed). *Organ transplantation and replacement.* Philadelphia: JB Lippincott Co.
2. Olson CO (1988). *Diagnosis and management of diabetes mellitus.* New York: Raven Press.
3. Kingham JD (1982). Diabetic retinopathy: recognition and management. In Bressler R and Johnson D (eds). *Management of diabetes mellitus.* Boston: PSG, Inc.
4. Deckert T (1988). Insulin-dependent diabetes mellitus and its complications. In Groth CG (ed). *Pancreatic transplantation,* Philadelphia: WB Saunders Co.
5. Lee S (1982). Management of diabetic renal disease. In Bressler R and Johnson D (eds). *Management of diabetes mellitus.* Boston PSG, Inc.
6. Foster DW (1983). Diabetes mellitus. In Petersdorf RG, Adams RO, Braunwald E, Isselbacher KJ, Martin JB and Wilson JD (eds). *Harrison's Textbook of internal medicine.* 10th ed. New York: McGraw-Hill Book Co.
7. Cahill GF, Etzwiler DD and Freinkel N (1976). Blood glucose control in diabetes. *Diabetes, 25,* 237-239.
8. Centers for Disease Control (1982). *Morbidity & Mortality Weekly Report,* February 26, *31*(7) (Issue).
9. Tchobroutsky G (1978). Relation of diabetic control to development of microvascular complications. *Diabetologia, 15*(3), 143-152.
10. Bloom A and Ireland J (1980). *A colour atlas of diabetes.* London: Wolfe Medical Publications, Ltd.
11. Rolles K (1987). Pancreatic and islet cell transplantation. In Catto G (ed). *Clinical transplantation: current practice and future prospects.* Lancaster, Pa: MTP Publications, Ltd.
12. Kelly W, Lillehei R, Merkel F, Idezuki Y and Goetz F (1967). Allotransplantation of the pancreas and duodenum along with the kidney in diabetic nephropathy. *Surgery, 61*(6), 827-837.
13. Najarian J, Kjellstrand C, Simmons R, Buselmeir T, Hartitzsch B and Goetz F (1973). Renal transplantation for diabetic glomerulosclerosis. *Annals of Surgery, 178*(4), 447-483.
14. Sutherland DER (1980). International human pancreas and islet transplant registry. *Transplantation Proceedings, 12*(4), 229.
15. Jonasson O, Reynolds W, Snyder G and Hoversten G (1977). Experimental and clinical therapy of diabetes by transplantation. *Transplantation Proceedings, 9*(1), 223-231.
16. Najarian J, Sutherland D, Matas A, Steffes M, Simmons R and Goetz F (1977). Human islet transplantation: a preliminary report. *Transplantation Proceedings, 9*(1), 233-236.
17. Sutherland DER, Moudry KC and Fryd DS (1989). Results of pancreas transplant registry. *Diabetes, 38*(1S), 46-54.
18. Smith JL, Wright FH, Schanbacher B and Corry RJ (1988). Improving patient and graft survival rates in pancreatic transplantation. *Transplantation Proceedings, 20*(1S), 866-867.
19. Gray DWR and Morris PJ (1988). Transplantation of isolated pancreas islets. In Groth CG (ed). *Pancreatic transplantation.* Philadelphia: WB Saunders Co.
20. Lafferty K, Prowse S and Simeonovic C (1984). Current status of experimental islet transplantation. *Transplantation Proceedings, 16,* 813-819.
21. Scharp DW (1984). Clinical feasibility of islet cell transplantation. *Transplantation Proceedings, 16,* 820-825.
22. Suthlerland DER (1987). Pancreas transplantation. *Diabetes Metabolism Reviews, 3*(4), 1061-1090.
23. Sutherland DER, Goetz FC and Najarian JS (1988). Experience with single pancreas transplantation compared with pancreas transplantation after a kidney transplantation; and with transplantation with pancreas grafts from living related compared with cadaveric donors. In Groth CG (ed). *Pancreatic transplantation.* Philadelphia: WB Saunders Co.
24. Nghiem DD and Corry J (1987). Technique of simultaneous renal pancreatoduodenal transplantation with urinary drainage of pancreatic secretion. *American Journal of Surgery, 153,* 405-406.
25. Dubernard JM, Martin X, Camozzi L and Sanseverino R (1988). Segmental pancreatic transplantation with ductal filling by polymer injection. In Groth CG (ed). *Pancreatic transplantation.* Philadelphia: WB Saunders Co.
26. Sutherland DER (1984). Selected issues of importance in clinical pancreas transplantation. *Transplantation Proceedings, 16*(3), 661-669.
27. Starzl TE and Tzakis AG (1988). Pancreatico-duodenal transplantation with enteric exocrine drainage. In Groth CG (ed). *Pancreatic transplantation.* Philadelphia: WB Saunders Co.
28. Corry RJ and Nghiem DD (1986). Transplantation of the intact pancreas organ: enteric drainage of the intact pancreas gland. *Transplantation and Immunology Letter, 3*(1), 1-4.
29. Corry RJ, Wright FH and Smith JL (1988). Whole organ pancreas transplantation. *Transplantation Proceedings, 20*(3S), 420-425.
30. Corry RJ (1987). University of Iowa experience in pancreatic transplantation. *Transplantation Proceedings, 19*(4S4), 37-39.
31. Sutherland DER and Moudry KC (1988). Pancreas transplant registry. In Groth CG (ed). *Pancreatic transplantation.* Philadelphia: WB Saunders Co.
32. Prieto M, Sutherland DER, Fernandez-Cruz L, Heil JB and Najarian JS (1987). Diagnosis of rejection in pancreas transplantation. *Transplantation Proceedings, 19,* 2348-2349.
33. Fernandez-Cruz L, Esmatges E, Andreu J, Targarona EM, Prieto M and Gil-Vernet J (1987). Advantages and disadvantages of urinary tract diversion in clinical pancreas transplantation. *Transplantation Proceedings, 19*(5), 3895-3898.

17

Bone Marrow Transplantation

Jane C. Clark and *Jennifer S. Webster*

Bone marrow transplantation, the transfer of hematopoietic cells from the bone marrow of one living organism into another living organism, has generated some of the most critical technologic and biologic challenges in the field of transplantation. With organ and tissue transplantation, challenges are twofold: (1) mechanical tissue and organ replacement and (2) immunosuppression of the host to prevent tissue rejection. With bone marrow transplantation, biologic replacement of cellular elements of the marrow is required.

In other types of transplantation, the recipient tissue or organ is removed and replaced by donor tissue or organ. In bone marrow transplantation, bone marrow cannot be removed physically from the recipient. Either marrow-toxic doses of chemicals or radiation are delivered to clear the marrow spaces of cellular elements of the hematopoietic system. Thus the potential damage to other organ systems by the chemicals and/or radiation given for marrow ablation is an additional risk of the procedure.

Immunosuppression of both the host and the donor marrow is required. Host immunosuppression allows donor marrow to engraft, while donor marrow immunosuppression minimizes the risk of the graft recognizing the host as foreign. With the transplantation of bone marrow, the length of time required to establish complete functioning of the transplanted tissue increased from minutes and hours to weeks.

Therefore care of the bone marrow transplant patient presents the added challenges of (1)

achieving adequate destruction of the recipient marrow, (2) balancing donor marrow and recipient immunosuppression, and (3) developing relatively long-term procedures for supporting the marrow recipient until engraftment and reconstitution of the bone marrow can occur. In the following sections, indications for and the historical implications of the challenges presented by bone marrow transplantation will be discussed.

INDICATIONS

Bone marrow transplantation has become a viable option in the treatment of selected patients with primary bone marrow failure and diseases of the bone marrow. Also, transplantation is indicated as a marrow rescue procedure from toxic and therapeutic effects of radiation therapy and chemotherapy.

Primary marrow failure occurs when one or more elements of the hematopoietic system fails to proliferate or differentiate into mature, functional, cellular elements. Examples of primary marrow failure include aplastic anemia and severe combined immune deficiency (SCID).

In addition to primary marrow failure, *diseases of the bone marrow* may inhibit the proliferation and/or differentiation of elements of the hematopoietic system. Leukemia, lymphoma, and multiple myeloma are examples of diseases of the marrow for which transplantation may be used as a therapeutic modality.

One of the most exciting applications of

marrow transplantation has been in *marrow rescue* for patients exposed, either accidently or therapeutically, to marrow-lethal doses of radiation therapy and/or chemotherapy. Marrow transplantation has played a role in the treatment of individuals exposed to marrow-lethal doses of radiation, such as in victims of radiation accidents. Marrow rescue has provided an option for more aggressive chemotherapy, which previously had been limited by the marrow toxicity of antineoplastic agents for patients with breast cancer, neuroblastoma, brain tumors, and lung cancer.

HISTORICAL PERSPECTIVE

The first attempt to transplant bone marrow therapeutically occurred in 1891 when Brown-Séquard administered a marrow preparation orally to treat nutritional deficits in a patient with leukemia. Despite this unsuccessful attempt, bone marrow preparations delivered via intramedullary and intravenous routes were used subsequently to treat anemia from a variety of causes; however, long-term therapeutic effects did not occur.[1,2]

The Atomic Age of the 1940s resulted in an increased interest in the application of bone marrow transplantation to treat the lethal effects of radiation exposure. Jacobsen et al (1949) and Lorenz et al (1951) demonstrated that mice could be protected against the lethal effects of irradiation by shielding the spleen,[3] a blood-forming organ, or by parenteral infusion of a bone marrow preparation.[4]

In the 1950s bone marrow transplantation was attempted in humans. Many of the donor marrows never engrafted, and recipients died from bleeding and infection. For those patients in whom engraftment occurred, virtually all died from graft-versus-host disease (GVHD).[1]

Historical complications of bone marrow transplantation

Early efforts at bone marrow transplantation in humans resulted in death for the majority of patients. Factors contributing to the high mortality seen in the early marrow transplantation can be grouped in three categories: (1) patient-related factors, (2) marrow-related factors, and (3) supportive care factors.

Patient-related factors include those characteristics of the patient which contributed to the failure of the marrow transplant. Patients selected for marrow transplantation suffered from marrow failure resulting from radiation accidents or disease, such as aplastic anemia or recurrent leukemia. Conventional methods of therapy had been exhausted. Patients were debilitated and often entered the transplant period with compromised respiratory, cardiovascular, hepatic, and renal systems, fulminating primary disease or infection, and inadequate marrow ablation. Most patients succumbed to infection, bleeding, and organ failure in the immediate posttransplant period before engraftment. For patients treated for leukemia who survived the initial transplant period, long-term survival was limited by recurrence of disease. Inadequate marrow ablation before transplantation was implicated.[2,5]

Marrow-related factors include those factors which contributed to the lack of reconstitution of the donor marrow in the recipient or the rejection of the donor marrow by the recipient. Early efforts at marrow collection lacked specificity with respect to the number of cells required to allow establishment of an immunocompetent donor marrow in the recipient. Lack of knowledge about the histocompatibility complex system resulted in the transplantation of marrow between donors and recipients with major human leukocyte antigen (HLA) incompatibilities. Death occurred in the immediate posttransplant period as a result of lack of donor-marrow engraftment and GVHD.

Supportive care factors include those factors which contributed to the support of the recipient during the interval between the pretransplant marrow ablation and reconstitution of the donor marrow in the recipient. Although pancytopenia occurred with regularity in patients who received marrow ablation, blood component therapy was either not available (granulocyte and platelet transfusions) or used infrequently (red cell transfusions) during early attempts at marrow transplantation.[1]

Limited availability of antimicrobial agents and the lack of empirical antimicrobial therapy in the absence of confirmed infectious organisms resulted in death from bacterial, fungal, and viral infections. In addition to lack of supportive blood component and antimicrobial therapy, bone marrow transplant recipients required prolonged intravenous therapy and nutritional support. Yet peripheral vascular access was problematic and was a limitation of supportive therapy.

In summary, early bone marrow transplantation was limited by lack of knowledge about the significance of donor-recipient compatibility, inadequate ablation of diseased recipient marrow, insufficient pharmacologic agents to ablate diseased marrow and to treat infections, and inadequate techniques for long-term vascular access. However, with scientific and technologic advances within the past 30 years and increased

interest in transplantation in general, bone marrow transplantation now is used successfully to treat a variety of diseases and to rescue the marrow from marrow-lethal exposure to physical and chemical substances.

TYPES OF BONE MARROW TRANSPLANT

Bone marrow for transplantation may be obtained from three major sources. An *autologous* transplant occurs when marrow is collected from a person, stored, and reinfused to the same person at a later time. An *allogeneic* transplant occurs when marrow is collected from a genetically nonidentical donor and transfused to a marrow recipient. For an allogeneic transplant, the donor may be related or unrelated. At the

Table 17-1 Comparison of bone marrow transplants

Type of transplant survival estimates	Eligibility	Disadvantages	Advantages
Autologous	Marrow free of detectable tumor Malignancy expected to respond to increased doses of antineoplastic agents Able to tolerate recovery procedure and period of immunosuppression	Potential tumor contamination	Readily available Genetically identical marrow No risk of GVHD
Allogeneic	HLA-MLC compatible donor Malignancy expected to respond to increased doses of antineoplastic agents *or* ability to ablate remaining diseased recipient marrow	Limited availability of HLA-MLC compatible donors Risk of GVHD	Lack of tumor contamination
Syngeneic	Genetically identical donor Malignancy expected to respond to increased doses of antineoplastic agents *or* ability to ablate remaining diseased recipient marrow	Rare availability of genetically identical donors Low risk of GVHD	Lack of tumor contamination

present time, the majority of allogeneic transplant donors are relatives of the recipient. Siblings of the recipient are the most potentially compatible donors for allogeneic marrow transplantation. A special case of donor-related transplantation, a *syngeneic* transplant, occurs with the donation of marrow from a genetically identical twin to the recipient. A comparison of the relative advantages and disadvantages of the major types of bone marrow transplantation are presented in Table 17-1.

Autologous transplantation represents the least risk in that the marrow is readily available, genetically identical, and carries no risk of GVHD. In contrast, allogeneic transplantation, especially from a nonrelated donor, presents the greatest risk to the recipient particularly with respect to GVHD.

With the increased application of marrow transplantation in both treatment of disease and marrow rescue, particularly in oncology, the use of nonrelated marrow donors has emerged as a potential approach. Since only about 35% to 40% of patients in need of a bone marrow transplant have an HLA-identical sibling donor,[6] interest has grown in establishing a registry of potential, nonrelated, HLA-matched donors. Because of the multiplicity of possible HLA-loci combinations, an extensive registry is required to identify completely HLA-matched donors. Several registries have been established recently in North America and Europe in spite of the obvious difficulties.[7,8] Thus the possibility of marrow transplantation has become a reality for patients who have no siblings or related marrow donors.

The ideal bone marrow transplant scenario

The ideal marrow for transplantation would be from a completely identical HLA donor, contain sufficient numbers of stem cells to ensure engraftment, and be capable of eliciting an immunologic response in the recipient, yet not resulting in severe GVHD. The ideal marrow recipient would be a person with either marrow failure or marrow disease in remission, intact and functional major organ systems, and adequate psychosocial and financial resources to cope with transplant therapy. However, in reality, the circumstances under which a bone marrow transplant is planned are less than ideal. The selection of recipients and donors for bone marrow transplantation results in a series of compromises from the ideal scenario.

CRITERIA FOR SELECTION OF A BONE MARROW RECIPIENT

The availability of a suitable marrow donor is the essential criterion for selection as a bone marrow recipient. In addition, the patient's underlying disease, age, concurrent health problems, psychosocial profile, and economic resources are considered.

Availability of donor marrow

Criteria for selection of bone marrow donors are based on genetic compatibility with the recipient as determined by HLA and mixed lymphocyte culture (MLC) testing. A thorough review of histocompatibility is presented in Part One of the text. Loci A, B, C, and DR compatibility is detected by serologic testing (HLA), whereas D loci compatibility is determined by mixing samples of the donor and recipient lymphocytes in culture and observing the degree of reaction (MLC). Mutual nonreactivity between the lymphocytes of the donor and recipient is desired. In the ideal donor the main genetic loci (A, B, C, D, and DR) are compatible with those of the recipient. Children inherit one chromosome 6 containing the HLA complex from each parent; therefore siblings of the recipient have the greatest likelihood of HLA-MLC compatibility.[9] For patients in need of transplant and without an HLA-MLC matched donor, marrow mismatched at one HLA loci is being transplanted. Although survival appears to be comparable, the incidence and severity of graft-versus-host disease is increased with marrow not matched at all major HLA loci.[7]

Disease status

Bone marrow transplantation has been used primarily to treat aplastic anemia and a variety of leukemias. For each type of disease, prognostic factors associated with disease status and previous therapy assist the transplant team to identify candidates at risk for morbidity and mortality from the procedure. These prognostic factors are weighed with other criteria, such as

Table 17-2 Comparison of allogeneic bone marrow transplant and chemotherapy outcomes

AML (actuarial survival at 3 to 5 years)		
Timing of transplant	BMT (%)	Chemotherapy (%)
First complete remission		
Age <30 years	50-70	20-40
Age >30 years	30-45	10-35
Initial relapse or second complete remission	30	<10
Advanced disease	10-20	0

From Champlin R (1988). Acute myelogenous leukemia: biology and treatment. *Mediguide to Oncology, 8*(4), 1-9.

age and concurrent health problems, to select patients for transplantation in whom the potential benefits of the procedure outweigh the potential risks.

Age

Age is a factor in evaluation of bone marrow recipients. Since the morbidity and mortality associated with marrow transplantation increase dramatically with age, the majority of transplant centers prefer to accept patients under 30 years of age.

To evaluate the relative survival by age and treatment, controlling for diagnosis, Champlin[10] compared patients with acute myelocytic leukemia treated with allogeneic bone marrow transplantation and chemotherapy (Table 17-2).

In patients under 30 years of age, the results of bone marrow transplantation were similar to or better than those resulting from chemotherapy[10]; therefore routine use of bone marrow transplantation in patients under 30 years of age was recommended. However, the timing of transplantation during the course of disease for patients greater than 30 years of age remains controversial.

General health status

For most patients, by the time bone marrow transplantation is considered as a treatment option, profound assaults on the integrity of the cardiovascular, respiratory, renal, and hepatic systems have occurred as a result of previous therapy. Evaluation of crucial body systems by physical examination, x-ray studies, and biochemical assays is included in the pretransplant bone marrow transplantation workup. Significant renal, hepatic, respiratory, and/or cardiovascular dysfunction resulting from either previous therapy or age may eliminate a patient from consideration as a transplant candidate.

Psychosocial profile

The psychosocial profile is essential for screening potential marrow recipients and planning care. The majority of transplant centers include a psychosocial and/or psychiatric evaluation as a part of the pretransplant workup. Evaluation of the recipient includes coping styles used when facing life stressors and disease, past psychiatric history, social support systems, and personal and financial resources.[11] Psychiatric history and current psychiatric problems may exclude a candidate from bone marrow transplantation. More commonly, fears and phobias related to the transplant procedure are identified and serve as a database for planning care before, during, and after the transplant procedure. The evaluation serves the following important functions:[12]

1. To introduce the patient and family to the hospital, transplant unit, and staff
2. To familiarize the staff with questions the patient and family have about the transplant procedure and to allow time for exchange of information
3. To identify resources and coping skills of the patient and family as a basis for planning care

The selection of a patient as a marrow recipient implies patient, family, and health care personnel and system commitment of time and resources to the transplant. The cost of a transplant includes both direct and indirect costs. With respect to direct costs, the average inpatient hospital expenditures for a bone marrow transplant range from $50,000 to $150,000. In addition, the costs of follow-up medical care, continued immunosuppressive and supportive therapies, and rehabilitation may be significant. Although bone marrow transplantation is recognized as an acceptable therapy by most insurance carriers for the treatment of leukemias and aplastic anemia, use of marrow transplant for the rescue from toxic effects of other therapy is still considered experimental, and coverage is limited or nonexistent. In addition to limited insurance coverage, the issue of cumulative insurance limits arises. By the time that most patients reach marrow transplantation, insurance coverage limits may have been reached.[5] Thus the patient and significant others are faced with the dilemma of incurring a significant financial burden in the form of loans, mortgages, and/or loss of property to meet the economic demands of the procedure.

For patients with limited or no medical insurance, marrow transplantation is not as realistic. Although many transplant centers have resources to assume the costs of transplantation in the acute care setting for indigent patients, the substantial costs of follow-up care remain an unresolved dilemma.

Indirect cost estimates are not available for the loss of time from work for the patient and significant others, nor the increase in insurance premiums, transportation, and housing associated with bone marrow transplantation. Although the direct and indirect costs of marrow transplantation are high, for most potential marrow recipients the costs of continued medical therapy without the hope for cure may result in comparable health care bills.[5]

In summary, selection of patients as marrow recipients depends on the availability of a donor marrow, disease and health status, age, and psychosocial profile. By carefully evaluating each potential marrow recipient using the identified criteria, patients may be selected in whom the potential benefits of marrow transplant outweigh the potential negative consequences of the procedure and morbidity and mortality may be diminished.

CRITERIA FOR SELECTION OF BONE MARROW DONOR

Donors for bone marrow transplantation differ from those for organ transplantation in several ways. First, the bone marrow donor is required to provide a minimal volume of marrow which the body can replace in days. Second, the bone marrow donor undergoes a minor versus a major surgical procedure to harvest the marrow. Third, the potential complications from marrow donation are limited. Finally, the donor faces psychologic risks associated with the potential of the marrow to reject host tissues and result in lethal GVHD in the host.

Histocompatibility

Criteria for selection of bone marrow donors are based on genetic compatibility, as measured by HLA and MLC testing. In other types of transplants, an immunocompetent recipient receives immunoincompetent tissues and organs. Therefore the major concern is host rejection of the transplanted organ. In bone marrow transplantation, an immunoincompetent recipient receives an immunocompetent donor marrow. As the donor marrow engrafts and proliferation of immunocompetent cells such as T and B lymphocytes, granulocytes, and monocytes occurs, the risk increases of the donor marrow recognizing the recipient as foreign and attempting to reject recipient tissues. The degree to which the donor and recipient are HLA-MLC incompatible influences the incidence of GVHD and patient survival. Although every effort is made to select a compatible donor, histocompatibility does not guarantee the success of the transplant nor prevention of GVHD.

Health status

In addition to compatibility testing, a complete history is taken and the marrow donor undergoes a physical examination. To minimize the risks of donation, hepatic, renal, pulmonary, and cardiovascular status are evaluated before anesthesia for the marrow harvest. Donors are also screened for hepatitis, HIV antibody, syphilis, CMV antibody, ABO, and Rh compatibility to minimize the potential risks to the recipient.

Psychosocial profile

A psychosocial profile, conducted by a psychologist, nurse, social worker, or transplant coordinator, is included in the evaluation of the majority of bone marrow donors. Donor perceptions of the marrow harvest and transplant procedures, motivation for donating, relationships with the recipient and other members of the family, support and financial resources, and potential disruption of life-style by the long-term requirements of marrow donors are evaluated.[13]

Although data indicate that the physiologic consequences of marrow donation are minimal, Wolcott et al[14] reported a 10% to 20% incidence of negative experiences and feelings among a sample of 18 marrow donors whose recipients survived the transplant procedure. In addition, negative responses toward the transplant procedure and the relationship with the marrow recipient were inversely correlated with the perception of recipient well-being and health status.

For the donor whose recipient dies, regret and guilt for having donated the marrow often occur. Guilt is particularly evident when the recipient succumbs to the lethal effects of GVHD. Thus, regardless of the outcome of the transplant, pretransplant psychosocial evaluation is a critical process to elicit donor needs before, during, and after transplant.

Age

Age does not exclude an individual from being a marrow donor. However, age can influence the volume of marrow obtained. The total volume of marrow required is 10 ml/kg of donor body weight. Therefore, if the donor is small and young, the volume of marrow collected may not contain adequate numbers of stem cells to reconstitute an immunocompetent marrow in the recipient. In the case of minor donors, legal guardians or court-appointed child advocates have been recommended to protect the rights of the child.

In summary, the major criteria for marrow donation are HLA-MLC compatibility between the donor and recipient, ability to harvest an adequate volume of marrow for engraftment, and donor safety. Evaluation of HLA-MLC compatibility, health status, and psychosocial profile provide critical donor information for determining selection.[15]

PRETRANSPLANT PERIOD

Once a suitable donor has been identified, the actual transplant procedure is planned. A con-

ditioning protocol designed to prepare the recipient for marrow transplant is implemented.[16] Selection of a conditioning protocol, which may include ablative or therapeutic chemotherapy, total body or nodal radiation, or a combination of chemotherapy and radiation therapy, is based on the indications for the transplant, the type of transplant anticipated, and previous therapy. The length of the conditioning procedure varies from 4 to 8 days. Regardless of the type of conditioning procedure used, three critical outcomes have been identified: (1) ablation of recipient marrow, (2) implementation of strategies to decrease predictable morbidity, and (3) establishment of long-term venous access for supportive therapy.

Recipient marrow ablation

Marrow ablation with radiation therapy and/or chemotherapy is used to prepare the recipient to accept the donor marrow by destroying remaining immunocompetent recipient cells and by clearing the marrow spaces. In the case of diseased marrow, eradication of remaining disease is an additional goal. However, the goals of ablation vary with both the type of transplant planned and the condition being treated (Table 17-3).

Chemotherapy and radiation therapy, used alone or in combination, are the mainstays of

Table 17-3 Goals of ablative therapy

Goal	Type of transplant/condition
Destroy immuno-competent cells in recipient to decrease risks of GVHD	Allogeneic/syngeneic Primary marrow failure Diseases of bone marrow Marrow rescue
Destroy abnormal cells in the recipient marrow	Autologous/allogeneic/syngeneic Diseases of bone marrow
Treat underlying disease at marrow-toxic dose levels	Autologous Marrow rescue

Table 17-4 Antineoplastic agents used in marrow ablative therapy

	Potential side effects	
Agent	Immediate	Long-term
Busulfan	Leukopenia Thrombocytopenia	Pulmonary fibrosis
Carmustine (BCNU)	Bone marrow suppression Nausea Vomiting	Pulmonary fibrosis
Cyclophosphamide	Leukopenia Thrombocytopenia Nausea Vomiting Alopecia Hemorrhagic cystitis	Pulmonary fibrosis Cardiotoxicity Sterility
Cytosine arabinoside (Cytarabine)	Leukopenia Thrombocytopenia Nausea Vomiting Stomatitis Diarrhea Neurologic toxicity	Sterility
Etoposide (VP-16)	Leukopenia Thrombocytopenia Alopecia Hypotension Anaphylaxis	

marrow ablation. Marrow-lethal doses of chemotherapy are given to the recipient before the infusion of donor marrow. Schedules for administration of ablative chemotherapy differ with various protocols. Specific antineoplastic agents commonly used in ablative chemotherapy and potential immediate and long-term side effects are presented in Table 17-4.

The nurse is responsible for administering the antineoplastic agents, teaching the patient and family strategies to decrease potential side effects, monitoring for immediate and long-term consequences of the therapy, and reporting significant side effects of therapy to the physician.

In addition to ablative chemotherapy, marrow recipients also may receive marrow-lethal doses of radiation therapy either to lymph node–bearing areas alone or to the total body. The dose of radiation delivered ranges from 750 to 1500 rads, given as either a single dose or fractionated doses over 3 to 4 days. The potential destructive effects of radiation therapy on normal organs are significant, ranging from pulmonary and cardiac fibrosis to hepatic necrosis.

In summary, the first goal of the conditioning procedure, ablation of the recipient marrow, is accomplished through delivery of marrow-lethal doses of chemotherapy and/or radiation therapy. The immediate effects of the ablative therapy are to prepare the recipient to receive the donor marrow and/or to eradicate residual disease. However, long-term effects of the conditioning therapies pose significant hurdles for the transplant recipient both in terms of morbidity and mortality.

Strategies to decrease predictable morbidity

Regardless of the type of transplant, predictable morbidity, such as bleeding and infection, will occur. Strategies to decrease the incidence of predictable morbidity are critical elements of the conditioning procedure. Infection resulting from prolonged immunosuppressive therapy is the most frequent cause of morbidity, is life-threatening because of the immunoincompetence of the recipient, and often is not recognized because of the inability of the recipient to exhibit a clinical inflammatory or immune response. Endogenous organisms, such as gram-negative and gram-positive bacteria of the gastrointestinal tract, are implicated in the majority of infections.

General strategies to decrease the incidence of infection include dental evaluation, gastrointestinal and vaginal sterilization, skin and oral care protocols, and implementation of a protective isolation or a laminar air-flow environment. A discussion of the nursing responsibilities with each strategy follows.

Dental evaluation. The oral cavity is a source of endogenous organisms. For most recipients, transplantation occurs after extensive primary therapy during which routine dental surveillance and care of the oral cavity and teeth may have been neglected. Thus dental evaluation is crucial both in decreasing the incidence of infection during marrow transplantation and increasing the success of gut sterilization procedures by decreasing the number of organisms harbored in the oral cavity.

Goals of the dental evaluation include identification of preexisting dental problems, treatment for selected dental problems, and prophylactic treatment of the oral cavity. The dental evaluation includes a thorough oral examination as well as x-ray evaluation. The issue of dental manipulation before marrow transplantation is of concern with respect to preexisting pancytopenia associated with previous therapy and/or disease. In marrow recipients in remission from disease or with a primary solid tumor, granulocytes and platelets should be adequate to allow dental manipulation without increasing transplant morbidity. However, since any form of dental manipulation may be a source of bacteremia, prophylactic antibiotics immediately before and for several days after dental procedures are recommended.[17]

The most common finding in the pretransplant dental evaluation is the accumulation of plaque and food particles on the teeth and under the gingiva. Accumulation of plaque and food particles may be treated by oral prophylaxis, a soft-bristled tooth brush moistened with hot water, soft wet gauze, or a moistened toothette. The virogousness with which plaque and food particles are removed will be determined in part by the platelet count and immunocompetence of the recipient.

Orthodontic or prosthodontic appliances are deterrents to adequate oral hygiene as well as potential sources of irritation and ulceration to the oral mucosa. Removal of such devices before marrow transplantation is recommended. Psychologic responses of patients may prohibit removal of prosthodontic appliances for the duration of the transplant period. In such cases, patients are encouraged to remove the appliances as much as tolerated.

Patients with dental caries pose a problem in terms of conditioning for marrow transplant. Caries likely to result in pulp involvement should be treated with temporary or permanent restoration. If the pulp is infected, the tooth should be extracted. Care is taken to remove the tooth with the least trauma possible and to close the wound properly to limit bleeding and the possibility of postextraction wound infection.[17]

In addition to the obvious prophylactic treatment of preexisting dental conditions, the pretransplant evaluation provides an opportunity for the marrow recipient and nurse to be instructed in oral care techniques required during the transplant and to establish rapport with the dentist. As an integral member of the transplant team, the dentist will be involved in care planning for the recipient throughout the transplant and posttransplant periods. Thus coordination of care protocols between the dentist and nurse is mandatory.

Gastrointestinal and vaginal sterilization. Infectious complications early in the course of bone marrow transplantation result from both exogenous and endogenous organisms. Endogenous organisms most commonly implicated are those found in the respiratory and gastrointestinal tracts. To decrease the number of viable endogenous organisms capable of overgrowth in the immunosuppressed host, sterilization of the gut and vagina may be recommended.[1]

Gastrointestinal sterilization consists of an oral preparation of nonabsorbable antibiotics, such as gentamycin, vancomycin, neomycin, and/or nystatin, which is swirled in the mouth and swallowed. Doses and schedules of administration for the oral preparation vary. The effectiveness of gut sterilization procedures depends on the ability of the patient to hold the preparation in the mouth for contact with the oral organisms and to tolerate swallowing the oral preparation for contact with organisms in the remainder of the gastrointestinal tract.

In addition to gut sterilization, vaginal sterilization is suggested to decrease endogenous organisms in female marrow recipients. Douches with povidone-iodine solutions are administered according to transplant protocol. Although the goal of both gastrointestinal and vaginal sterilization is to decrease the risk of infection, sterilization procedures are not without the risk of suprainfection.

Skin and oral care protocols. In addition to dental evaluation and gastrointestinal and vaginal sterilization, skin and oral care protocols are initiated as primary prevention strategies against infection. Skin care protocols generally include daily bathing with an antibacterial soap and perineal cleansing after each voiding and bowel movement with a povidone-iodine solution diluted with sterile water.

Oral care protocols have three major components: (1) removal of food and mucoid debris from the teeth and gingiva, (2) maintenance of oral mucosal integrity and moisture, and (3) administration of prophylactic oral antibiotics (Table 17-5).

Table 17-5 Components of an oral care protocol

Component	Nursing interventions	Medical interventions
Removal of debris	Brush teeth 4 times a day, after each meal and at bedtime Use soft-bristled toothbrush rinsed with hot water, moistened sterile gauze or toothette Use a nonirritating dentifrice such as baking soda and/or a fluoride toothpaste Rinse mouth with cleansing solution such as 1:4 hydrogen peroxide and water; baking soda and water (1 tsp in 500 ml); and then with sterile water.	
Maintenance of mouth integrity	Avoid chemical, physical, and thermal irritants Avoid alcohol and tobacco use Remove dental prosthetics Avoid hot foods and liquids	
Moisture	Rinse mouth with water every 2 hours while awake and when awakened during the night Drink a minimum of 3000 ml of fluid each day if possible	IV fluids for hydration
Prophylactic oral antibiotics		Clotrimazole troche 10 mg or nystatin 5 ml orally every 4 hours

Although the oral care protocol appears simple, compliance with recommended procedures among transplant patients is low. Concurrent stomatitis, mucositis, and generalized fatigue may result in the patient not assuming responsibility for meticulous oral care. Then the nurse or a family member must implement the protocol if the benefits of oral care in reducing infection from endogenous organisms are to be realized.

Protective environment. The final strategy used to decrease the risk of infection from exogenous organisms is the use of a protective environment. Several types of protective environments are available: isolation, reverse isolation, laminar air-flow in a clean environment, and laminar air-flow in a sterile environment.[18] The type of protective environment employed for bone marrow transplantation varies from institution to institution and remains a controversial issue with respect to cost-benefit ratio for patient care and personnel demands.

Although cost-benefit ratio, effectiveness in preventing infection, psychologic side effects, and effects on quality of life and survival have been identified as factors germane to defining the relative benefits of a conventional isolation room versus a laminar air-flow environment, survival becomes the decisive factor. Empirical data indicate that although the number of infections can be reduced in the immunocompromised patient with the use of a laminar air-flow unit, survival for patients with leukemia was not significantly different from that for patients treated in a conventional room with reverse isolation precautions.[19] Yet Buckner et al,[20] in a study of patients with aplastic anemia treated in conventional rooms versus laminar air-flow units, found that the severity of GVHD was significantly less and long-term survival was significantly greater for patients treated in the laminar air-flow environments. Other clinical trials are in progress to distinguish those bone marrow transplant patients for whom laminar air-flow environments make a significant contribution to survival.

Vascular access for long-term supportive therapy. Since long-term supportive therapy in the form of blood components, antimicrobials, nutritional support, and immunosuppressive agents is required after transplantation, vascular access is critical. Double- or triple-lumen silastic catheters are placed into the right atrium through a subcutaneous tunnel on the anterior chest before initiation of the conditioning radiation and/or chemotherapy.[21] Because the catheter insertion procedure breaks the natural skin barrier as well as provides a direct intravascular

Table 17-6 Components of a standard catheter care protocol

Component	Nursing interventions
Examination of catheter	Assess the exit site and catheter tract for signs/symptoms of infection: redness, swelling, pain, or exudate. Assess for obvious catheter displacement Report changes to physician
Maintenance of a clean and dry occlusive dressing	Change catheter dressing every other day and as necessary Use sterile technique in changing dressing Clean around catheter exit site with an antimicrobial solution (e.g., povidone-iodine) Apply an occlusive dressing
Maintenance of catheter patency	Flush catheter with heparin solution 100 U/ml daily when not used for infusions Flush catheter with normal saline between infusions of different solutions Flush catheter with normal saline after collecting blood samples

route for infectious organisms, meticulous care of the central catheter is required. A standard catheter care protocol is presented in Table 17-6. In general, the catheter care protocol is designed to maintain a clean, dry environment at the catheter insertion site, to maintain catheter patency, and to monitor for signs and symptoms of catheter malfunction and infection.

THE TRANSPLANT PROCEDURE

Once the conditioning protocol has been completed, the recipient is ready to receive the transplanted marrow. For patients receiving an allogeneic or syngeneic transplant, the process begins with the harvest of the donor marrow. In the case of autologous transplant, the process begins with thawing of the recipient marrow that has been harvested and cryopreserved before the procedure.

Marrow harvest

Marrow harvest is a technically simple procedure. With the donor under general anesthesia, two to three incisions are made in the skin over the posterior iliac crests using sterile technique. An aspiration needle is inserted into the puncture sites and marrow is aspirated in 2 ml to 5 ml aliquots. The total volume of marrow obtained is 10 ml/kg of donor body weight.[19] However, the volume of marrow collected is less critical than is the actual number of stem cells harvested. To improve the percentage of stem cells in the harvest, the anterior iliac crests and sternum are often used in addition to the posterior iliac crests for multiple aspirations. In most centers, four times the number of cells required for reconstitution are harvested to increase engraftment rates.[22] In the case of autologous marrow harvest, frequently a volume of marrow is removed from the donor to provide a "backup" quantity for infusion should engraftment of the first marrow infusion not occur. The harvested marrow is added to a heparinized tissue culture medium and filtered through steel screens to remove particles of fat and bone.

Whole blood that circulates through the marrow sinuses constitutes the majority of marrow volume aspirated during the harvest. Since volumes ranging from 400 ml to 1000 ml may be collected during the harvest, an autophlebotomy of the donor is performed usually at least 1 week before the marrow donation. During the procedure, the donor receives the autotransfusion of whole blood to replace harvested blood.

Marrow processing

In allogeneic and syngeneic transplants, donor marrow is transferred to blood transfusion bags at the time of harvest. If the donor is a different ABO blood type from the recipient, red blood cell removal or T cell depletion may be required. However, in most cases the marrow is available for infusion within a few hours after donation.

Autologous marrow is centrifuged to remove the buffy coat, nucleated cells, and stem cells. Although clinical remission generally is a criterion for bone marrow transplantation, the assumption is made that viable tumor cells exist within the collected marrow. Therefore collections from individuals with malignant diseases of or involving the marrow usually are purged before cryopreservation.

Purging is the removal of residual malignant cells from the marrow through physical separation and immunologic or pharmacologic in vitro treatment of the harvested marrow.[23] Although purging of the marrow is recommended to decrease the recurrence of malignant disease, the process is not without risk. Data indicate that marrow purging is correlated with a 5- to 7-day delay of engraftment.[24] However, the clinical significance of marrow purging on survival continues to be debated.

Once necessary manipulation of the marrow is complete, the buffy coat is treated with a chemical solvent, dimethylsulfoxide (DMSO). DMSO protects the stem cells from lysis during the freezing process. Then the marrow is suspended in a plasma and tissue culture medium and frozen at temperatures varying from $-40°$ C to $-196°$ C. Frozen marrow can be stored for 6 years or longer.

Care of the donor

Care of the marrow donor is focused on immediate postoperative care, preparation for discharge, and long-term psychologic responses to marrow donation. Immediate postoperative care includes monitoring the donor for signs and symptoms of untoward effects of anesthesia, applying pressure dressings over puncture sites, and assessing pressure dressings for evidence of bleeding for the first 3 to 4 hours after the donation. Pain or soreness at the puncture sites is the most common sequela of marrow donation. Mobility may be limited for several days as a result of discomfort at the puncture sites and stiffness in the lower back. Symptoms improve significantly within 24 hours, although residual effects may endure for up to a week.

Few complications are associated with marrow donation. However, complications other than those related to anesthesia may occur after the donor has been discharged from the hospital. Therefore discharge teaching becomes an important aspect of care after marrow donation.

Donors complain primarily of discomfort at the puncture sites and fatigue after marrow donation. Comfort measures including mild analgesics, warm compresses, and rest for several days are usually sufficient to manage the complaints. Most donors are seen in a follow-up visit several days after the procedure. Donor hemoglobin and hematocrit levels are evaluated. In addition to discomfort and fatigue, infection and scarring of puncture sites and fever, pain, redness, swelling, or exudate at the puncture sites may occur. Should discomfort and fatigue persist or signs and symptoms of infection occur, the donor should be instructed to notify the physician.

Emotionally, the donor may require supportive care. Most donors identify strongly with and feel responsible for the well-being of the recipient. If the marrow fails to engraft or the recipient dies from a complication associated with the transplant, the donor may have profound feelings of failure and guilt. Anticipatory guidance with respect to the emotional responses commonly experienced by marrow donors may be indicated.

Marrow infusion

For patients receiving allogeneic and syngeneic transplants, the donor marrow is brought directly from the harvesting procedure to the recipient for infusion. For patients receiving autologous transplants, the frozen marrow is thawed in the transfusion bag in a sterile saline bath to body temperature. Procedures for thawing cryopreserved marrow may vary, and review of institutional policies and procedures is advised.

The actual marrow infusion is a simple procedure and is usually uneventful. The marrow, which resembles a whole blood transfusion, is infused through a nonfiltered administration set through a peripheral or central venous access. Rates of infusion vary with the volume of marrow and the policies of the institution. However, marrow infusions usually extend over a maximum of 4 hours.

The critical factor for thawed marrow is to infuse the volume as quickly as possible to decrease the risk of cell deterioration related to exposure to the DMSO preservative. Often the thawed marrow will be drawn into large syringes and infused by intravenous push through a central catheter.

COMPLICATIONS OF MARROW INFUSION

Although complications from the marrow infusion occur infrequently, the nurse must be aware of potential problems and monitor the patient closely. Fluid overload and pulmonary complications related to microscopic emboli and allergic reactions to donor granulocytes in the marrow are considered critical sequelae of marrow infusion. The majority of complications of marrow infusion occur within the first hour. Therefore assessments of the patient should be completed every 15 minutes for the first hour and every 30 minutes for the remainder of the infusion. Complications of marrow infusion include allergic reactions, fluid overload, and pulmonary emboli. Allergic reactions are most commonly seen in allogeneic and syngeneic transplant patients, whereas fluid overload and microscopic pulmonary emboli may be seen in any type of marrow transplant. The nurse must be cognizant of the potential sequelae of marrow infusion, teach the patient and family about significant symptoms to report, and monitor the patient closely during and immediately after the infusion.

A final unpleasant but less serious side effect of autologous marrow infusion is often neglected in descriptions of the transplant procedure but can be distressing for the marrow recipient. As the autologous marrow is infused through the central catheter, DMSO, the chemical solvent, is excreted through the lungs. A pungent, garliclike odor and taste are described by the marrow recipient. The patient may become nauseated from the strong taste and smell. The taste sensation usually subsides within a few minutes after completion of the infusion, but the smell may linger in the room for days. Antiemetics are used to treat nausea and vomiting and hard candy is offered to reduce the unpleasant taste.

Posttransplant care of the marrow recipient

Nursing care of the patient who has received a bone marrow transplant is complex, challenging, and requires a systematic, flexible approach. The condition of the patient varies from day to day and from hour to hour. Complications may occur simultaneously, may have similar manifestations, may cause other complications, or may exacerbate other complications.[25] The clinical condition of the recipient demands close observation, immediate assessment of any patient complaint, and evaluation of *subtle* changes in the patient. Common responses experienced by the marrow recipient will be discussed with respect to acute complications of the conditioning regimen, acute complications of the transplant, and long-term complications of both the conditioning regimen and transplant.

Complications related to the conditioning regimen. Many of the common problems seen after transplantation are a direct result of the conditioning regimen, either radiation therapy and/or chemotherapy, required before transplant. These responses are predictable; therefore, efforts to minimize the effects and vigilant evaluation of the effectiveness of care are instituted early in the course of the treatment.[26,27]

Gastrointestinal complications. Gastrointestinal (GI) complications result from both chemotherapy and radiation therapy used in conditioning regimens. Common manifestations, including anorexia, nausea, vomiting, diarrhea, stomatitis, and mucositis, occur early in the

course of transplantation and may continue for several weeks. GI complications become significant in long-term survival of the bone marrow recipient, because secondary complications, including nutritional deficits, fluid and electrolyte imbalance, and alteration in comfort, may result in morbidity or mortality. Nursing interventions, medical interventions, and potential secondary complications from GI complications are presented in Table 17-7.[28]

Pancytopenia. Pancytopenia resulting from the cytotoxic effects of chemotherapy and radiation therapy poses profound risks to the bone marrow recipient during the pretransplant and posttransplant period. Severe thrombocytopenia and granulocytopenia place the recipient in jeopardy for bleeding and infection, respectively, and therefore constitute potentially life-threatening complications.[28] In addition, anemia depletes the recipient of energy and may severely limit activity in general. Nursing interventions, medical interventions, and potential secondary complications from anemia, thrombocytopenia, and granulocytopenia are presented in Table 17-8.[29]

Venoocclusive disease. Venoocclusive disease (VOD), which involves occlusion of hepatic blood flow resulting in albumin- and sodium-rich fluid collection in the peritoneal cavity, occurs as a result of fibrous deposits in the terminal hepatic venules and sinusoids. First described in 1979, VOD is considered a potentially life-threatening complication of radiation and chemotherapy used in conditioning procedures for bone marrow transplantation. VOD occurs in nearly 20% of allogeneic and autologous transplant patients.[30] Nursing interventions, medical interventions, and potential secondary complications of VOD are presented in Table 17-9. Of patients developing VOD, 45% eventually die of progressive liver dysfunction.[30]

Pulmonary complications. Damage to lung tissue may occur as a result of (1) the conditioning procedure, (2) opportunistic infections, (3) GVHD, and/or (4) vascular abnormalities (Table 17-10).[31] Timing of onset in relation to the transplant is important in the differential diagnosis of pulmonary complications. Pulmonary complications may result in mortality even in the

Table 17-7 Management of GI complications

Complication	Potential secondary complications	Nursing interventions	Medical interventions
Anorexia	Nutritional deficits	Consult dietitian Identify well-tolerated, favorite foods Serve small, frequent meals/supplements	Nutritional support
Nausea	Nutritional deficits	Remove food coverings outside room Serve cold rather than warm or hot foods Bland diet Emesis basin within reach	Nutritional support Routine antiemetics Serum electrolytes, BUN, creatinine Fluid/electrolyte replacement
Vomiting	Nutritional deficits Fluid/electrolyte imbalances	Record character, quality, and volume of emesis Provide comfort measures during vomiting episodes Monitor for side effects of antiemetics	Fluid/electrolyte replacement
Diarrhea	Nutritional deficits Fluid/electrolyte imbalances Weakness/fatigue Perineal irritation	Record character, quality, and amount of diarrhea Cleanse perineal area after each stool Assess for signs/symptoms of dehydration Weigh daily	Antidiarrheals Bacterial, fungal, viral cultures
Stomatitis	Nutritional deficits Secondary infection Bleeding	Institute oral care protocol Record condition of oral cavity daily Offer soft, cool, bland foods/fluids Monitor for side effects of analgesics	Topical and systemic analgesics Antibiotics/antifungals Culture lesions
Mucositis	Nutritional deficits Ineffective airway clearance	Encourage oral fluids Gently suction thick mucous secretions	Fluid management

Table 17-8 Management of pancytopenia

Complication	Potential secondary complications	Nursing interventions	Medical interventions
Anemia	Fatigue Decreased role performance Decreased activity level	Implement energy conservation strategies Assist with ambulation as needed Plan for valued activities in daily routine	Complete blood counts Irradiated red blood cell transfusion Hgb/Hct <8/25
Granulocytopenia	Infection	Teach personal hygiene measures: Oral, perineal, skin care protocols Implement caregiver/visitor handwashing protocol/masks Monitor for signs/symptoms of infection Cough, fever, pain, diarrhea, agitation, white patches in mouth, urinary frequency or burning Assess wound, vascular access device insertion sites, mucous membranes, and skin daily Assess vital signs every 4 hours Report signs/symptoms to physician Assess and report signs/symptoms of toxic effects of antimicrobial therapy	Routine screening cultures Fever workup for T >101°F Chest x-ray examination, urine and blood cultures Antibacterial, antifungal, and antiviral drugs Irradiated granulocyte transfusions
Thrombocytopenia	Bleeding Oral mucosa Bladder Rectum Abdomen Brain Potential for injury	Monitor platelet count Assess for petechiae/ecchymoses on extremities; bleeding from oral mucosa, bladder, rectum, nose, sputum Apply pressure to bone marrow biopsy and venipuncture sites Assess for changes in mental status Avoid invasive procedures: IM injections, enemas, rectal suppositories, catheters Avoid potentially traumatic conditions: constipation, flossing, shaving with a straight-edged razor	Platelet count Laxatives to prevent constipation Avoid aspirin-containing medications Irradiated platelet transfusions for platelet count <30,000 or frank bleeding Medroxyprogesterone acetate (Depo-Provera)/contraceptives

Table 17-9 Management of venoocclusive disease

Complication	Potential secondary complications	Nursing interventions	Medical interventions
Impaired hepatic blood flow	Hepatic congestion Ascites Sodium/water retention Intravascular volume depletion Renal insufficiency Hepatocyte death	Serial I&Os Serial weights Serial abdominal girth measurements Sodium/water restriction Monitor for postural hypotension	Maintenance of intravascular volume: Packed red cell transfusions Albumin Diuretics Hemodialysis
Impaired hepatic function	Jaundice Altered metabolism Coagulopathy Encephalopathy	Limit patient activity Assess for signs/symptoms of hemorrhage Assess for neurologic and mental status changes Implement methods to decrease itching: cool compresses, lanolin-based lotion, oatmeal baths Implement methods to decrease scratching: gloves, trim fingernails Monitor for signs/symptoms of drug toxicity	Antipruritics Coagulation studies Liver function tests Platelet transfusions Peak/trough levels of drugs metabolized by liver/kidneys

face of a successful transplant; therefore interventions to prevent the occurrence of bacterial, fungal, and viral infections in the lung should be implemented. Prophylactic antimicrobial therapy, modified doses of chemotherapy and radiation, and immunization have been shown to reduce the incidence of pulmonary problems after transplantation.[31]

Infections. Localized and systemic infection from bacterial, viral, fungal, and protozoal organisms continue to be significant problems in the posttransplant management of the marrow recipient.[32] A pattern of occurrence for infections has been described (Table 17-11).[33] Thus prophylactic antimicrobial therapy may be planned to coincide with high risk periods for specific infections. A complete discussion of the most common organisms associated with posttransplant morbidity may be found in Chapter 3.

Acute complications of the transplant procedure. Complications that result from the transplant procedure depend on the type of transplant. For recipients of autologous transplants, the lack of engraftment poses the greatest threat in terms of survival. For recipients of allogeneic and syngeneic transplants, lack of engraftment and GVHD pose the greatest threats to survival.

Lack of engraftment. Lack of engraftment of the donor marrow occurs in less than 15% of patients receiving allogeneic and syngeneic

Table 17-10 Pulmonary complications

Complication	Causative factor
Infectious pneumonitis	Cytomegalovirus Herpes simplex/ zoster virus Bacterial infections Fungal infections Protozoal infections
Noninfectious pneumonitis	Conditioning procedure Chemotherapy/ radiation Leukemic recurrence Transfusion reactions
Graft-versus-host disease	Bronchitis Obstructive airway disease Sinopulmonary infections Chronic aspiration
Pulmonary vascular abnormalities	Thrombi Emboli Endothelial thickening

Table 17-11 Timing of infections

Timing after transplant	Infectious organism
First month	Gram-negative bacteria Gram-positive bacteria Herpes simplex virus *Candida albicans* *Asperigillus* *Fusarium*
Second and third months	Herpes simplex virus Herpes zoster virus Cytomegalovirus
After third month	Herpes zoster virus *Pneumocystis carinii*

Adapted from McGlave P (1985, November 15). The status of bone marrow transplantation for leukemia. *Hospital Practice, 20,* 97-110.

transplants and in less than 5% of patients receiving autologous transplants. Lack of engraftment occurs primarily because of infusion of inadequate numbers of stem cells and/or inadequate preparation of the recipient marrow. Lack of engraftment is determined by serial marrow aspirates and biopsies after the transplant procedure. Usually cellular precursors will begin to appear in the bone marrow by 21 days after transplant. Should engraftment not occur, the patient is faced with going through another transplant procedure or death as a result of infection and/or bleeding.

Graft-versus-host disease. GVHD is a complication of allogeneic bone marrow transplant, occurring in 40% to 50% of recipients receiving HLA-matched, MLC-nonreactive donor marrow. GVHD occurs when donor immunocompetent T lymphocytes, infused with the marrow donation or through blood products from the donor, recognize immunoincompetent recipient tissues as foreign and attempt to destroy them. The skin, liver, and GI tract are the main target organs of GVHD.[34]

The skin is the most common organ of involvement and often is the first organ to demonstrate changes specific to GVHD. The skin reaction usually begins as a fine, maculopapular, erythematous rash on the palms of the hands and the soles of the feet. As the reaction progresses, generalized erythroderma, wet desquamation, blistering, and loss of superficial skin layers may occur (Table 17-12). Differential diagnosis of skin reactions related to GVHD include skin changes associated with radiation therapy, antimicrobial therapy, and steroid treatment. A skin biopsy is needed to confirm GVHD involvement.[34-36]

GVHD with liver involvement results in both physical and laboratory changes. Although patients with mild liver involvement may be asymptomatic, alkaline phosphatase and serum bilirubin levels generally are elevated. In addition, physical symptoms of right upper quadrant pain, hepatomegaly, and jaundice may occur. Differential diagnoses associated with GVHD with liver involvement include venoocclusive disease and hepatitis. Confirmation of GVHD with liver involvement is made by liver biopsy, although the risk of postbiopsy bleeding and

Table 17-12 Clinical staging of acute GVHD

Stage	Skin	Liver	Gastrointestinal tract
+	Maculopapular rash <25% of body surface	Bilirubin 2-3 mg/100 ml	>500-1000 ml diarrhea per day
+ +	Maculopapular rash 25%-50% of body surface	Bilirubin >3-6 mg/100 ml	>1000-1500 ml diarrhea per day
+ + +	Generalized erythroderma	Bilirubin >6-15 mg/100 ml	>1500 ml diarrhea per day
+ + + +	Generalized erythroderma with bullous formation and desquamation	Bilirubin >15 mg/100 ml	Severe abdominal pain, with or without ileus

Adapted from Thomas ED, Storb R, Clift RA, Fefer A, Johnson FL, Neiman PE, Lerner KG, Glucksberg H and Buckner CD (1974). Bone marrow transplantation. *New England Journal of Medicine, 292*(17), 895-902.

false negative results must be considered. Severity of liver involvement is staged based on increasingly elevated serum bilirubin levels (see Table 17-12).

In addition to skin and liver involvement, GVHD may also involve the GI tract. Green, watery diarrhea, abdominal cramping, nausea, vomiting, and anorexia may be the initial symptoms. As the severity increases, villi in the GI tract are destroyed and the intestinal mucosa sloughs. Absorption in the GI tract is diminished and transit time decreases, resulting in a copious volume of diarrhea, fluid and electrolyte imbalances, malabsorption syndrome, a change from guaiac-negative to -positive stool, and occasionally a massive GI bleed. Confirmation of GI involvement with GVHD is made by rectal biopsy, although the dangers of bleeding and infection in the immunocompromised patient are critical considerations. Severity of GI involvement is staged based on increasing volumes of diarrhea and/or ileus and pain levels (see Table 17-12).[37]

Care of the patient with GVHD requires acute observation skills, documentation of serial changes in the condition of the patient, and evaluation of patient responses to the disease and therapy. Specific nursing and medical interventions in the management of GVHD are described in Table 17-13. Nursing care of the patient is focused on detection of early symptoms of GVHD, support of patient comfort, and implementation of the medical plan of care.[38]

Although significant improvements have been made in both histocompatibility testing and prophylactic treatment, GVHD is considered to pose a major threat to successful bone marrow transplantation. GVHD poses a threat to life in the acute stage, during the first 100 days after transplantation. In addition, quality of life for the recipient may be compromised in the chronic stage, after the first 100 days. Prolonged severe skin involvement and immobility may result in scarring, loss of skin elasticity, and disfigurement as well as contractures. The debilitating effects of prolonged diarrhea are severe weight loss, fluid and electrolyte imbalances, and potential denuding of perineal skin. Chronic involvement of the liver with GVHD produces compounding morbidity factors such as bleeding, altered drug metabolism, and ascites. Therefore efforts focused on both the primary and secondary prevention of GVHD have been instituted.

Primary prevention of GVHD has been through improvements in histocompatibility testing and inactivation of donor T lymphocytes either by suppressing proliferation or inhibiting

Table 17-13 Management of signs and symptoms of GVHD

Organ involved	Stage	Nursing interventions	Medical interventions
Skin	+ + + + + + + + + +	Institute measures to promote comfort Oatmeal baths, calamine lotion, cool compresses, loose clothing to decrease itching Institute measures to decrease risks of injury Discourage scratching; keep fingernails short; apply loose cotton gloves Institute measures to maintain moisture in skin Lubricate skin with ½ mineral oil, ½ A & D ointment after bath Institute measures to promote comfort Bed cradle to prevent contact with bed clothing and decrease friction, pressure, and shearing forces Institute measures to prevent secondary complications Apply sterile petroleum gauze over blistering to prevent infection Range of motion exercises to prevent contractures	Analgesics Antipruritics Immunosuppressive agents Antibiotic creams Pigskin grafts
Gastrointestinal tract		Institute measures to minimize irritation to bowel Consult dietician for foods low in residue, nonirritating to bowel, high in protein and calories Institute measures to detect secondary complications Record volume and characteristics of diarrhea Serial weight measures Guaiac stools Monitor for signs and symptoms of dehydration Decreased skin turgor, dryness of mucous membranes Monitor for signs and symptoms of electrolyte imbalance Monitor serum K^+, Na^+ levels, weakness, fatigue Institute measures to decrease risks of infection Perineal hygiene after each bowel movement Skin protector to anus and perineum after each bowel movement Institute measures to decrease discomfort Sitz bath, warm water bottle to abdomen for cramping	Immunosuppressive agents Antidiarrheals Fluid and electrolyte replacement Nutritional support Blood loss replacement
Liver		Monitor liver function Institute measures to decrease discomfort from skin irritation Monitor responses to drug therapy with potential hepatotoxicity	

Table 17-14 Pharmacologic agents used in the prevention and treatment of GVHD

Agent	Route of administration	Potential side effects	General nursing considerations
Methotrexate	IV/oral	Marrow suppression Mucosal ulceration Rash Pruritis Photosensitivity	Teach patient/family regarding potential side effects of immunosuppressive therapy Administer immunosuppressive agents as prescribed by physician Monitor for signs and symptoms of side effects of therapy Report occurrence of side effects to physician Institute measures to promote safety and comfort Assess for signs and symptoms of infection in an immunocompromised patient
Antithymocyte globulin	IV	Anaphylaxis Chills and fever	
Cyclosporine	IV/oral	Drug interactions Renal toxicity Hepatic toxicity GI disturbances Hirsutism Burning of soles and palms	
Corticosteroids	IV/oral	Euphoria Insomnia Hyperglycemia Fluid retention Hypertension Adrenal insufficiency GI irritation	

the T lymphocyte from recognizing the host cells as foreign through the use of methotrexate, antithymocyte globulin (ATG), or cyclosporine.[39] Secondary prevention (i.e., measures to minimize GVHD once active) has focused on suppression of inflammatory and immune responses through the use of steroids, ATG, cyclosporine, and monoclonal antibodies. Pharmacologic agents used in primary and secondary prevention of GVHD, routes of administration, potential side effects, and nursing considerations are presented in Table 17-14.

• • •

In summary, although the actual bone marrow transplant is a technologically simple procedure, the care of the recipient in the critical days and months before and after the transplant is intricate and paradoxic. The conditioning procedure and the sequelae of the transplant potentially affect every major system in the body in the immediate and long-term posttransplant periods. In addition, bone marrow transplantation is a paradoxic treatment. The transplant is required because of a nonfunctional bone marrow; the patient is at risk for infection and bleeding from prolonged marrow suppression from the conditioning procedures; and posttransplant care is focused on immunosuppression of the donor marrow to prevent development of an immune response to recipient tissues. Care provided to the bone marrow transplant recipient, donor, and family requires sensitivity to physical as well as psychosocial issues, an understanding of the rationale for the procedure, expert clinical assessment skills to detect subtle changes in the condition of the patient, competence in the performance of care activities, and development of collegial relationships with a spectrum of health care professionals to ensure coordination of services.

PREPARATION FOR DISCHARGE

Discharge criteria after bone marrow transplant are based on the ability of the patient/family to mobilize personal and community resources to meet the physical and psychosocial demands of the posttransplant period. Criteria may include that the patient and family be able to do the following:

- Describe the rationale for the bone marrow transplant procedure
- Demonstrate competence in self-care activities
- Identify community resources available for managing home and follow-up care
- Discuss plans for reintegration of personal, family, and community life
- Identify signs and symptoms of recurrence and/or long-term sequelae that require professional assistance for management

Yet the time of discharge can be confusing and anxiety provoking for the patient and family.[12] The expert teaching and counseling skills of the nurse will be required to prepare the patient and family to assume responsibility for care required after discharge.

At the time of discharge patients still may be nauseated, easily fatigued, and coping with skin changes related to radiation therapy or GVHD. Skin discoloration, dryness, flaking, or rash may be present. The patient does not feel as well as anticipated and may be discouraged by the physical and psychosocial responses to the transplant. Discouragement may be reinforced by the need for continued supportive therapy such as blood transfusions, nutritional support, and continued social isolation.[40,41]

Some patients may be returning to a living situation without family support. The patient will require assistance from community agencies and a special effort by the health care team to ensure that patient needs can be met within the home. A skilled nursing care facility may be required as a bridge between leaving the acute care hospital and returning to independent living.

For patients returning home, concerns related to the transition from acute care to home care may be expressed by family members, such as confidence in their ability to meet the needs of the patient, what to do in case of an emergency, availability of knowledgeable health care resources in the local community, and the slow progress of the patient with respect to nutritional intake and activity levels.[41]

The health care team has a responsibility to hear the concerns of both patients and family members, to acknowledge the anxiety and stress aroused by the pending discharge, and to plan systematically for the transition with the patient, family, and community resources. Coordination is essential among members of the health care team, the physician, nurse, social worker, nutritional support personnel, and physical therapy staff.

A variety of issues, including medical follow-up, supportive care, self-care skills, and adaptation to the consequences of transplantation, need to be addressed before discharge. The patient will need continued medical outpatient follow-up, perhaps as frequently as two to three times a week initially. Close observation is necessary because of the risks of GVHD, infection, failure to thrive, and the need for further blood component therapy. Immediate outpatient follow-up may require the patient and family to remain within an accessible distance of the hospital or to be referred to a physician able to manage the posttransplant care within the local community. The social worker can assist the patient and family to find lodging near the outpatient clinic. Many transplant centers have hotels for housing patients and families for the first 100 days after the transplant procedure.

As a consequence of the physical, nutritional, or immunosuppression status of the patient, continued supportive care may be necessary. Physical therapy, nutritional support, and/or antimicrobial therapy may be required at home. In many cities, skilled nursing care agencies are available and well equipped to manage the spectrum of home intravenous therapies required for the posttransplant patient. The nurse and social worker coordinate with the physician apropriate referrals within the community for continued supportive care.

The patient and family are faced with assuming responsibility for self-care at the time of discharge from the acute care setting. Self-care skills include activities of daily living—bathing, toileting, feeding, and dressing. Medication administration, management of vascular access devices and continuing health care needs, monitoring for side effects of the conditioning procedure and transplant, and decision-making regarding symptoms that should be reported to

the health care team are also required. In addition, resumption of valued roles and responsibilities and adaptation to the outcomes of the transplant procedure are long-term objectives.

Since a year may be needed for the patient to establish a completely immunocompetent marrow, the risk of infection will continue to be a threat to health.[42] After discharge, meticulous personal hygiene measures will be required. Daily baths, oral care after eating and before bedtime, and perineal hygiene after toileting will remain the focus of an infection prevention regimen.

Transplant patients will often be discharged on a variety of medications such as antimicrobials and immunosuppressive agents. If complications have occurred as a result of the transplant, the list of discharge medications may be longer. The patient and family must be confident in their ability to master medication administration at home—giving the correct medication, at the proper dose level, and within the scheduled timeframe. Nowhere is the accuracy of medication administration more crucial than in the immunosuppressive regimen to prevent GVHD. In addition to administration, the patient and family will now assume the monitoring function of the nurse with respect to the common side effects of medication. Discharge medications should be reviewed with patients and family members before discharge, written drug information and schedules of administration provided, and community resources identified should questions arise.

Because continued supportive therapy may be required, the patient will be discharged with a vascular access device in place. Although many patients and families will be adept at caring for the devices because of previous therapy, the home care becomes more critical in the posttransplant period with respect to the risk of infection. In addition to daily care, the patient and family will be required to know how to manage the device in case of an emergency (e.g., occlusion or breakage). Return demonstration of care techniques and emergency care is essential to evaluate the competency of the patient and family. Should concerns be ex-

---

POTENTIAL LONG-TERM CONSEQUENCES OF BONE MARROW TRANSPLANTATION

Chronic GVHD
  Infection
  Contractures
  Failure to thrive
Endocrine abnormalities
  Primary ovarian/testicular failure
  Hypothyroidism
  Deceleration of growth
Cataracts
Recurrence of disease
Pulmonary complications
  Infection
  Obstructive lung disease
  Restrictive lung disease
Neurologic complications
  Personality changes
  Ataxia
  Photophobia
Second malignancies

---

pressed by the patient and family or the nurse with respect to the ability of the patient or family to care for the vascular device, referral to a home health care agency may be made.

Although the patient may have experienced immediate side effects of the conditioning procedure and transplant, both procedures have long-term consequences for which the patient and family must monitor closely. Long-term consequences of the conditioning procedure and transplant are included in the box above.

The nurse may be involved in the education of patients and families on the consequences of the transplant procedure and long-term followup care; therefore knowledge of signs and symptoms of latent effects of transplantation is essential.

In addition to monitoring for signs and symptoms, the patient and family also assume decision-making responsibilities about symptoms to report to the health care team. To facilitate accurate decision-making, a written list of critical symptoms to be reported should be included in discharge teaching. Screening questions about the critical symptoms should be included with the history and physical examination in subsequent follow-up visits.

For most bone marrow transplant recipients, discharge from the acute care hospital will be the culmination of 4 to 6 weeks of treatment after a previous extended illness. During the illness before the transplant procedure, many patients will have relinquished valued roles and responsibilities within the family, the workplace or school, and the community. Although the activities immediately after discharge will continue to focus on the patient in the "sick role," efforts should be made to encourage the patient to assume as much independence and control as possible, to begin to assume valued roles and activities within the immediate family, and to plan a future life with significant others.

SUMMARY

Bone marrow transplantation is a viable treatment option for an increasing number of patients. Although technically a simple procedure, the pretransplant and posttransplant care of the donor, recipient, and family requires the expertise and coordination of services of a spectrum of health care professionals. The nurse assumes pivotal roles as educator, counselor, care provider, and manager throughout the transplant experience. For some patients the consequence of bone marrow transplant will be death—for others, survival. By developing knowledge, skills, and positive attitudes toward marrow transplantation, the nurse is able to assist the patient and family to adapt to either consequence within a caring and supportive relationship.

Bone marrow transplantation continues to evolve as the knowledge of immunology and disease expands, selection of conditioning protocols becomes more individualized, and the support of the patient in the posttransplant period becomes more systematic and refined.[43] The rapidly changing field of transplantation offers the nurse opportunities for continued personal and professional growth.

REFERENCES

1. Freedman SE (1988). An overview of bone marrow transplantation. *Seminars in Oncology Nursing, 4*(1), 3-8.
2. Thomas ED, Storb R, Clift RA, Fefer A, Johnson FL, Neiman PE, Lerner KG, Glucksberg H and Buckner CD (1975, April 17). Bone marrow transplantation. *New England Journal of Medicine, 292*(16), 832-842.
3. Jacobson LO, Marks EK, Robson MJ, Gaston E and Zirkle RE (1949). Effect of spleen protection on mortality following x-irradiation. *Journal of Laboratory and Clinical Medicine, 34,* 1538-1543.
4. Lorenz E, Uphoff D, Reid TR and Shelton E (1951). Modifications of irradiation injury in mice and guinea pigs by bone marrow injections. *Journal of National Cancer Institute, 12,* 197-201.
5. Thomas ED (1987). Bone marrow transplantation. *CA: A Journal for Clinicians, 37,* 291-301.
6. Bortin MM and Rimm AA (1986). Increasing utilization of bone marrow transplantation. *Transplantation, 42*(3), 229-234.
7. McCullough J, Rogers G, Dahl R, Therkelsen D, Kamstra L, Crisham P, Kline W, Bowman R, Scott E, Halagan N, Williams J and Sandler SG (1986). Development and operation of a program to obtain volunteer bone marrow donors unrelated to the patient. *Transfusion, 26*(4), 315-323.
8. McElligott MC, Menitove JE and Aster RH (1986). Recruitment of unrelated persons as bone marrow donors: A preliminary experience. *Transfusion, 26*(4), 309-314.
9. Dudjak L (1984). HLA typing: implications for nurses. *Oncology Nursing Forum, 11*(5), 30-36.
10. Champlin R (1988). Acute myelogenous leukemia: biology and treatment. *Mediguide to Oncology, 8*(4) 1-9.
11. Folsom TL and Popkin MK (1986). Current and future perspectives on psychiatric involvement in bone marrow transplantations. *Psychiatric Medicine, 4*(3), 319-329.
12. Lesko LM (1985). Psychological aspects of bone marrow transplantation. *The Candlelighters Childhood Cancer Foundation Progress Report, V* (Special Issue), 11-12.
13. Ruggiero MR (1988). The donor in bone marrow transplantation. *Seminars in Oncology Nursing, 4*(1), 9-14.
14. Wolcott DL, Wellisch DK, Fawzy FT and Landsverk J (1986). Psychological adjustment of adult bone marrow transplant donors whose recipient survives. *Transplantation, 41*(4), 484-488.
15. Wiley FM and Decuir-Whalley S (1983). Allogeneic bone marrow transplantation for children with acute leukemia. *Oncology Nursing Forum, 10*(3), 49-53.
16. Mueller SK (1982). Bone marrow transplant teaching and documentation tool. *Oncology Nursing Forum, 9*(2), 57-63.
17. Lasser SD, Camitta BM and Needleman HL (1977). Dental management of patients undergoing bone marrow transplantation for aplastic anemia. *Oral Surgery, 43*(2), 181-189.
18. Nuscher R, Baltzer L, Repinec DA, Almquist G, Barrett J, LaBombardi S, DeMao JD, Diver ME, Field BA, Lee MC, Mamora J, Pizzo B, Sheehy BN, Sullivan M and Tierney J (1984, June). Bone marrow transplantation: a lifesaving option. *American Journal of Nursing,* 764-772.
19. Zaia JA and Forman SJ (1987). Management of the bone marrow transplant recipient. In Parrillo JE and Masur H (eds). *The critically ill immunosuppressed patient: diagnosis and management* (pp 381-413). Rockville, Md: Aspen Publishers.
20. The Seattle Bone Marrow Transplant Team: Buckner CD, Clift RA, Sanders JE, Meyers JD, Counts GW, Farewell VT, Thomas D (1978). Protective environment for marrow transplant recipients: a prospective study. *Annals of Internal Medicine, 89*(6), 893-901.
21. Hutchinson MM and King AH (1983). A nursing perspective on bone marrow transplantation. *Nursing Clinics of North America, 18*(3), 511-522.
22. Cogliano-Shutta NA, Broda EJ and Gress JS (1985). Bone marrow transplantation: an overview and comparison of autologous, syngeneic, and allogeneic treatment modalities. *Nursing Clinics of North America, 20*(1), 49-66.
23. Schryber S, Lacasse CR and Barton-Burke M (1987). Autologous bone marrow transplantation. *Oncology Nursing Forum, 14*(4), 74-79.
24. Ciobanu N (1986). Bone marrow transplantation for treatment of malignancies. *Mediguide to Oncology, 6*(1) 1-5.
25. Ford R and Ballard B (1988). Acute complications after bone marrow transplantation. *Seminars in Oncology Nursing, 4*(1), 15-24.
26. Corcoran-Buchsel P (1986). Long-term complications of allogeneic bone marrow transplantation: nursing implications. *Oncology Nursing Forum, 13*(6), 61-70.
27. Nims JW and Strom S (1988). Late complications of bone marrow transplant recipients: nursing care issues. *Seminars in Oncology Nursing, 4*(1), 47-54.
28. Hutchinson MM and Itoh K (1982). Nursing care of the patient undergoing bone marrow transplantation for acute leukemia. *Nursing Clinics of North America, 17*(4), 697-710.
29. O'Quin T and Moravec C (1988). The critically ill bone marrow transplant patient. *Seminars in Oncology Nursing, 4*(1), 25-30.
30. Jones RJ, Kamthorn SKL, Lee KSK, Beschorner WE, Vogel VG, Grochow LB, Braine HG, Vogelsang GB, Sensenbrenner LL, Santos GW and Saral R (1987). Venoocclusive disease of the liver following bone marrow transplantation. *Transplantation, 44*(6), 778-783.
31. Krowka MJ, Rosenow EC and Hoagland HC (1985). Pulmonary complications of bone marrow transplantation. *Chest, 87*(2), 237-245.
32. Meyers JD (1988). Prevention and treatment of cytomegalovirus infection after marrow transplantation. *Bone Marrow Transplantation, 3,* 95-104.

33. McGlave PB (1985). The status of bone marrow transplantation for leukemia. *Hospital Practice, 20,* 97-110.

34. Deeg HJ and Storb R (1986). Acute and chronic graft-versus-host disease: clinical manifestations, prophylaxis, and treatment. *Journal of National Cancer Institute, 76*(6), 1325-1328.

35. Saurat JH (1981). Cutaneous manifestations of graft-versus-host disease. *International Journal of Dermatology, 20*(4), 249-256.

36. McConn R (1987). Skin changes following bone marrow transplantation. *Cancer Nursing, 10*(2), 82-84.

37. Thomas ED, Storb R, Clift RA, Fefer A, Johnson FL, Neiman PE, Lerner KG, Glucksberg H and Buckner CD (1975, April 24). Bone marrow transplantation. *New England Journal of Medicine, 292*(17), 895-902.

38. de la Montaigne M, de Mao J, Nuscher R and Stutzer CA (1981). Standards of care for the patient with "graft-versus-host disease" post bone marrow transplant. *Cancer Nursing, 4,* 191-198.

39. Klemm P (1985). Cyclosporin A: use in preventing graft versus host disease. *Oncology Nursing Forum, 12*(5), 25-31.

40. Corcoran-Buchsel P and Parchem C (1988). Ambulatory care of the bone marrow transplantation patient. *Seminars in Oncology Nursing, 4*(1), 41-46.

41. Haberman MR (1988). Psychosocial aspects of bone marrow transplantation. *Seminars in Oncology Nursing, 4*(1), 3-8.

42. Witherspoon RP (1986). Suppression and recovery of immunologic function after bone marrow transplantation. *Journal of National Cancer Institute, 76*(6), 1321-1324.

43. Thomas ED (1988). The future of marrow transplantation. *Seminars in Oncology Nursing, 4*(1), 74-78.

Appendixes

A

AACN Position Statement: Roles and Responsibilities of Critical Care Nurses in Organ and Tissue Transplantation

Since 1954 when the first renal transplant was performed, there has been a dramatic increase in the demand for organs for transplantation. In 1984 alone, there were 24,000 cornea transplants, 7,000 kidney transplants, 350 heart transplants, 300 liver transplants, 90 pancreas transplants, and 30 heart/lung transplants performed in the United States. Advances in surgical techniques, a better understanding of the immune system, development of new and more effective immunosuppressive drugs, and better organ preservation techniques have made it possible to transplant a larger number and an increased variety of organs.

The major limiting factor in organ transplantation is the shortage of available organs. Although approximately 20,000 individuals become potential donors in the United States each year, only about 2,500 actually become donors. The organ shortage is not due to an inadequate supply of potential cadaveric donors; it is largely due, instead, to the failure of health care professionals to identify potential donors and initiate the organ donation process in a timely manner.

□ Adopted by the AACN Board of Directors, June 1986. Reprinted with permission of the American Association of Critical Care Nurses, Newport Beach, Calif.

Whereas,

- Technological, immunological, and surgical advances have made organ and tissue transplantation a therapeutic modality for many patients with end-stage organ disease,
- Technological, immunological, and surgical advances have resulted in an increase in the demand for transplantable organs and tissues,
- Organ and tissue transplantation has been shown to save lives, restore sight, and improve quality of life in many patients with end-stage organ disease,
- Success rates for heart, liver, and kidney transplantation have increased significantly in this decade,
- Thousands of Americans could potentially benefit from organ and tissue transplantation,
- The majority (95%) of potential organ donors die in critical care units,
- Of the potential organ and tissue donors each year in the United States, only approximately 15% actually donate organs and tissues,
- Critical care nurses are the major care givers to potential donors, recipients, and families,

- Critical care nurses are the vital link for the patient and family in relation to the organ and tissue donation and transplantation process,
- Critical care nurses may be responsible for approaching family members of potential organ and tissue donors,
- Families in the immediate period of grief, after hearing the diagnosis of brain death for a loved one, are preoccupied with their loss and often do not think of organ donation,
- Eight out of ten grieving families do consent to organ or tissue donation when asked,
- There are personal, professional, cultural, social, religious, and ethical considerations pertaining to organ and tissue transplantation,
- National attention has been given to access and distribution of transplantable organs and tissues,
- Legislation has addressed the lack of donor organs and tissues,
- A sophisticated mechanism does exist in the United States for the procurement of donor organs and tissues,

Therefore, be it hereby resolved that, in accordance with personal beliefs and values, the critical care nurse shall

- Collaborate with health care professionals and families in donor identification and care, the organ and tissue procurement process, and recipient care,
- Develop knowledge and awareness of the personal, professional, cultural, social, religious, and ethical issues related to organ and tissue transplantation,
- Develop knowledge and awareness of local, state, and national legislation relevant to organ and tissue transplantation,
- Provide support needed by families of potential and actual organ and tissue donors,
- Participate in the implementation of standards for care of potential donors, recipients, and families,
- Participate in the selection process of potential recipients,
- Participate in endeavors designed to advance the science and art of transplantation nursing.

B

AACN Position Statement: Required Request and Routine Inquiry: Methods to Improve the Organ and Tissue Donation Process

Remarkable progress in the field of organ and tissue transplantation has increased the demand for the number and variety of organs and tissues. Aproximately 20,000 individuals may be potential donors in the United States each year, but only about 2,500 actually become donors.

The major limiting factor in organ and tissue transplantation is the shortage of available organs and tissues. The organ and tissue shortage is due to the failure of health care professionals to identify potential donors and to initiate the organ donation process, rather than an inadequate supply of donors.

The values of contemporary society govern the ethical framework for a voluntary system of organ donation. These values include:

- Saving lives and improving the quality of life.
- Respecting individual autonomy.
- Promoting a sense of community through acts of generosity.
- Showing respect for the donor patient.
- Showing respect for the wishes of the family.

The Uniform Anatomical Gift Act (1968) created the legal framework for a voluntary system of organ and tissue donation. This act established the legal right of all adult Americans to make known, prior to death, their wishes regarding organ and tissue donation. In the absence of such direction, the decision to donate organs and tissues is the right of the family members. The limitations of this voluntary process have recently led to an increase in legislation regarding required request.

Whereas, required request legislation directs hospitals to develop policies so that all patients and their families and the families of deceased patients can be informed about the possibility of donating organs and tissues, and

Whereas, such a policy assists the health care professional during the initiation process of organ and tissue donation, and

Whereas, such a policy gives *all* an opportunity to consider organ and tissue donation, and

Whereas, required request legislation and policies of routine inquiry offer the patient and the family members the right to choose between voluntary donation and refusal, and

Whereas, the rights of the patient and the family members are best served by the participation of the critical care nurse in the development, implementation, and evaluation of standardized policies, and

Whereas, by providing the necessary direction for inquiry of the patient and family members, required request legislation and pol-

□ Adopted by the AACN Board of Directors, December 1986. Reprinted with permission of the American Association of Critical Care Nurses, Newport Beach, Calif.

icies of routine inquiry facilitate the role of the critical care nurse who is the primary care giver to potential organ and tissue donors, recipients, and their families;

Therefore, be it hereby resolved that, the American Association of Critical-Care Nurses strongly supports legislation for required request;

Be it further resolved that, the American Association of Critical-Care Nurses recommends that institutions adopt policies that standardize the process of routine inquiry concerning organ and tissue donation;

Be it further resolved that, the critical care nurse shall, in accordance with personal beliefs and values, participate in the development, implementation, and evaluation of the hospital's policy.

Index